T0226397

Pediatric Anesthesiology

Editors

ALAN JAY SCHWARTZ
DEAN B. ANDROPOULOS
ANDREW DAVIDSON

ANESTHESIOLOGY CLINICS

www.anesthesiology.theclinics.com

Consulting Editor
LEE A. FLEISHER

March 2014 • Volume 32 • Number 1

ELSEVIER

1600 John F. Kennedy Boulevard • Suite 1800 • Philadelphia, Pennsylvania, 19103-2899

http://www.theclinics.com

ANESTHESIOLOGY CLINICS Volume 32, Number 1
March 2014 ISSN 1932-2275, ISBN-13: 978-0-323-28694-7

Editor: Jennifer Flynn-Briggs
Developmental Editor: Susan Showalter

Anesthesiology Clinics (ISSN 1932-2275) is published quarterly by Elsevier Inc., 360 Park Avenue South, New York, NY 10010-1710. Months of issue are March, June, September, and December. Periodicals postage paid at New York, NY and at additional mailing offices. Subscription prices are $160.00 per year (US student/resident), $330.00 per year (US individuals), $400.00 per year (Canadian individuals), $533.00 per year (US institutions), $674.00 per year (Canadian institutions), $225.00 per year (Canadian and foreign student/resident), $455.00 per year (foreign individuals), and $674.00 per year (foreign institutions). To receive student and resident rate, orders must be accompanied by name of affiliated institution, date of term, and the *signature* of program/residency coordinator on institutions letterhead. Orders will be billed at individual rate until proof of status is received. Foreign air speed delivery is included in all *Clinics'* subscription prices. All prices are subject to change without notice. POSTMASTER: Send address changes to *Anesthesiology Clinics,* Elsevier Health Sciences Division, Subscription Customer Service, 3251 Riverport Lane, Maryland Heights, MO 63043. Customer Service (orders, claims, online, change of address): Elsevier Health Sciences Division, Subscription Customer Service, 3251 Riverport Lane, Maryland Heights, MO 63043. Tel:1-800-654-2452 (U.S. and Canada); 314-447-8871 (outside U.S. and Canada). Fax: 314-447-8029. E-mail: journalscustomerservice-usa@elsevier.com (for print support); journalsonlinesupport-usa@elsevier.com (for online support).

Reprints. For copies of 100 or more of articles in this publication, please contact the Commercial Reprints Department, Elsevier Inc., 360 Park Avenue South, New York, NY 10010-1710. Tel.: 212-633-3874; Fax: 212-633-3820; E-mail: reprints@elsevier.com.

Anesthesiology Clinics, is also published in Spanish by McGraw-Hill Inter-americana Editores S. A., P.O. Box 5-237, 06500 Mexico D. F., Mexico.

Anesthesiology Clinics, is covered in *MEDLINE/PubMed (Index Medicus), Current Contents/Clinical Medicine, Excerpta Medica, ISI/BIOMED,* and *Chemical Abstracts.*

Printed and bound by CPI Group (UK) Ltd, Croydon, CR0 4YY

Contributors

CONSULTING EDITOR

LEE A. FLEISHER, MD, FACC, FAHA
Robert D. Dripps Professor and Chair of Anesthesiology and Critical Care, Professor of Medicine, Perelman School of Medicine, University of Pennsylvania School of Medicine, Philadelphia, Pennsylvania

EDITORS

ALAN JAY SCHWARTZ, MD, MSEd
Director of Education & Program Director, Pediatric Anesthesiology Fellowship, Department of Anesthesiology and Critical Care Medicine, The Children's Hospital of Philadelphia; Professor of Clinical Anesthesiology and Critical Care, Perelman School of Medicine University of Pennsylvania, Philadelphia, Pennsylvania

DEAN B. ANDROPOULOS, MD, MHCM
Chief of Anesthesiology, Texas Children's Hospital; Professor, Anesthesiology and Pediatrics, Baylor College of Medicine, Houston, Texas

ANDREW DAVIDSON, MBBS, MD, FANZCA
Associate Professor, Royal Children's Hospital, Parkville, Melbourne, Victoria, Australia

AUTHORS

RICHARD J. BANCHS, MD
Assistant Professor of Anesthesiology, Department of Anesthesiology (MC515), University of Illinois Medical Center, Children's Hospital University of Illinois, Chicago, Illinois

DAVID BUCK, MD, MBA
Advanced Fellow Quality Improvement and Safety, Department of Anesthesiology, Cincinnati Children's Hospital, Cincinnati, Ohio

KATRIN CAMPBELL, MD
Assistant Professor of Anesthesiology and Pediatrics, Director, Division of Sedation, Texas Children's Hospital, Baylor College of Medicine, Houston, Texas

NICHOLAS P. CARLING, MD
Assistant Professor of Pediatrics and Anesthesiology; Director of Neuroanesthesia, Texas Children's Hospital, Baylor College of Medicine, Houston, Texas

NICHOLAS M. DALESIO, MD
Assistant Professor, Division of Pediatric Anesthesiology, Department of Anesthesiology and Critical Care Medicine, Johns Hopkins University School of Medicine, Baltimore, Maryland

SABINA DICINDIO, DO
Department of Anesthesiology and Critical Care Medicine, Nemours/Alfred I. duPont Hospital for Children, Wilmington, Delaware; Assistant Professor of Anesthesiology, Department of Anesthesiology, Jefferson Medical College, Thomas Jefferson University, Philadelphia, Pennsylvania

JOHN E. FIADJOE, MD
Assistant Professor, Department of Anesthesiology and Critical Care, Children's Hospital of Philadelphia, Perelman School of Medicine at the University of Pennsylvania, Philadelphia, Pennsylvania

ROBERT H. FRIESEN, MD
Professor, Department of Anesthesiology, University of Colorado School of Medicine, Colorado

CHRIS D. GLOVER, MD
Assistant Professor of Pediatrics and Anesthesiology; Director of the Acute Pain Service, Texas Children's Hospital, Baylor College of Medicine, Houston, Texas

C. DEAN KURTH, MD
Professor, Department of Anesthesiology, Cincinnati Children's Hospital, University of Cincinnati College of Medicine, Cincinnati, Ohio

MARY LANDRIGAN-OSSAR, MD, PhD
Senior Associate in Perioperative Anesthesia, Department of Anesthesiology, Perioperative and Pain Medicine, Boston Children's Hospital, Instructor of Anaesthesia, Harvard Medical School, Boston, Massachusetts

GREGORY J. LATHAM, MD
Assistant Professor, Department of Anesthesiology and Pain Medicine, Seattle Children's Hospital, University of Washington School of Medicine, Seattle, Washington

JERROLD LERMAN, MD, FRCPC, FANZCA
Clinical Professor of Anesthesiology, Department of Anesthesia, Women and Children's Hospital of Buffalo, SUNY at Buffalo, Bufffalo; Department of Anesthesia, Strong Medical Center, University of Rochester, Rochester, New York

ERICA P. LIN, MD, FAAP
Assistant Professor of Clinical Anesthesia & Pediatrics, Department of Anesthesiology, Cincinnati Children's Hospital Medical Center, University of Cincinnati College of Medicine, Cincinnati, Ohio

ANDREAS W. LOEPKE, MD, PhD, FAAP
Associate Professor of Clinical Anesthesia & Pediatrics, Department of Anesthesiology, Cincinnati Children's Hospital Medical Center, University of Cincinnati College of Medicine, Cincinnati, Ohio

JAGROOP MAVI, MD
Assistant Professor, Clinical Anesthesia and Pediatrics, Department of Anesthesia, Cincinnati Children's Hospital Medical Center, Cincinnati, Ohio

CRAIG D. MCCLAIN, MD, MPH
Senior Associate in Perioperative Anesthesia, Department of Anesthesiology, Perioperative and Pain Medicine, Boston Children's Hospital, Assistant Professor of Anaesthesia, Harvard Medical School, Boston, Massachusetts

DAVID L. MOORE, MD
Associate Professor, Clinical Anesthesia and Pediatrics, Department of Anesthesia, Cincinnati Children's Hospital Medical Center, Cincinnati, Ohio

AMOD SAWARDEKAR, MD
Assistant Professor of Anesthesiology, Department of Pediatric Anesthesiology, Ann & Robert H. Lurie Children's Hospital of Chicago, Feinberg School of Medicine, Northwestern University, Chicago, Illinois

DEBORAH A. SCHWENGEL, MD
Assistant Professor, Division of Pediatric Anesthesiology, Department of Anesthesiology and Critical Care Medicine; Department of Pediatrics, Johns Hopkins University School of Medicine, Baltimore, Maryland

RAVI SHAH, MD
Assistant Professor of Anesthesiology, Department of Pediatric Anesthesiology, Ann & Robert H. Lurie Children's Hospital of Chicago, Feinberg School of Medicine, Northwestern University, Chicago, Illinois

SULPICIO G. SORIANO, MD, FAAP
Professor of Anaesthesia, Endowed Chair in Pediatric Neuroanesthesia, Department of Anesthesiology, Perioperative, and Pain Medicine, Boston Children's Hospital, Harvard Medical School, Boston, Massachusetts

STEPHEN STAYER, MD
Professor of Anesthesiology and Pediatrics, Medical Director of Perioperative Services, Associate Chief, Pediatric Anesthesiology, Texas Children's Hospital, Baylor College of Medicine, Houston, Texas

TRACEY L. STIERER, MD
Assistant Professor, Departments of Anesthesiology and Critical Care Medicine, and Otolaryngology-Head and Neck Surgery, Johns Hopkins University School of Medicine, Baltimore, Maryland

PAUL A. STRICKER, MD
Assistant Professor, Department of Anesthesiology and Critical Care, Children's Hospital of Philadelphia, Perelman School of Medicine at the University of Pennsylvania, Philadelphia, Pennsylvania

SANTHANAM SURESH, MD, FAAP
Anesthesiologist-in Chief, Professor of Anesthesiology & Pediatrics, Department of Pediatric Anesthesiology, Ann & Robert H. Lurie Children's Hospital of Chicago, Feinberg School of Medicine, Northwestern University, Chicago, Illinois

MICHAEL SURY, MB, BS, FRCA, PhD
Department of Anaesthesia, Great Ormond Street Hospital, London, United Kingdom

MARY C. THEROUX, MD
Pediatric Anesthesiologist and Director of Research, Anesthesiology Division, Department of Anesthesiology and Critical Care Medicine, Nemours/Alfred I. duPont Hospital for Children, Wilmington, Delaware; Professor of Anesthesiology and Pediatrics, Jefferson Medical College, Thomas Jefferson University, Philadelphia, Pennsylvania

LAURA TORRES, MD
Associate Professor of Anesthesiology and Pediatrics, Chair, Sedation Oversight Committee, Texas Children's Hospital, Baylor College of Medicine, Houston, Texas

MARK D. TWITE, MB BChir
Associate Professor, Department of Anesthesiology, University of Colorado School of Medicine, Colorado

ANNA VARUGHESE, MD, MPH
Associate Professor, Department of Anesthesiology, Cincinnati Children's Hospital, University of Cincinnati College of Medicine, Cincinnati, Ohio

BRITTA S. VON UNGERN-STERNBERG, MD, PhD, DEAA, FANZCA
Chair of Pediatric Anesthesia, Department of Anesthesia and Pain Management, Princess Margaret Hospital for Children; Winthrop Professor, Chair of Pediatric Anesthesia, School of Medicine and Pharmacology, The University of Western Australia, Perth, Australia

Contents

Preoperative anxiolysis is important for children scheduled for surgery. The nature of the anxiety depends on several factors, including age, temperament, past hospitalizations, and socioeconomic and ethnic backgrounds. A panoply of interventions effect anxiolysis, including parental presence, distraction, and premedication, although no single strategy is effective for all ages. Emergence delirium (ED) occurs after sevoflurane and desflurane in preschoolage children in the recovery room. Symptoms usually last approximately 15 minutes and resolve spontaneously. The Pediatric Anesthesia Emergence Delirium [PAED] scale is a validated scale to diagnose ED and evaluate therapeutic interventions for ED such as propofol and opioids.

The volume of pediatric invasive and noninvasive procedures outside the operating room continues to increase. The acuity and complexity of patient clinical condition has resulted in the expansion of the anesthesiologist's role in remote sites. The anesthesia provider must ensure patient safety by assuring appropriate patient preparation, having available required equipment for monitoring and rescue, planning careful sedation/anesthesia management, continuing vigilance and observation into the recovery phase, and requiring strict discharge criteria. A quality improvement program for the department of anesthesiology should review anesthetic and sedation outcomes of patients both inside and outside the operating room.

This article focuses on common respiratory complications in the postanesthesia care unit (PACU). Approximately 1 in 10 children present with respiratory complications in the PACU. The article highlights risk factors and at-risk populations. The physiologic and pathophysiologic background and causes for respiratory complications in the PACU are explained and suggestions given for an optimization of the anesthesia management in the perioperative period. Furthermore, the recognition, prevention, and treatment of these complications in the PACU are discussed.

There are 3 surgical procedures that patients with cerebral palsy (CP) undergo that may be considered major procedures: femoral osteotomies combined with pelvic osteotomies, spine fusion, and intrathecal baclofen pump implant for the treatment of spasticity. Many complications are known to occur at a higher rate in this population, and some may be avoided with prior awareness of the preoperative pathophysiology of the patient with CP.

neuronal cell death and subsequent learning and memory impairment. Several cohort studies in neonates with significant comorbidities requiring surgical procedures early in life have also demonstrated abnormal neuro-developmental outcomes. This article provides an overview of the currently available data from both animal experiments and human clinical studies regarding the effects of sedatives and anesthetics on the developing brain.

Children need cardiac catheterization to establish the diagnosis and monitor the response to treatment when undergoing drug therapy for the treatment of pulmonary arterial hypertension (PAH). Children with PAH receiving general anesthesia for cardiac catheterization procedures are at significantly increased risk of perioperative complications in comparison with other children. The most acute life-threatening complication is a pulmonary hypertensive crisis. It is essential that the anesthesiologist caring for these children understands the pathophysiology of the disease, how anesthetic medications may affect the patient's hemodynamics, and how to manage an acute pulmonary hypertensive crisis.

The technique of choice for surgical correction of pectus excavatum is the Nuss procedure, a minimally invasive technique in which rigid metal bars are placed transthoracically beneath the sternum and costal cartilages until permanent remodeling of the chest wall has occurred. Intraoperatively, anesthesia focuses on three areas: the potential for catastrophic blood loss caused by perforation of large capacitance vessels and the heart, the potential for malignant arrhythmias, and the consequences of bilateral iatrogenic pneumothoraces. Postoperatively, analgesia is institutionally dependent and controversial, based on usage and type of regional anesthesia. The necessity of multimodal analgesic techniques creates a common ground across different hospital systems.

Children with cancer undergo a host of surgeries and procedures that require anesthesia during the various phases of the disease. A safe anesthetic plan includes consideration of the direct effects of tumor, toxic effects of chemotherapy and radiation therapy, the specifics of the surgical procedure, drug-drug interactions with chemotherapy agents, pain syndromes, and psychological status of the child. This article provides a comprehensive overview of the anesthetic management of the child with cancer, focuses on a systems-based approach to the impact from both tumor and its treatment in children, and presents a discussion of the relevant anesthetic considerations.

ANESTHESIOLOGY CLINICS

Preface

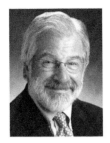 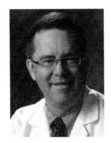 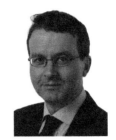

Alan Jay Schwartz, MD, MSEd   Dean B. Andropoulos, MD, MHCM   Andrew Davidson, MBBS, MD, FANZCA

Editors

Pediatric anesthesiology presents clinicians with recurring management issues that warrant review and updating. This issue of *Anesthesiology Clinics* provides "just what the doctor ordered" for a review of key topics in pediatric anesthesia patient care.

This issue is divided into 5 topical areas: (1) preanesthesia and postanesthesia considerations, (2) neurophysiology and neuroanesthesia, (3) cardiothoracic anesthesia, (4) regional anesthesia, and (5) practice management. The articles in each area are current considerations of patient care issues that have had an evergreen timeframe of interest.

As examples, Jerry Lerman and Richard Banchs offer a current perspective on preoperative anxiety and emergence agitation of pediatric patients and Steve Stayer brings us up to date on safe, effective, and efficient sedation of children in the nonoperating room environment. Sulpicio Soriano and Andreas Loepke present a most timely consideration of anesthetic neurotoxicity. Paul Stricker and John Fiadjoe review the high acuity care of children undergoing craniofacial surgery. The article devoted to regional anesthesia originates from Santhanam Suresh and Jennifer Rhodes, placing focus on the use of ultrasound to enhance safe care of children. Last, Dean Kurth, Anna Varughese, and David Buck remind readers about the modern day concern with quality assurance, also providing information from the Wake Up Safe initiative. There are 15 articles in total covering many of the "hot topics" about which readers are eager to learn.

We encourage you to read these up-to-date articles on some of the key issues confronting pediatric anesthesiologists and get the latest word on safe anesthetic management!

Alan Jay Schwartz, MD, MSEd
Department of Anesthesiology and Critical Care Medicine
The Children's Hospital of Philadelphia
34th Street and Civic Center Boulevard
Room 9327
Philadelphia, PA 19104-4399, USA

Anesthesiology Clin 32 (2014) xiii–xiv
http://dx.doi.org/10.1016/j.anclin.2013.11.002
1932-2275/14/$ – see front matter © 2014 Elsevier Inc. All rights reserved.

anesthesiology.theclinics.com

Dean B. Andropoulos, MD, MHCM
Texas Children's Hospital
6621 Fannin Street
Houston, TX 77030, USA

Andrew Davidson, MBBS, MD, FANZCA
Royal Children's Hospital
Flemington Road
Parkville
Melbourne, Victoria
3052 Australia

E-mail addresses:
schwartza@email.chop.edu (A.J. Schwartz)
dbandrop@texaschildrens.org (D.B. Andropoulos)
andrew.davidson@rch.org.au (A. Davidson)

Preoperative Anxiety Management, Emergence Delirium, and Postoperative Behavior

Richard J. Banchs, MD[a], Jerrold Lerman, MD, FRCPC, FANZCA[b,c],*

KEYWORDS

- Anxiety • Children • Distraction • Emergence delirium • Parental presence
- Pediatric • Premedication

KEY POINTS

- Preoperative anxiolysis is of utmost importance for children undergoing surgery.
- Preoperative educational materials, parental presence at induction of anesthesia (PPIA), distraction, and pharmacologic interventions are effective anxiolytics.
- Emergence delirium (ED) resurfaced with the newer insoluble anesthetics, sevoflurane and desflurane, as a nuisance and potentially serious sequela in young children in the recovery room.
- Research and investigation into the treatments of ED was stymied by the absence of a validated scale for ED until the Pediatric Anesthesia Emergence Delirium (PAED) scale was published.
- Causative factors for ED have not yet been elucidated, but several strategies have been described to attenuate ED, including propofol infusion and use of α2-agonists, opioids, and others.

INTRODUCTION

As the views and understanding of the factors that affect a child's anesthetic experience evolve, preoperative anxiety, postoperative behavior, and parental participation in the child's health care experience have become important considerations. In

[a] Department of Anesthesiology (MC515), University of Illinois Medical Center, Children's Hospital University of Illinois, 1740 West Taylor Street, Suite 3200 West, Chicago, IL 60612-7239, USA; [b] Department of Anesthesia, Women and Children's Hospital of Buffalo, SUNY at Buffalo, 219 Bryant Street, Buffalo, NY 14222, USA; [c] Department of Anesthesia, Strong Medical Center, University of Rochester, 601 Elmwood Avenue, Rochester, NY 14642, USA
* Corresponding author. Department of Anesthesia, Women and Children's Hospital of Buffalo, SUNY at Buffalo, 219 Bryant Street, Buffalo, NY 14222.
E-mail address: jerrold.lerman@gmail.com

Anesthesiology Clin 32 (2014) 1–23
http://dx.doi.org/10.1016/j.anclin.2013.10.011   anesthesiology.theclinics.com
1932-2275/14/$ – see front matter © 2014 Elsevier Inc. All rights reserved.

children, preoperative anxiolysis is important not only for compassionate reasons but also for improving postoperative behavior such as ED. Parents and society expect not only effective but also patient- and family-centered care. This review summarizes the current state of the art of perioperative management of children.

PREOPERATIVE ANXIETY
Framework

Parental separation and induction of anesthesia is one of the most stressful experiences for a child undergoing a surgical procedure. Stress may be manifested not only during the induction period but also during the postoperative period.[1] Although all children are vulnerable to stress, preschool children and toddlers aged 1 to 6 years seem to be the most vulnerable. Evidence suggests that children who are anxious in the holding area and during the induction experience a greater distress during the immediate postoperative period.[1–4] Preoperative anxiety is an independent predictor for postoperative negative behaviors.[2] Common postoperative negative behavior include nightmares, waking up crying, separation anxiety, and temper tantrums,[2,5] whereas more serious behavioral changes such as new-onset enuresis are uncommon.[5] The risk of postoperative negative behavior is 3.5-fold greater in children who experienced preoperative anxiety.[2] Of these children, 67% will develop negative behaviors on the first day after surgery, 45% on the second day, and 23% within 2 weeks.[2] Negative behaviors persist for up to 6 months in 20% of the children and for up to 1 year in 7.3% of the children.[5] In addition to a surgical procedure, any other health care encounter that proves to be traumatic may increase the likelihood of an anesthesia phobia when the child returns to the hospital. How perioperative anxiety affects later emotional and intellectual development remains unclear, but negative memories of hospitalizations and anesthetic care may persist well into adulthood.[6]

Measuring preoperative anxiety in a child is challenging. However, quantifying the degree of anxiety experience by a child may be a worthy pursuit to understand the magnitude of the problem and to stratify appropriate therapeutic interventions to mitigate its effects. Several scales have been developed to measure preoperative anxiety and have been used for both clinical and research purposes. However, because self-reporting scales are unsuitable for preverbal children, there are currently no scales for children younger than 2 years. Clinical parameters such as heart rate and blood pressure have been used in the past to assess anxiety, but these clinical parameters have shown a low validity and reliability. Plasma cortisol concentrations[7] after induction have also been used to quantify perioperative anxiety, but these are also insensitive measurements and impractical for every pediatric clinical practice.

Factors that Contribute to Preoperative Anxiety

Several factors contribute to preoperative anxiety and postoperative behavioral changes in children, including age, gender, temperament and ethnicity, previous hospital experience, type of anesthetic induction, type of surgery, and postoperative pain.

Age

The studies of the effects of age on anxiety during the induction of anesthesia have yielded inconsistent results. Younger children seem to be more anxious at separation from their parents[8] and less cooperative during induction of anesthesia than older children.[9,10] They also suffer from a greater incidence of postoperative behavioral disturbances,[9,11,12] which may last up to 6 months after surgery.[5] However, an observational study of 2122 children undergoing ambulatory surgery determined that distress at induction did not vary significantly with age.[13] Infants younger than 1 year may or may not express anxiety on separation from their parents and, depending on the infants, may be easily distracted. Paradoxically, another study noted that children older than 7 years were actually more anxious in the preoperative holding area than those aged 4 to 7 years, although anxiety was not measured during induction of anesthesia.[5] The inconsistent results regarding the relationship between anxiety and distress and age may, in part, be attributed to imprecise metrics that were used to measure the anxiety in children, a paucity of prospective randomized controlled trials, and small sample sizes.

Perioperative anxiety in children may depend primarily on their stages of development.[14] Each age group roughly correlates with a stage of development, and each stage manifests different psychological issues that require different and specific therapeutic approaches.[14] Infants are less likely to experience separation anxiety, children 1 to 3 years experience separation anxiety but respond positively to distraction and comforting measures,[14] and children aged 4 to 6 years seek explanations and a desire to maintain control of their environment. Furthermore, older children between the ages of 7 and 12 years have strong desires to be involved in the decision-making process.[14] Adolescents fear losing face and are concerned with their inability to cope.[14] The last 2 age groups respond well to explanations, to maintain control of events, and to preserve their privacy and independence as coping mechanisms to decrease anxiety.[14]

Gender
Gender has not been found to be a factor involved in preoperative anxiety or in postoperative behavioral problems in prepubescent children.[5,12]

Temperament and ethnicity
Perioperative anxiety is influenced by a child's temperament. Temperament is the behavioral makeup of a child that influences the reaction to surrounding stimuli and stressful environments. Four temperament components have been identified: emotionality, activity, sociability, and impulsivity.[15] Temperament has been measured using the EASI scale (emotionality, activity, sociability, impulsivity scale), which is an observer-based measurement tool that uses the parents to assess their child's temperament.[15] Parents score each of 5 patterns of behavior between 1 and 5 for a total score between 5 and 25. In a prospective study of 183 children aged 2 to 10 years undergoing elective surgery, situational anxiety of the mother, temperament and age of the child, and quality of previous medical encounters significantly correlated with preoperative anxiety.[5] Previous surgery, premedication, and lack of enrollment in a day care were predictors of child's anxiety at separation from the parents.[5] The Post-hospitalization Behavior Questionnaire (PHBQ) is a tool to assess behavioral changes in children after health care encounters. The PHBQ is a parental questionnaire that includes 27 items in 6 categories: general anxiety, separation anxiety, sleep anxiety, eating disturbances, aggression toward authority, apathy, and withdrawal.[16] Each item is graded on a scale from 1 to 5. Low scores indicate a positive behavioral change and high scores indicate a negative behavioral change. The PHBQ has good test validity and reliability, although it has not been studied in all age groups and is subject to parental bias.

Recent evidence suggests that cultural differences, including language and ethnicity, may contribute to changes in behavior, specifically behavior during the recovery period.[17]

Previous hospital experience
A previous health care experience may influence a child's preoperative level of anxiety. Children who have had previous negative health care encounters experience

greater anxiety in the holding area and at separation from parents.[5,12,18] Reducing a child's anxiety during the preoperative period may not only benefit the current perioperative process but also decrease anxiety at subsequent anesthesia encounters. Stressful life experiences close in time to a hospital admission can also affect how a child reacts to anesthesia and the overall surgical experience.

Type of anesthesia

The effects of the type of anesthesia induction on preoperative anxiety and other behaviors are unclear. In children aged 2 to 7 years who were premedicated with midazolam, anxiety was least in those anesthetized by inhalational anesthesia compared with an intravenous (IV) or rectal induction with methohexitone.[19] Postoperative behavior was similar among the 3 groups, although negative memories occurred more frequently in the inhalational group compared with the other 2 groups. At present, there is insufficient evidence to determine whether one type of anesthesia decreases perioperative anxiety any more or less than another.

Type of surgery

Whether the type of surgery influences the incidence of preoperative anxiety and postoperative behavior is unclear. Several studies concluded that the type of surgery does not increase the risk of postoperative maladaptive behaviors,[9,12,13,20] whereas other studies found that surgery of the genitourinary system[2] and inpatient surgery[18] were associated with an increased risk of postoperative behavioral changes. Preoperative anxiety is similar for elective and emergency procedures.[13] The effect of postoperative pain on the risk of postoperative maladaptive behavior is not well understood either. Using the PHBQ, one study found that pain was a significant predictor of behavioral changes that lasted up to 4 weeks,[19] whereas another reported a poor correlation between the severity of postoperative pain and behavioral changes.[5] The effect of the type of surgery on preoperative and postoperative anxiety and behavior remains unresolved.

INTERVENTIONS

The purpose of preoperative anxiolysis is to reduce a child's anxiety and decrease the risk of negative postoperative behavioral changes. Preoperative anxiolysis also improves cooperation during induction and may contribute to increased parental satisfaction. Several strategies have been used to reduce preoperative anxiety, including PPIA, preoperative educational programs, sedative premedication, and distraction techniques. Additional studies are needed to determine the optimal intervention for each age group. Several tools have been used to assess preoperative anxiety. The Yale Preoperative Anxiety Score (YPAS) is an observer assessment tool designed for children between the ages of 2 and 6 years. The YPAS has shown good validity and reliability in several clinical trials.[21] A modified version of the YPAS, the modified Yale Preoperative Anxiety Score (mYPAS), has been developed for children between the ages of 5 to 12 years. The mYPAS is based on the total score from 5 behavioral categories: the child's activity, facial expressions, alertness and arousal, vocalization, and interaction with adults. The mYPAS has shown good validity and intraobserver and interobserver reliability in numerous clinical trials.[22] Cooperation of a child during the induction phase of anesthesia has also been used as a surrogate measure of anxiety. The Induction Compliance Checklist (ICC) measures the cooperation of a child using a checklist of 10 items.[23] The ICC has excellent interobserver and intraobserver variability, but the validity of this scale to measure preoperative anxiety has not been validated. A visual analog scale has also been used to assess cooperation of a child at induction.

PPIA

PPIA is a common practice in many countries but more common in Europe than in the United States. In a survey of US and UK anesthesiologists, 58% of US anesthesiologists agreed with PPIA but in only 5% of the cases were parents routinely allowed in the operating room.[24] In contrast, 84% of British anesthesiologists allowed PPIA in more than 75% of the cases. Contrary to US anesthesiologists, most British anesthesiologists believed that PPIA decreased children's anxiety, increased their cooperation, and benefited both the parent and the anesthesia provider.[24] Fear of litigation has often been cited as an impediment to PPIA. Apart from isolated anecdotal cases, there is no evidence to support the notion that PPIA increases the risk of a lawsuit should an untoward event occur. Safety has also been cited as an impediment to PPIA.[25,26] Concerns over the safety of a child during PPIA are generally not substantive, although even when PPIA is routinely practiced, unusual circumstances may occur.[7,27] Acceptance of PPIA is mainly a function of a provider's experience, expertise, and available operating room logistical support. The level of anxiety of an experienced anesthesiologist is not increased by the presence of a parent at induction.[7] The unavailability of an induction room or of an operating room staff member to accompany the parent back to the holding area is often cited as the main cause preventing the routine presence of parents at induction. Several studies concluded that perioperative anxiety is decreased by the presence of a parent during induction.[28–30] However, these studies have been criticized for their lack of randomization and the use of tools to assess anxiety that had not been previously validated.[28–30] A total of 8 additional trials assessed PPIA, and none showed a significant difference in anxiety or cooperation during induction when parents were present.[31] One study showed that PPIA was significantly less effective than midazolam in reducing children's anxiety at induction.[31] In a study using a visual analog score for cooperation,[7] PPIA did not improve cooperation in children during induction. PPIA does not affect anxiety in infants younger than 1 year.[32] In 2 studies of PPIA and preoperative anxiety in the holding area, on entering the operating room and during induction of anesthesia, the investigators found no correlation between parental presence and anxiety.[7,10] A single measurement after induction showed reduced plasma cortisol levels in children of calm parents, shy and inhibited children, and in children older than 4 years.[7] PPIA does not reduce the risk of postoperative behavioral changes as determined by the PHBQ,[10,28,29] even with 6-month follow-up evaluations.[7]

Several reasons may in part explain the lack of effect of PPIA on preoperative anxiety.

1. First, many studies have not addressed high anxiety levels experienced by parents, which are known to affect a child's anxiety level and overall temperament.[10]
2. The simple presence of a parent may be insufficient to decrease a child's anxiety.
3. Even if a parent were present, the lack of a specific active role for the parent may actually contribute to the child's anxiety.[33]

It has also been shown that parents experience preoperative anxiety when they witness their child in distress.[34,35] Parent anxiety has been well documented using a visual analog score and the State Trait Anxiety Inventory (STAI), which is a gold standard for measuring anxiety in adults. There are several sources of anxiety for parents. These include the following:

1. Concerns about how their child reacts to a new environment
2. Concerns about their child's well-being
3. Concerns on witnessing their child's loss of consciousness and immobility[34–36]

4. Concerns that they are abandoning their child when they leave the operating room after the induction

Parents who are particularly vulnerable to experiencing anxiety during PPIA include

1. The parents of young children
2. Parents of a single child
3. Parents in the health care field[35–37]
4. Mothers of a child undergoing a surgical procedure[34,36,37]

If given a choice, parents generally prefer to accompany their child during the induction of anesthesia, regardless of their level of anxiety.[35] Parents believe their presence benefits their child. However, parental anxiety could actually negatively affect their child. Using the Global Mood Scale and the STAI, several studies have shown that children of anxious parents experience more anxiety than those of calm parents.[5,10] A child's anxiety in the holding area and after separation from the parent is greater if the parent is anxious.[5] A child of an anxious parent is 3.2 times more likely to have persistent behavioral problems up to 6 months after a surgical procedure, compared with a child of a calm parent.[5]

Although the role of PPIA in decreasing a child's anxiety during induction is still debated, what is clear is that PPIA does not decrease the parent's level of anxiety. In a study of parental anxiety, the level of anxiety was the same when measured in the holding area (control group) or after PPIA (intervention group).[10] Some anxious parents found that separation from their child actually relieved their own anxiety.[10] Only parents who were calm before induction of anesthesia felt less anxious when participating in their child's induction.[10] A single study demonstrated that PPIA reduces parental anxiety, but this study has been criticized for a lack of randomization.[30] In the current environment of family-centered care, many advocate for parental involvement in all aspects of a child's hospital experience as a strategy to increase overall parental satisfaction. However, even this assertion has been challenged as 2 studies noted that satisfaction with the perioperative experience did not improve with PPIA.[7,32]

PREOPERATIVE PREPARATION PROGRAMS

Preoperative preparation programs to decrease preoperative anxiety have had mixed results, stemming from the inherent immaturity and lack of reliability in children and the variability of interventions needed to successfully address every age group, temperament, and baseline personality.[38] In a study of 143 children aged 2 to 6 years, children who were randomized to the preoperative interactive book exhibited greater anxiety on the day of surgery but fewer behavioral changes 2 weeks after surgery than those who received the routine preoperative treatment.[39] Parents in the intervention group reported that preoperative interactive book helped their child (87%) and themselves (83%). Children who were randomized to routine preoperative preparation were significantly more aggressive postoperatively than those who received the interactive teaching book preoperatively. In another study, children were randomized to either a preoperative preparation program that consisted of information, a tour and role play with child-life specialists, or no intervention. The anxiety of the children in the preoperative period was significantly less in the intervention group but did not reach statistical significance for the induction and postoperative periods.[39,40] Children aged 2 to 3 years, those who were emotionally labile and those with previous hospital experience, were more anxious after the preoperative preparation program. Children older than 6 years were least anxious if they participated in the preoperative preparation program more than 5 days before surgery and most anxious if they participated

1 day before surgery.[39] Anxiety increased in children younger than 8 years who had a previous hospital experience and who viewed a preoperative videotape of hospital-related material the night before their surgery compared with those who viewed a nonmedical video.[41,42] Children older than 8 years did not experience this increase in anxiety. Younger children become more anxious after participating in preoperative preparation programs because they have difficulty distinguishing fantasy from reality. Reality-based preparation programs may sensitize young children undergoing surgical procedures.[33] To stratify the effects of different interventions on perioperative anxiety, one study compared the effects of a tour of the operating room plus a videotape plus role play with a tour of the operating room and video and with a tour alone in children aged 2 to 12 years.[40] Those who participated in a tour of the operating room plus a videotape plus role play exhibited reduced anxiety in the holding area compared with the other 2 groups.[40] However, beyond the holding area, the interventions did not affect perioperative anxiety.[40] The investigators also determined that preoperative preparation program exerted no effect on postoperative behavior in children 2 weeks after their surgical experience.

Anxiety has also been measured in children after their parents read to them an age-appropriate interactive teaching book explaining the anesthesia process 1 to 3 days before surgery.[43] Perioperative anxiety in the study and control groups was similar. The investigators reported a significant decrease in aggressive behavior after surgery in the teaching book group compared with the control group.[43]

Children who have undergone a psychological intervention-targeted behavioral strategy for surgery supervised by a pediatric psychologist are less anxious and more cooperative in the preoperative period and during the induction of anesthesia than controls.[44] This psychological program has also shown to be more efficient in reducing a mother's anxiety and increasing her satisfaction.

A novel preoperative preparation program is the ADVANCE family-centered behavioral preparation program which is an acronym for Anxiety-reduction, Distraction, Video modeling and education, Adding parents, No excessive reassurance, Coaching, and Exposure/shaping.[45] This program is a multicomponent behavioral preparation program that in addition to standard preoperative management provides strategies and instructions to reduce preoperative anxiety, teach parents distraction techniques, video modeling and education before the day of surgery, PPIA, avoid excessive reassurance at induction of anesthesia, coach to reinforce the skills needed to succeed during induction, and exposure/shaping to familiarize the child with induction by mask.[45] The effectiveness of ADVANCE, family-centered behavioral preparation, on preoperative anxiety and postoperative outcome measures was compared with PPIA alone, oral midazolam, and control groups.[45] Anxiety in parents and children in the ADVANCE group was significantly less than that in the other 3 groups in the holding area. Furthermore, anxiety in children in the ADVANCE group was less than in those in the control and PPIA groups during induction of anesthesia.[45] Anxiety and compliance in children in both the ADVANCE and midazolam groups were similar during induction of anesthesia. In terms of postoperative recovery, the incidence of ED and analgesic requirements in the recovery room in children in the ADVANCE group were less than those in the other groups. Discharge times for children in the ADVANCE group were less compared with times in the 3 other groups.[45] In a postscript, the investigators conceded that a major obstacle in operating a program like ADVANCE was the large operational costs.

The effects of information or preparation programs for parents have also been studied. In a randomized study, discussing either routine or detailed anesthetic risk information and discussion regarding their child's anesthetic did not affect anxiety levels before the surgical intervention, on the day of surgery in the holding area, after separation from their child, or immediately after the intervention.[46] The results were unaffected by both parental educational level and baseline parental anxiety.

Preoperative preparation programs to decrease preoperative anxiety in children can also reduce parental anxiety.[43] Parents who watched a preanesthetic video to facilitate parental education and anxiolysis before pediatric ambulatory surgery were less anxious compared with the control group.[47] Preoperative preparation programs also increase parental satisfaction.[43] For example, children of parents who had acupuncture demonstrated more anxiolysis and were more cooperative during the induction of anesthesia compared with those whose parents had sham acupuncture.[31] Moreover, the parents who received acupuncture were significantly less anxious than parents in the sham group.[31] However, in 2 trials that reported the impact of audiovisual aids on preoperative and postoperative outcomes, preoperative videos did not significantly affect the anxiety of either the child or the parent.[31]

PERIOPERATIVE INTERVENTIONS

The perioperative dialogue is a holistic intervention aimed at reducing perioperative anxiety in children. Perioperative dialogue is based on the beneficial effects of dialogue and continued support throughout the perioperative encounter.[48,49] In children undergoing ambulatory surgery, perioperative dialogue reduces perioperative anxiety as determined by salivary cortisol concentrations and decreases postoperative morphine consumption.[49]

PHARMACOLOGIC ANXIOLYSIS
Midazolam

The use of pharmacologic premedication varies widely among practices, age groups, and geographic location.[24] The most commonly used agent for anxiolysis is midazolam. The major appeal of oral midazolam stems from its safety record, effectiveness, and reliability in reducing preoperative anxiety in children. The only substantive drawback of oral midazolam is its bitter taste, which may cause children to refuse to finish drinking it or to cause them to expectorate it.

Randomized controlled trials have established midazolam's effectiveness as a preoperative anxiolytic in children.[50–57] The dose of oral midazolam has not been clearly understood over the ages of children who need it, and this has led to underdosing or prolonged times to reach maximum effect. Most clinicians administer doses of 0.5 mg/kg without regard for the child's age. The dose of oral midazolam for anxiolysis, analogous to inhalational anesthetics, increases with decreasing age. That is, a dose of 0.5 mg/kg will suit children aged 3 to 5 years, but for children aged 1 to 3 years, doses as large as 0.75 or 1 mg/kg may be required to achieve anxiolysis in 95% of children. This point has been studied from at least 2 perspectives, the pharmacologic and the neurobehavioral.[58,59] To ensure a greater than 95% success in anxiolysis for children 3 years or younger, a dose of 0.75 mg/kg should be administered. This dose usually achieves a maximum effect within 10 to 15 minutes. For older children, an oral dose of 0.4 mg/kg is suitable for children 6 years or older and a dose of 0.3 mg/kg for those 10 years or older.

In addition to decreasing perioperative anxiety, midazolam decreased the incidence of negative behavioral changes, including separation anxiety and postoperative eating disturbances,[57] although in one study, it actually increased negative postoperative behaviors.[56] Preoperative midazolam may decrease the incidence of negative behavior by 2 postulated mechanisms, either by reducing preoperative anxiety or by causing anterograde amnesia.[60] Midazolam has been shown to confer anterograde amnesia in as little as 10 minutes.[60] No serious complications have been reported after oral midazolam administration in doses between 0.2 and 1.0 mg/kg,[50,51,53–57] although 2 children experienced dysphoric reactions after 0.75 and 1.0 mg/kg oral midazolam.[52] Children with sleep-disordered breathing undergoing tonsillectomy have been given premedication with oral midazolam, 0.5 mg/kg, without serious sequelae. In an observational study, one of the 70 children who were enrolled experienced a transient desaturation to 77% for 5 seconds, awakening from the midazolam spontaneously, without stimulation or other intervention.[61]

The effects of midazolam on the quality of emergence, discharge times, and postoperative behavioral disturbances have also been studied yielding conflicting results.[62] Oral midazolam in a dose of 0.5 to 0.75 mg/kg delayed recovery from anesthesia in 3 studies,[50–52] but another study found no delay in recovery and hospital discharge after 0.2 to 0.3 mg/kg of oral midazolam in surgeries lasting 10 minutes.[54] In a study that compared oral midazolam, 0.5 mg/kg, with PPIA, children who received midazolam were less anxious on entering the operating room and at induction of anesthesia compared with those with PPIA.[23] The times to recover from anesthesia and the incidence of negative behavioral changes were similar in the 2 groups.[23] Parental anxiety was significantly less when children who received midazolam were separated from their parents. In children undergoing an inhalational induction, oral midazolam was more effective in reducing preoperative anxiety than PPIA.[23] When oral midazolam (0.5 mg/kg) was compared with oral midazolam plus PPIA,[63] the incidence of perioperative anxiety was similar in the 2 groups. Parental anxiety postinduction was reduced and satisfaction with the perioperative process increased in the midazolam/PPIA group compared with the midazolam only group.

Midazolam has also been administered intranasally (IN) in a dose of 0.2 to 0.3 mg/kg in a 0.5 mL volume, with a time to peak effect of 15 minutes but a 2.5-hour elimination half-life.[64,65] The most serious problem with this route of administration is a burning sensation in the nasopharynx after recovery from anesthesia. Midazolam has also been administered sublingually, rectally, and intramuscularly (IM), although these routes offer no particular advantages in children.

Midazolam interacts synergistically with propofol to reduce the propofol requirements during induction of anesthesia, a characteristic attributed to midazolam's effects on the γ-aminobutyric acid (GABA) receptors.[63] Midazolam also provides more favorable conditions for inserting laryngeal mask airways in the presence of propofol.[66] Both characteristics have been cited as advantages to using midazolam for anxiolysis in the perioperative period.

Other Pharmacologic Agents

Clonidine, dexmedetomidine,[67] ketamine, and sufentanil have all been used as anxiolytics in the preanesthetic period. Clonidine is an α2-adrenergic agonist with analgesic, anxiolytic, and sedative properties and decreases the anesthetic and postoperative analgesic requirements.[68] Despite these properties, children who were scheduled for tonsillectomy surgery and who were premedicated with clonidine (4 μg/kg) exhibited more anxiety during separation from their parents, increased opioid requirements postoperatively, and greater postoperative pain scores compared with those who were premedicated with oral midazolam (0.5 mg/kg).[69] In a meta-analysis of 10 studies of healthy children undergoing ambulatory surgery who were premedicated with oral clonidine, a dose of 2 to 4 μg/kg decreased both anxiety at induction of anesthesia and the incidence of ED.[70] This meta-analysis neither addressed the effects of preoperative clonidine for surgeries of prolonged duration nor did it stratify for confounding factors such as the effects of clonidine on postoperative nausea and vomiting (PONV).[70] The major advantages of the α2-agonists include an absence of respiratory depression and fewer paradoxic reactions compared with midazolam. However, there are several major disadvantages of clonidine use, including its slow onset of action (>60 minutes), prolonged duration of action, and its sedation effects. At a dose of 4 μg/kg, the clinical effects and peak blood concentration of oral clonidine occur at 60 and 90 minutes, respectively.[69] This slow onset of action precludes the use of clonidine in many busy ambulatory pediatric anesthesia practices.

Dexmedetomidine is another α2-adrenergic agonist that has also been used for preoperative anxiolysis. Its α2 receptor specificity is 8-fold greater than for clonidine, reducing the frequency of side effects.[71,72] Despite dexmedetomidine's slow onset time (30–60 minutes), its duration of action (85 minutes) is less than that of clonidine, which makes it a candidate for use in ambulatory surgery. IN dexmedetomidine has also been used for premedication in children. IN dexmedetomidine, 1 μg/kg, provides more effective sedation than oral midazolam, 0.5 mg/kg,[71,73] or oral dexmedetomidine, 1 μg/kg. In a dose response study of IN dexmedetomidine, 2 μg/kg provided better sedation in children 5 to 8 years old than 1 μg/kg. In children 1 to 4 years old, 1 or 2 μg/kg provided equivalent anxiolysis.[74] To further exploit combination premedications, the combination of IN dexmedetomidine (2 μg/kg) and oral ketamine (3 mg/kg) provided easy separation from their parents, accepted IV cannulation, and did not lead to side effects and postoperative complications when compared with smaller doses of IN dexmedetomidine, larger doses of ketamine, and oral ketamine alone (5 mg/kg).[75]

Ketamine has been developed as a premedication for cognitively impaired children who are uncooperative and for healthy unimpaired children. For cognitively impaired children, IM ketamine, 2 to 5 mg/kg, is administered from a stock solution of 100 mg/mL. It has an onset time of approximately 10 minutes. The children should be seated on a gurney before IM ketamine is administered to avoid having to lift the child from the recumbent position once the child is completely unconscious. Oral ketamine (5–6 mg/kg) was developed as an alternative to oral midazolam, although emesis has proven to be a problem with ketamine.[76] Some prefer a 50–50 mixture of midazolam (0.3 mg/kg) and ketamine (3 mg/kg) to mitigate the side effects of the medications.[77]

IN sufentanil (2 μg/kg) is an effective premedication, although one study reported a 23% incidence of desaturation (<90%).[78] Chest wall rigidity occurred in 45% of children after administration of 4.5 μg/kg IN.[79]

ADDITIONAL NONPHARMACOLOGIC STRATEGIES

Several nonpharmacologic strategies have been found to be effective for anxiolysis in children. Clowns, hypnosis, low sensory stimulation, and handheld video games all reduce preoperative anxiety. In a systematic review of 17 trials involving 1796 children, anxiolysis after several nonpharmacologic strategies was evaluated.[31] Video games given to children in the preoperative period significantly reduced anxiety at induction compared with no intervention or premedication. Clowns have also been shown to reduced anxiety in children. In contrast, hypnosis and music therapy did not reduce anxiety at induction of anesthesia.[31] PPIA caused no anxiolysis in 8 trials and was significantly less effective as an anxiolytic than oral midazolam in one study.[31] Other distraction techniques such as playing with a favorite toy, viewing animated cartoons, listening to humorous stories, role playing, creative reinterpretation of the environment, and magic tricks reduced anxiety and increased the level of cooperation compared with controls.[80–82] Certain provider behaviors have been shown to exacerbate anxiety. Repetitive reassurance, excessive talk, apologizing, and adult-appropriate medical explanations all increase perioperative anxiety in children,[83] although parental reassurance may not prove to be as harmful as originally believed.[84] Other language such as empathy, distraction, and assurance may be effective to promote coping.[83] To address this issue and to train health care providers to improve their behaviors, the Provider-Tailored Intervention for Perioperative Stress (P-TIPS) was developed to promote children's coping and decrease behaviors that may exacerbate children's distress. In a trial of the effectiveness of P-TIPS, the rate of desired behaviors increased and the rate of undesired behaviors decreased in participants compared with control.[85] Furthermore, parents who were in contact with trained providers also demonstrated an increase in their rates of desired versus undesired behaviors.[85] The study of the effectiveness of P-TIPS in preventing anxiety and improving the recovery process (in terms of postoperative pain, recovery room stay, nausea and vomiting, ED, maladaptive behavioral change, and parental anxiety and satisfaction) in children undergoing surgery is currently underway.[86]

ED
Definition and Incidence

ED is a complex of perceptual disturbances and psychomotor agitation that occurs most commonly in preschool-aged children in the early postanesthetic period. The term ED is often used interchangeably with emergence agitation and postanesthetic excitement. For the purposes of this review, the authors refer to this complex as ED.

ED has been defined as a dissociated state of consciousness[87] in a child who is crying, inconsolable, and thrashing. In this state, children typically do not recognize familiar objects or people such as parents or caregivers.[87] It occurs in the recovery room, in the early recovery period. Wells reported paranoid ideation as a component of ED in an adult and children.[88] In general, combative behavior more aptly describes the behavior found in children with ED rather than restlessness and incoherence.[89] The authors define ED as "a disturbance in a child's awareness of and attention to his/her environment with disorientation and perceptual alterations including hypersensitivity to stimuli and hyperactive motor behavior in the immediate postanesthesia period."[90] The time course of ED usually begins as the child awakens from general anesthesia (typically in the first 30 minutes of recovery), lasts 5 to 15 minutes, and resolves spontaneously. The incidence of ED ranges from 5.3% to 50% and depends on several factors: the metric used to measure it, age group, anesthetic technique, and type of surgery.[91]

ED is a cause for concern because it may result in injury to the child, disruption of the surgical site, and accidental removal of the IV catheter and surgical drains. In addition, a child experiencing ED requires extra nursing care and may require the use of supplemental sedatives that may delay discharge from the recovery room. The underlying cause of ED has not been clearly elucidated. Several factors have been suggested as potential causes of ED, including factors related to patient characteristics, anesthetic technique, and type of surgery.

Assessment Tools

More than 16 rating scales have been used to measure ED. The lack of consensus on a single tool with which to assess ED demonstrates the inherent difficulty in interpreting maladaptive behavior in small children, and especially in children who are not able to verbalize pain or anxiety. Most scales assess emotional distress and agitation, which are associated features rather than core features of a true ED.[92] Crying, agitation, and lack of cooperation have been included in several scales, but these behaviors are not specific to ED. They may also characterize children who are in pain, as many are after surgery, or who are frightened during the early emergence period from general anesthesia.[90] These behaviors do overlap with behaviors measured in behavioral pain scales such as the Faces Legs Activity Cry and Consolability scale, the Children's and Infants' Postoperative Pain Scale, and the Children's Hospital of Eastern Ontario Pain Scale.[92] Hence, it is fair to state that agitation does not always indicate ED. However, agitation and thrashing requiring restraint[93,94] are the most frequently used parameters to define ED in children.[95–97]

The PAED scale was developed to specifically assess ED in young children. It consists of 5 psychometric items: the child makes eye contact with the caregiver, purposeful movement, awareness of the surroundings, restlessness, and whether the child is inconsolable. Items are each scored on a scale from 0 to 4. When the total score exceeds 10, ED is likely present, although some have suggested that a score greater than 12 more likely confirms ED. The PAED scale has good reliability and validity, having been used in more than 90 studies to date.[90] A PAED score of 5 does not mean there is half a chance of ED, but rather any score less than the threshold of 10 (or 12) has no meaning in terms of ED. PAED has been compared with other scores[98,99] with variable results.[100]

Efforts have been undertaken to further refine the behaviors associated with ED. Activity; nonpurposefulness; eyes averted, stared, or closed; no language; and nonresponsivity appears to be significantly associated with ED.[92] These behaviors are not significantly associated with pain or tantrum and are believed to reflect the true Diagnostic and Statistical Manual of Mental Disorders IV/V diagnostic criteria for delirium. A logistic regression showed that eyes averted or stared and nonpurposefulness were significant predictors of ED, whereas no language and activity did not significantly predict ED.[92]

Causative Factors

Age

Children between the ages of 2 and 5 years are more likely to experience ED on recovery from general anesthesia, with no gender predilection.[95] The psychological immaturity of a child's nervous system and the rapid awakening from general anesthesia in an unfamiliar environment may be responsible for the genesis of ED.[95] It has also been proposed that delirium in children and in the elderly may have a similar pathway.[101] Immaturity of the cholinergic centers and the hippocampus and low levels of neurotransmitters may provide an explanation for the susceptibility of younger children to ED.[101] It has been suggested that the GABA$_A$ receptor could be excitatory rather than inhibitory in early infancy, explaining this paradoxic reaction to anesthesia in young children. As the child matures, the GABA$_A$ receptor transforms into an inhibitory neurotransmitter, and the reaction no longer occurs, as in the adult.[102] These receptors could be excitatory rather than inhibitory in early infancy because of a switch from high to low chloride content in the neurons.[102] Other evidence, however, provides a conflicting view leaving the mechanism behind the ED behavior unexplained.[103]

Preoperative anxiety and temperament

Preoperative anxiety has been associated with an increased likelihood of a restless recovery and postoperative maladaptive behaviors. However, a clear relationship between preoperative anxiety and ED has not been established. The odds of experiencing ED increases 10% for each increment of 10 points in a child's preoperative anxiety score (mYPAS).[104] The odds ratio of having new-onset postoperative maladaptive behavior is 1.43 for children with marked ED, as compared with children with no symptoms of ED.[104] A 10-point increase in the preoperative anxiety scores increase the odds that a child will have a new-onset maladaptive behavior after surgery by 12.5%.[104] Despite these data, a statistically significant relationship between preoperative anxiety and postoperative maladaptive behaviors such as ED remains unconfirmed.[104]

It is likely that the underlying emotional temperament of a child determines his responses to outside stimuli and the degree to which preoperative anxiety and postoperative agitation are manifested. Children who are emotional, impulsive, or withdrawn[104] are at increased risk for developing ED.

Anesthetic technique

ED has been reported in children after both inhalational and intravenous anesthesia. Sevoflurane, desflurane, isoflurane,[5,16,20,51] and to a lesser extent halothane[93,105] have all been implicated as causative agents for ED. Most of the intravenous agents (midazolam, remifentanil, propofol, ketamine, and barbiturates) have also been associated with ED, although the incidence with these latter agents is far less than it is with inhalational anesthetics. Research into the etiology of ED has been made difficult when investigators have selected a surgical model that is associated with pain in the recovery room, a behavior that is often difficult to distinguish from ED, and when scales are used to diagnose ED that have not been validated to measure ED.

In children undergoing magnetic resonance imaging (MRI), the incidence of ED after use of sevoflurane may be up to 7-fold greater than with that of halothane. ED occurs more commonly after ether inhalational anesthetics than after alkanes like halothane,[89,94–97,106–115] suggesting that this is a class action. Considering that the electroencephalogram changes that are associated with sevoflurane are similar to those observed with either desflurane or isoflurane[116] but different from halothane,[117] it is possible that ED is related to the interference with the balance between neuronal synaptic inhibition and excitation in the central nervous system produced by the ether anesthetics.[118]

Sevoflurane has been shown to potentiate $GABA_A$-receptor-mediated inhibitory postsynaptic currents at high concentrations and to block these currents at low concentrations.[119] This biphasic effect of sevoflurane on $GABA_A$–receptor-mediated postsynaptic currents may be a contributing factor to the genesis of ED in young children.[120]

Specific brain metabolites may also contribute to ED in young children. The metabolic signature of sevoflurane shows greater brain concentrations of lactate and glucose than that of propofol. Lactate and glucose correlate positively and total creatine negatively with ED.[121] The association between ED and serum lactate concentration suggests that anesthesia-induced enhanced cortical activity in the unconscious state "may interfere with rapid return to coherent brain connectivity patterns required for normal cognition upon emergence of anesthesia."[121]

Several other factors have also been implicated as causes of ED. Depth of anesthesia[122] and rapid awakening[112,114,123–127] were postulated as contributing factors, but subsequent studies determined they were not associated with ED. Although some have suggested that the type of surgery (such as head and neck) may be associated with ED, there is no evidence to support this claim either.[128]

Pain

The presence of postoperative pain may contribute to the genesis of ED in preschool-aged children. Several studies reported that the incidence of ED in children decreased after analgesic/sedatives were administered intraoperatively. For example, the incidence of ED in children who were anesthetized with halothane or sevoflurane decreased 3- to 4-fold when ketorolac was administered intraoperatively.[111] Similarly, ED was prevented when fentanyl, 1 or 2.5 μg/kg, was administered intraoperatively to children undergoing ambulatory surgery, although the fentanyl preserved the rapid recovery associated with desflurane anesthesia.[98,129] The incidence also decreased after IN fentanyl was administered intraoperatively.[99,130] The incidence of ED decreased after administration of clonidine 3 μg/kg IV or via the caudal space[131] or 2 μg/kg IV[132] and dexmedetomidine 0.2 μg/kg IV. The possibility that these analgesics sedate the child to prevent or attenuate ED rather than provide pain relief has not been clarified. To further investigate the role of pain in this phenomenon, the incidence of ED has been determined in children aged 1 and 6 years undergoing inguinal hernia repair. Two studies demonstrated that agitation occurred significantly more frequently after use of sevoflurane anesthesia than that of halothane anesthesia despite the presence of an effective but preemptive caudal block.[95,97] Similarly, the incidence of ED after sevoflurane or desflurane was similar when analgesia was provided by a caudal block.[133] However, to completely remove pain as a confounding variable, the incidence of ED was determined in children undergoing diagnostic MRI. ED occurred in 33% of young children anesthetized with sevoflurane compared with 0% of those anesthetized with halothane.[96] The same group determined that the incidence of ED decreased from 56% to 12% when IV fentanyl, 1 μg/kg, was administered to children anesthetized with sevoflurane for MRI 10 minutes before discontinuation of the anesthetic suggesting the sedative effect of fentanyl may be contributory to attenuating ED.[129]

Inadequate pain control remains a potential cause of or contributor to the incidence of ED after brief surgical procedures for which the peak analgesic effect of the agent administered is delayed until the child is awake.[111] Although pain cannot be entirely excluded as a contributing factor to the presence of ED, current evidence suggests the influence of other mechanisms in the cause of ED. It is likely that several factors combined and specific characteristics of a child's temperament contribute to the development of ED.

PREVENTION AND TREATMENT OF ED

The only strategy that could prevent ED from occurring at all is to use a total intravenous anesthetic approach for the anesthetic procedure. The authors generally use a propofol infusion, supplemented with opioids and/or midazolam, with analgesia provided by either a regional block or opioid. This approach may be supplemented with nitrous oxide as well. Using this technique, the incidence of ED approaches zero.

Propofol, either as a single bolus or administered as an infusion has been shown to decrease the incidence of ED after sevoflurane anesthesia.[134,135] Preoperative administration of midazolam may decrease the incidence of ED,[69,94] although the evidence is still conflicting.[103,134,136] Clonidine[137,138] and dexmedetomidine[139,140] have also been noted to decrease the incidence of ED. Clonidine may exert its effect centrally by reducing the noradrenaline content in adrenergic areas of the brain observed with all the inhaled anesthetics. This increase in noradrenaline content is prominent during sevoflurane or isoflurane anesthesia and persists in some areas of the brain during the recovery phase.[132] Magnesium sulfate infusion reduces the incidence of ED during tonsillectomy in children with a number needed to treat of 3.[141] Chloral hydrate has not shown to decrease the incidence of ED.[142] Preemptive analgesia with opioids, ketorolac, and α2-agonists and regional anesthesia have all been shown to decrease the incidence of ED in children. Their effects may be due to combinations of analgesia and sedation.[97,98,111,131,132,143–146] Melatonin,[147] oxycodone,[148] oral ketamine,[149] and oral transmucosal fentanyl citrate[150] have also been used to decrease the incidence of ED. Remifentanil[151,152] however, has yielded conflicting effects on the incidence of ED. A meta-analysis[134] of the pharmacologic prevention of ED after sevoflurane and desflurane in children reported that propofol, ketamine, fentanyl, and preoperative analgesia successfully prevented ED.

The decision to treat ED in the recovery room is often influenced by the severity and duration of the symptoms and by concerns over the safety of the child, disruption of the surgical site, and the accidental removal of IV access and drains. There is no evidence, however, that if left untreated ED has long-term sequelae in children. However, steps should be taken to protect the child from self-injury and to provide a quiet and dark environment where the child can recover. Parental presence has not been shown to affect either the incidence or the severity of ED, except in one study.[153] If parents are present during ED, they should be appropriately reassured and be made aware that the situation is self-limiting and that the child will return to his or her normal behavior in due course. If treatment of ED becomes necessary, a single bolus of propofol (0.5–1.0 mg/kg IV),[134,135,154] fentanyl (1–2.5 μg/kg IV),[129,143] or dexmedetomidine (0.5 μg/kg IV)[134,139,140] has been successful in decreasing the severity and duration of the episode.

REFERENCES

1. Schwartz BH, Albino JE, Tedesco LA. Effects of psychological preparation on children hospitalized for dental operations. J Pediatr 1993;102:634–8.
2. Kain ZN, Wang SM, Mayes LC, et al. Distress during the induction of anesthesia and postoperative behavioral outcomes. Anesth Analg 1999;88:1042–7.
3. Eckenhoff JE. Relationship of anesthesia to postoperative personality changes in children. Am J Dis Child 1958;86:587–91.
4. Meyers E, Muravchick S. Anesthesia induction techniques in pediatric patients: a controlled study of behavioral consequences. Anesth Analg 1977;56:538–42.
5. Kain ZN, Mayes LC, O'Connor TZ, et al. Preoperative anxiety in children, predictors and outcomes. Arch Pediatr Adolesc Med 1996;150:1238–45.
6. Vessey JA, Bogetz MS, Dunleavey MF, et al. Memories of being anesthetized as a child. Anesthesiology 1994;81:A1384.
7. Kain ZN, Mayes LC, Caramico LA, et al. Parental presence during induction of anesthesia. A randomized controlled trial. Anesthesiology 1996;84:1060–7.
8. Vetter TR. The epidemiology and selective identification of children at risk for preoperative anxiety reactions. Anesth Analg 1993;77:96–9.
9. Kotiniemi LH, Ryhanen PT, Moilanen IK. Behavioural changes in children following day-case surgery: a 4-week follow-up of 551 children. Anaesthesia 1997;52:970–6.
10. Bevan JC, Johnston C, Tousignant G. Preoperative parental anxiety predicts behavioural and emotional responses to induction of anaesthesia in children. Can J Anaesth 1990;37:177–82.
11. Visintainer MA, Wolfer JA. Psychological preparation of surgical pediatric patients; the effect on children's and parents' stress responses and adjustment. Pediatrics 1975;56:187–202.
12. Kotiniemi LH, Ryhanen PT, Moilanen IK. Behavioural changes following routine ENT operations in two to ten year old children. Paediatr Anaesth 1996;6:45–9.
13. Holm-Knudsen RJ, Carlin JB, McKenzie IM. Distress at induction of anaesthesia in children. A survey of incidence, associated factors and recovery characteristics. Paediatr Anaesth 1998;8:383–92.

14. McGraw T. Preparing children for the operating room: psychological issues. Can J Anaesth 1994;41:1094–103.
15. Buss AH, Plomin R, Willerman L. The inheritance of temperaments. J Pers 1973; 41:513–24.
16. Vernon DT, Schulman JL, Foley JM. Changes in children's behavior after hospitalisation. Am J Dis Child 1966;111:581–93.
17. Fortier MA, Tan ET, Mayes LC, et al. Ethnicity and parental report of postoperative behavioral changes in children. Paediatr Anaesth 2013;23:422–8.
18. Lumley MA, Melamed BG, Abeles LA. Predicting children's presurgical anxiety and subsequent behavior changes. J Pediatr Psychol 1993;18:481–97.
19. Kotiniemi LH, Rhyanen PT. Behavioural changes in children's memories after intravenous, inhalation and rectal induction of anaesthesia. Paediatr Anaesth 1996;6:201–7.
20. Thompson RH, Vernon DT. Research on children's behavior after hospitalization: a review and synthesis. J Dev Behav Pediatr 1993;14:28–35.
21. Kain ZN, Mayes LC, Cicchetti DV, et al. Measurement tool for preoperative anxiety in young children: the Yale preoperative anxiety scale. Child Neuropsychol 1995;1:203–10.
22. Kain ZN, Mayes LC, Cicchetti DV, et al. The Yale preoperative anxiety scale: how does it compare with a 'gold standard'? Anesth Analg 1997;85:783–8.
23. Kain ZN, Mayes LC, Wang S, et al. Parental presence during induction of anesthesia versus sedative premedication. Which intervention is more effective? Anesthesiology 1998;89:1147–56.
24. Kain ZN, Mayes LC, Bell C, et al. Premedication in the United States: a status report. Anesth Analg 1997;84:427–32.
25. Bowie JR. Parents in the operating room? Anesthesiology 1993;78:1192–3.
26. Johnson YJ, Nickerson M, Quezado ZM. An unforeseen peril of parental presence during induction of anesthesia. Anesth Analg 2012;115:1371–2.
27. Gauderer MW, Lorig JL, Eastwood DW. Is there a place for parents in the operating room? J Pediatr Surg 1989;24:705–7.
28. Schulman JL, Foley JM, Vernon DT, et al. A study of the effect of the mother's presence during anesthesia induction. Pediatrics 1967;39:111–4.
29. Hannallah RS, Rosales JK. Experience with parents' presence during anaesthesia induction in children. Can J Anaesth 1983;30:286–9.
30. Cameron JA, Bond MJ, Pointer SC. Reducing the anxiety of children undergoing surgery: parental presence during anaesthetic induction. J Paediatr Child Health 1996;32:51–6.
31. Yip P, Middleton P, Cyna AM, et al. Nonpharmacological interventions for assisting the induction of anaesthesia in children. Evid Based Child Health 2011;6: 71–134.
32. Palermo TM, Tripi PA, Burgess E. Parental presence during anaesthesia induction for outpatient surgery of the infant. Paediatr Anaesth 2000;10:487–91.
33. Watson AT, Visram A. Children's preoperative anxiety and postoperative behaviour. Paediatr Anaesth 2003;13:188–204.
34. Shirley PJ, Thompson N, Kenward M, et al. Parental anxiety before elective surgery in children. A British perspective. Anaesthesia 1998;53:956–9.
35. Ryder IG, Spargo PM. Parents in the anaesthetic room. A questionnaire survey of parents' reactions. Anaesthesia 1991;46:977–9.
36. Vessey JA, Bogetz MS, Caserza CL, et al. Parental upset associated with participation in induction of anaesthesia in children. Can J Anaesth 1994;41: 276–80.

37. Litman RS, Berger AA, Chhibber A. An evaluation of preoperative anxiety in a population of infants and children undergoing ambulatory surgery. Paediatr Anaesth 1996;6:443–7.
38. Litman RS. Allaying anxiety in children. When a funny thing happens on the way to the operating room. Anesthesiology 2011;115:4–5.
39. Kain ZN, Mayes LC, Caramico LA. Preoperative preparation in children: a cross-sectional study. J Clin Anesth 1996;8:508–14.
40. Kain ZN, Caramico LA, Mayes LC, et al. Preoperative preparation programs in children: a comparative examination. Anesth Analg 1998;87:1249–55.
41. Melamed BG, Dearborn M, Hermecz DA. Necessary considerations for surgery preparation. Age and previous experience. Psychosom Med 1983;45:517–25.
42. Faust J, Melamed BG. Influence of arousal, previous experience and age on surgery preparation of same day surgery and in-hospital pediatric patients. J Consult Clin Psychol 1984;52:359–65.
43. Margolis JO, Ginsberg B, Dear GD, et al. Paediatric preoperative teaching: effects at induction and postoperatively. Paediatr Anaesth 1998;8:17–23.
44. Cuzzocrea F, Gugliandolo MC, Larcan R, et al. A psychological preoperative program: effects on anxiety. Paediatr Anaesth 2013;23:139–43.
45. Kain ZN, Caldwell-Andrews AA, Mayes LC, et al. Family-centered preparation for surgery improves perioperative outcomes in children. Anesthesiology 2007;106:65–74.
46. Kain ZN, Wang SM, Caramico LA, et al. Parental desire for perioperative information and informed consent: a two-phase study. Anesth Analg 1997;84:299–306.
47. Cassady JF, Wysocki TT, Miller KM, et al. Use of a preanesthetic video for facilitation of parental education and anxiolysis before pediatric ambulatory surgery. Anesth Analg 1999;88:246–50.
48. Linberg S. From fear to confidence: children with a fear of general anaesthesia and the perioperative dialogue for dental treatment. J Adv Perioperat Care 2006;2:143–51.
49. Wennstrom B, Tornhage CJ, Nasic S, et al. The perioperative dialogue reduces postoperative stress in children undergoing day surgery as confirmed by salivary cortisol. Paediatr Anaesth 2011;21:1058–65.
50. Feld LH, Negus JB, White PF. Oral midazolam preanesthetic medication in pediatric outpatients. Anesthesiology 1990;73:831–4.
51. Parnis SJ, Foate JA, Van Der Walt JH, et al. Oral midazolam is an effective premedication for children having day-stay anaesthesia. Anaesth Intensive Care 1992;20:9–14.
52. McMillan CO, Spahr-Schopfer IA, Sikich N, et al. Premedication of children with oral midazolam. Can J Anaesth 1992;39:545–50.
53. McCluskey A, Meakin GH. Oral administration of midazolam as a premedicant for paediatric day-case anaesthesia. Anaesthesia 1994;49:782–5.
54. Davis PJ, Tome JA, McGowan FX, et al. Preanesthetic medication with intranasal midazolam for brief pediatric surgical procedures. Anesthesiology 1995;82:2–5.
55. Gillerman RG, Hinkle AJ, Green HM, et al. Parental presence plus oral midazolam decreases frequency of 5% halothane inductions in children. J Clin Anesth 1996;8:480–5.
56. McGraw T, Kendrick A. Oral midazolam premedication and postoperative behaviour in children. Paediatr Anaesth 1998;8:117–21.
57. Kain ZN, Mayes LC, Wang SM, et al. Postoperative behavioral outcomes in children: effects of sedative premedication. Anesthesiology 1999;90:758–65.

58. Coté CJ, Cohen IT, Suresh S, et al. A comparison of three doses of a commercially prepared oral midazolam syrup in children. Anesth Analg 2002;94:37–43.
59. Kain ZN, MacLaren J, McClain BC, et al. Effects of age and emotionality on the effectiveness of midazolam administered preoperatively to children. Anesthesiology 2007;107:545–52.
60. Kain ZN, Hofstadter MB, Mayes LC, et al. Midazolam – effects on amnesia and anxiety in children. Anesthesiology 2000;93:676–84.
61. Francis A, Eltaki K, Bash T, et al. The safety of preoperative sedation in children with sleep-disordered breathing. Int J Pediatr Otorhinolaryngol 2006;70:1517–21.
62. Rosenbaum A, Kain ZN, Larsson P, et al. The place of premedication in pediatric practice. Paediatr Anaesth 2009;19:817–28.
63. Kain ZN. Premedication and parental presence revisited. Curr Opin Anaesthesiol 2001;14:331–7.
64. Kogan A, Katz J, Efrat R, et al. Premedication with midazolam in young children: a comparison of four routes of administration. Paediatr Anaesth 2002;12:685–9.
65. Chiaretti A, Barone G, Rigante D, et al. Intranasal lidocaine and midazolam for procedural sedation in children. Arch Dis Child 2011;96:160–3.
66. Bhaskar P, Mailk A, Kapoor R, et al. Effect of midazolam premedication on the dose of propofol for laryngeal mask airway insertion in children. J Anaesthesiol Clin Pharmacol 2010;26:503–6.
67. Davidson A, McKenzie I. Distress at induction: prevention and consequences. Curr Opin Anaesthesiol 2011;24:301–6.
68. Nishina K, Mikawa K, Shiga M, et al. Clonidine in paediatric anaesthesia. Paediatr Anaesth 1999;9:187–202.
69. Fazi L, Jantzen E, Rose J, et al. A comparison of oral clonidine and oral midazolam as preanesthetic medications in the pediatric tonsillectomy patient. Anesth Analg 2001;92:56–61.
70. Dahmani S, Brasher C, Stany I, et al. Premedication with clonidine is superior to benzodiazepines. A meta-analysis of published studies. Acta Anaesthesiol Scand 2010;54:397–402.
71. Yuen VM, Hui TW, Irwin MG, et al. A comparison of intranasal dexmedetomidine and oral midazolam for premedication in pediatric anesthesia: a double-blinded randomized controlled trial. Anesth Analg 2008;106:1715–21.
72. Yuen VM. Dexmedetomidine: perioperative applications in children. Paediatr Anaesth 2010;20:256–64.
73. Yuen VM, Hui TW, Irwin MG, et al. Optimal timing for the administration of intranasal dexmedetomidine for premedication in children. Anaesthesia 2010;65:922–9.
74. Yuen VM, Hui TW, Irwin MG, et al. A randomised comparison of two intranasal dexmedetomidine. Anaesthesia 2012;67:1210–6.
75. Jia JE, Chen JY, Hu X, et al. A randomized study of intranasal dexemedetomidine and oral ketamine for premedication in children. Anaesthesia 2013;68:944–9.
76. Gutstein HB, Johnson KL, Heard MB, et al. Oral ketamine preanesthetic medication in children. Anesthesiology 1992;76:28–33.
77. Funk W, Jakob W, Riedl T, et al. Oral preanesthetic medication for children: double-blind randomized study of a combination of midazolam and ketamine vs midazolam or ketamine alone. Br J Anaesth 2000;84:335–40.
78. Henderson JM, Brodsky DA, Fisher DM, et al. Pre-induction of anesthesia in pediatric patients with nasally administered sufentanil. Anesthesiology 1988;68:671–5.

79. Karl H, Keifer AT, Rosenberger JL, et al. Comparison of the safety and efficacy of intranasal midazolam or sufentanil for preinduction of anesthesia in pediatric patients. Anesthesiology 1992;76:209–15.
80. Lee J, Lee J, Lim H, et al. Cartoon distraction alleviates anxiety in children. Anesth Analg 2012;115:1168–73.
81. Mifflin KA, Hackmann T. Streamed video clips to reduce anxiety in children. Anesth Analg 2012;115(5):1162–7.
82. Vagnoli L, Caprilli S, Robiglio A, et al. Clown doctors as treatment for preoperative anxiety in children: a randomized, prospective study. Pediatrics 2005; 116:e563–7.
83. Chorney JM, Tan ET, Kain AN. Adult-child interactions in the postanesthesia care unit: behavior matters. Anesthesiology 2013;118:834–41.
84. Martin SR, Chorney JM, Cohen LL, et al. Sequential analysis of mother's and father's reassurance and children's postoperative distress. J Pediatr Psychol 2013;38(10):1121–9.
85. Martin SR, Chorney JM, Tan EW, et al. Changing healthcare providers' behavior during pediatric inductions with an empirically based intervention. Anesthesiology 2011;115:18–27.
86. Kain Z. Healthcare provider behavior and children's perioperative distress. Available at: http://clinicaltrials.gov/show/NCT01878747. Accessed December 22, 2013.
87. Olympio MA. Postanesthetic delirium: historical perspectives. J Clin Anesth 1991;3:60–3.
88. Wells LT, Rasch DK. Emergence "delirium" after sevoflurane anesthesia: a paranoid delusion? Anesth Analg 1999;88:1308–10.
89. Voepel-Lewis T, Malviya S, Tait AR. A prospective cohort study of emergence agitation in the pediatric postanesthesia care unit. Anesth Analg 2003;96:1625–30.
90. Sikich N, Lerman J. Development and psychometric evaluation of the pediatric anesthesia emergence delirium scale. Anesthesiology 2004;100:1138–45.
91. Smessaert A, Schehr CA, Artusio JF. Observations in the immediate postanaesthesia period. II. Mode of recovery. Br J Anaesth 1960;32:181–5.
92. Malarbi S, Stargatt R, Howard K, et al. Characterizing the behavior of children emerging with delirium from general anesthesia. Paediatr Anaesth 2011;21: 942–50.
93. Cole JW, Murray DJ, McAllister JD, et al. Emergence behaviour in children: defining the incidence of excitement and agitation following anaesthesia. Paediatr Anaesth 2002;12:442–7.
94. Lapin SL, Auden SM, Goldsmith LJ, et al. Effects of sevoflurane anaesthesia on recovery in children: a comparison with halothane. Paediatr Anaesth 1999;9: 299–304.
95. Aono J, Ueda W, Mamiya K, et al. Greater incidence of delirium during recovery from sevoflurane in preschool boys. Anesthesiology 1997;87:1298–300.
96. Cravero J, Surgenor S, Whalen K. Emergence agitation in paediatric patients after sevoflurane anaesthesia and no surgery: a comparison with halothane. Paediatr Anaesth 2000;10(4):419–24.
97. Weldon BC, Bell M, Craddock T. The effect of caudal analgesia on emergence agitation in children after sevoflurane versus halothane anesthesia. Anesth Analg 2004;98:321–6.
98. Cohen IT, Hannallah RS, Hummer KA. The incidence of emergence agitation associated with desflurane anesthesia in children is reduced by fentanyl. Anesth Analg 2001;93:88–91.

99. Galinkin JL, Fazi LM, Cuy RM, et al. Use of intranasal fentanyl in children undergoing myringotomy and tube placement during halothane and sevoflurane anesthesia. Anesthesiology 2000;93:1378–83.
100. Bajwa SA, Fancza DC, Cyna AM. A comparison of emergence delirium scales following general anesthesia in children. Paediatr Anaesth 2010;20(8):704–11.
101. Martini DR. Commentary: the diagnosis of delirium in pediatric patients. J Am Acad Child Adolesc Psychiatry 2005;44:395–8.
102. Ben-Ari Y, Tseeb V, Raggozzino D, et al. Gamma-aminobutyric acid (GABA): a fast excitatory transmitter which may regulate the development of hippocampal neurones in early postnatal life. Prog Brain Res 1994;102:261–73.
103. Viitanen H, Annila P, Viitanen M, et al. Premedication with midazolam delays recovery after ambulatory sevoflurane anesthesia in children. Anesth Analg 1999; 89:75–9.
104. Kain ZN, Caldwell-Andrews AA, Maranets I, et al. Preoperative anxiety and emergence delirium and postoperative maladaptive behaviors. Anesth Analg 2004;99:1648–54.
105. Viitanen H, Annila P, Rorarius M, et al. Recovery after halothane anaesthesia induced with thiopental, propofol-alfentanil or halothane for day-case adenoidectomy in small children. Br J Anaesth 1998;81:960–2.
106. Moore JK, Moore EW, Elliott RA, et al. Propofol and halothane versus sevoflurane in paediatric day-case surgery: induction and recovery characteristics. Br J Anaesth 2003;90:461–6.
107. Keaney A, Diviney D, Harte S, et al. Postoperative behavioral changes following anesthesia with sevoflurane. Paediatr Anaesth 2004;14:866–70.
108. Cravero JP, Beach M, Dodge CP, et al. Emergence characteristics of sevoflurane compared to halothane in pediatric patients undergoing bilateral pressure equalization tube insertion. J Clin Anesth 2000;12:397–401.
109. Viitanen H, Baer G, Annila P. Recovery characteristics of sevoflurane or halothane for day-case anaesthesia in children aged 1–3 years. Acta Anaesthesiol Scand 2000;44:101–6.
110. Johannesson GP, Floren M, Lindahl SG. Sevoflurane for ENT-surgery in children. A comparison with halothane. Acta Anaesthesiol Scand 1995;39:546–50.
111. Davis PJ, Greenberg JA, Gendelman M, et al. Recovery characteristics of sevoflurane and halothane in preschool-aged children undergoing bilateral myringotomy and pressure equalization tube insertion. Anesth Analg 1999; 88:34–8.
112. Welborn LG, Hannallah RS, Norden JM, et al. Comparison of emergence and recovery characteristics of sevoflurane, desflurane and halothane in pediatric ambulatory patients. Anesth Analg 1996;83:917–20.
113. Hallen J, Rawal N, Gupta A. Postoperative recovery following outpatient pediatric myringotomy: a comparison between sevoflurane and halothane. J Clin Anesth 2001;13:161–6.
114. Lerman J, Davis PJ, Welborn LG, et al. Induction, recovery, and safety characteristics of sevoflurane in children undergoing ambulatory surgery. A comparison with halothane. Anesthesiology 1996;84(6):1332–40.
115. Valley RD, Ramza JT, Calhoun P, et al. Tracheal extubation of deeply anesthetized pediatric patients: a comparison of isoflurane and sevoflurane. Anesth Analg 1999;88:742–5.
116. Freye E, Bruckner J, Latasch L. No difference in electroencephalographic power spectra or sensory-evoked potentials in patients anaesthetized with desflurane or sevoflurane. Eur J Anaesthesiol 2004;21:373–8.

117. Constant I, Dubois MC, Piat V, et al. Changes in electroencephalogram and autonomic cardiovascular activity during induction of anesthesia with sevoflurane compared with halothane in children. Anesthesiology 1999;91:1604–15.
118. Yli-Hankala A, Vakkuri A, Sarkela M, et al. Epileptiform electroencephalogram during mask induction of anesthesia with sevoflurane. Anesthesiology 1999; 91:1596–603.
119. Olsen RW, Yang J, King RG, et al. Barbiturate and benzodiazepine modulation of GABA receptor binding and function. Life Sci 1986;39:1969–76.
120. Viitanen H, Tarkkila P, Mennander S, et al. Sevoflurane-maintained anesthesia induced with propofol or sevoflurane in small children: induction and recovery characteristics. Can J Anaesth 1999;46:21–8.
121. Zvi J, Li H, Makaryus R, et al. Metabolomic profiling of children's brains undergoing general anesthesia with sevoflurane and propofol. Anesthesiology 2012; 117(5):1062–71.
122. Liao WW, Wang JJ, Wu GJ, et al. The effect of cerebral monitoring on recovery after sevoflurane anesthesia in ambulatory setting in children: a comparison among bispectral index, A-line autoregressive index, and standard practice. J Chin Med Assoc 2011;74:28e36.
123. Picard V, Dumont L, Pellegrini M. Quality of recovery in children: sevoflurane versus propofol. Acta Anaesthesiol Scand 2000;44:307–10.
124. Uezono S, Goto T, Terui K, et al. Emergence agitation after sevoflurane versus propofol in pediatric patients. Anesth Analg 2000;91:563–6.
125. Cohen IT, Finkel JC, Hannallah RS, et al. Rapid emergence does not explain agitation following sevoflurane anaesthesia in infants and children: a comparison with propofol. Paediatr Anaesth 2003;13:63–7.
126. Grundmann U, Uth M, Eichner A, et al. Total intravenous anaesthesia with propofol and remifentanil in paediatric patients: a comparison with a desflurane-nitrous oxide inhalation anaesthesia. Acta Anaesthesiol Scand 1998;42:845–50.
127. Oh AY, Seo KS, Kim SD, et al. Delayed emergence process does not result in a lower incidence of emergence agitation after sevoflurane anesthesia in children. Acta Anaesthesiol Scand 2005;49:297–9.
128. Eckenhoff JE, Kneale DH, Dripps RD. The incidence and etiology of postanesthetic excitement. A clinical survey. Anesthesiology 1961;22:667–73.
129. Cravero JP, Thyr B, Beach M, et al. The effects of small dose fentanyl on pediatric patients after sevoflurane anesthesia without surgery. Anesthesia Analgesia 2003;97:364–7.
130. Finkel JC, Cohen IT, Hannallah RS, et al. The effect of intranasal fentanyl on the emergence characteristics after sevoflurane anesthesia in children undergoing surgery for bilateral myringotomy tube placement. Anesth Analg 2001;92: 1164–8.
131. Bock M, Kunz P, Schreckenberger R, et al. Comparison of caudal and intravenous clonidine in the prevention of agitation after sevoflurane in children. Br J Anaesth 2002;88:790–6.
132. Tesoro S, Mezzetti D, Marchesini L, et al. Clonidine treatment for agitation in children after sevoflurane anesthesia. Anesth Analg 2005;101:1619–22.
133. Locatelli BG, Ingelmo PM, Emre S, et al. Emergence delirium in children: a comparison of sevoflurane and desflurane anesthesia using the paediatric anesthesia emergence delirium scale. Paediatr Anaesth 2013;23(4):301–8.
134. Dahmani S, Stany I, Brasher C, et al. Pharmacological prevention of sevoflurane- and desflurane-related emergence agitation in children: a meta-analysis of published studies. Br J Anaesth 2010;104(2):216–23.

135. Kim MS, Moon BE, Kim H, et al. Comparison of propofol and fentanyl administered at the end of anaesthesia for prevention of emergence agitation after sevoflurane anaesthesia in children. Br J Anaesth 2013;110(2):274–80.
136. Cohen IT, Drewsen S, Hannallah RS. Propofol or midazolam do not reduce the incidence of emergence agitation associated with desflurane anaesthesia in children undergoing adenotonsillectomy. Paediatr Anaesth 2002;12:604–9.
137. Heinmiller LJ, Nelson LB, Goldberg MB, et al. Clonidine premedication versus placebo: effects on postoperative agitation and recovery time in children undergoing strabismus surgery. J Pediatr Ophthalmol Strabismus 2013;50(3):150–4.
138. Lerman J. Inhalation agents in pediatric anaesthesia - an update. Curr Opin Anaesthesiol 2007;20(3):221–6.
139. Shukry M, Clyde MC, Kalarickal PL, et al. Does dexmedetomidine prevent emergence delirium in children after sevoflurane-based general anesthesia? Paediatr Anaesth 2005;15:1098–104.
140. Ibacache ME, Muñoz HR, Brandes V, et al. Single-dose dexmedetomidine reduces agitation after sevoflurane anesthesia in children. Anesth Analg 2004; 98:60–3.
141. Abdulatif M, Ahmed A, Mukhtar A, et al. The effect of magnesium sulphate infusion on the incidence and severity of emergence agitation in children undergoing adenotonsillectomy using sevoflurane anaesthesia. Anaesthesia 2013;68: 1045–52.
142. Kil HK, Kim WO, Han SW, et al. Psychological and behavioral effects of chloral hydrate in day-case pediatric surgery: a randomized, observer-blinded study. J Pediatr Surg 2012;47(8):1592–9.
143. Cohen IT, Finkel JC, Hannallah RS, et al. The effects of fentanyl on the emergence characteristics after desflurane or sevoflurane anesthesia in children. Anesth Analg 2002;94:1178–81.
144. Kim D, Doo AR, Lim H, et al. Effect of ketorolac on the prevention of emergence agitation in children after sevoflurane anesthesia. Korean J Anesthesiol 2013; 64(3):240–5.
145. Aouad MT, Kanazi GE, Siddik-Sayyid SM, et al. Preoperative caudal block prevents emergence agitation in children following sevoflurane anesthesia. Acta Anaesthesiol Scand 2005;49:300–4.
146. Kim HS, Kim CS, Kim SD, et al. Fascia iliaca compartment block reduces emergence agitation by providing effective analgesic properties in children. J Clin Anesth 2011;23(2):119–23.
147. Samarkandi A, Naguib M, Riad W, et al. Melatonin vs midazolam premedication in children: a double-blind, placebo-controlled study. Eur J Anaesthesiol 2005; 22:189–96.
148. Murray DJ, Cole JW, Shrock CD, et al. Sevoflurane versus halothane: effect of oxycodone premedication on emergence behaviour in children. Paediatr Anaesth 2002;12:308–12.
149. Kararmaz A, Kaya S, Turhanoglu S, et al. Oral ketamine premedication can prevent emergence agitation in children after desflurane anesthesia. Paediatr Anaesth 2004;14:477–82.
150. Binstock W, Rubin R, Bachman C, et al. The effect of premedication with OTFC, with or without ondansetron, on postoperative agitation, and nausea and vomiting in pediatric ambulatory patients. Paediatr Anaesth 2004;14:759–67.
151. Dong YX, Meng LX, Wang Y, et al. The effect of remifentanil on the incidence of agitation on emergence from sevoflurane anaesthesia in children undergoing adenotonsillectomy. Anaesthesia Intensive Care 2010;38:718–22.

152. Shen X, Hu C, Li W. Tracheal extubation of deeply anesthetized pediatric patients: a comparison of sevoflurane and sevoflurane in combination with low-dose remifentanil. Paediatr Anaesth 2012;22(12):1179–84.
153. Yoo JB, Kim MJ, Cho SH, et al. The effects of pre-operative visual information and parental presence intervention on anxiety, delirium, and pain of post-operative pediatric patients in PACU. J Korean Acad Nurs 2012;42(3):333–41.
154. Chen J, Li W, Hu X, et al. Emergence agitation after cataract surgery in children: a comparison of midazolam, propofol and ketamine. Pediatr Anesth 2010;20: 873–9.

Anesthesia and Sedation Outside the Operating Room

Katrin Campbell, MD[a], Laura Torres, MD[b], Stephen Stayer, MD[c],*

KEYWORDS

- Pediatric • Anesthesia • Sedation • Procedure suite • Pediatric radiology
- Quality improvement

KEY POINTS

- The volume and clinical complexity of patients requiring procedures outside the operating room (OR) continues to increase.
- The demand for pediatric sedation is too great for pediatric anesthesiologists to exclusively deliver procedural sedation for healthy children outside the OR.
- The decision to deliver a general anesthetic with a secured airway versus deep sedation for most procedures outside the OR is based on special requirements for the procedure, the pain of the procedure, the child's comorbidities, and the experience and comfort of the anesthesiologist with deep sedation techniques.
- Risk related to sedation and anesthesia outside the OR can be broken down into inadequate sedation, oversedation/adverse response to sedatives, and failure to rescue.
- Hospital systems are benefited by anesthesiology participation and leadership of a sedation committee, whose charter is the oversight of effective, efficient, and safe sedation throughout the institution.

INTRODUCTION

The provision of anesthesia and sedation for children undergoing procedures outside the operating room (OR) continues to evolve. The volume of invasive and noninvasive procedures is increasing, as is the clinical complexity of patients requiring these procedures.[1] Practices strive to eliminate the use of physical restraints for painful and frightening procedures. In addition, the requirements for appropriate personnel to administer and monitor sedation have dramatically changed. It is no longer acceptable to administer a cocktail of meperidine, promethazine, and chlorpromazine in an unmonitored environment. As an example of growth, at our institution, 2578 patients

[a] Division of Sedation, Texas Children's Hospital, Baylor College of Medicine, 6621 Fannin St, Suite A300, Houston, TX 77030, USA; [b] Department of Pediatrics, Sedation Oversight Committee, Texas Children's Hospital, Baylor College of Medicine, 6621 Fannin St, Suite A300, Houston, TX 77030, USA; [c] Pediatric Anesthesiology, Texas Children's Hospital, Baylor College of Medicine, 6621 Fannin St, Suite A300, Houston, TX 77030, USA
* Corresponding author.
E-mail address: sstayer@bcm.tmc.edu

Anesthesiology Clin 32 (2014) 25–43
http://dx.doi.org/10.1016/j.anclin.2013.10.010
anesthesiology.theclinics.com

received anesthesia or deep sedation outside the OR in 2003, representing 11% of total cases; by 2012, that number had increased to 8695 (24% of cases).

In contrast to OR anesthesia, the approach to providing sedation and anesthesia outside the OR varies among institutions and even among different providers in the same institution.[2–7] Anesthesia providers are commonly requested to care for children who need sedation, but have significant comorbidities, such as obstructive sleep apnea, obesity, craniofacial abnormalities, and significant pulmonary or cardiac disease. Many (nonanesthesia) pediatric specialists provide procedural sedation, with similar goals of analgesia and immobility to optimize procedural conditions. In order to accomplish these goals, pediatric sedation practitioners administer sedative and anesthetic medications that produce deep sedation. There is controversy about the training and qualifications of sedation specialists. There is also controversy about the types and doses of anesthetic medications that they administer. Anesthesia departments have a responsibility to their institutions to ensure the safe and effective delivery of sedatives and anesthetics, no matter the location or the personnel, and federal authorities dictate that anesthesiologists should provide oversight and credentialing of sedation practices.[8,9] Failed sedations frustrate families and add cost, and therefore, sedation services must also develop practices to minimize this occurrence. The demand for pediatric sedation is too great for pediatric anesthesiologists to exclusively deliver this care. In addition, fellowship trained pediatric anesthesiologists are skilled in providing anesthetic management of children with life-threatening medical conditions undergoing complex surgical procedures (eg, a child undergoing repair of a diaphragmatic hernia while supported with extracorporeal membrane oxygenation). Using such highly trained specialists to provide sedation for an otherwise healthy child could be considered a wasteful use of resource.

GOALS

The goals for procedural sedation/anesthesia are[7]:

- First, ensure safety.
  - The anesthesia provider should be trained in administration of sedative medications and rescue from adverse events.
  - The anesthesia provider is not the individual performing the procedure.
  - The anesthesia provider administers medications and monitors and records vital signs.
  - Careful monitoring should continue after the procedure until discharge criteria have been met.
- Minimize pain and discomfort.
- Minimize psychological discomfort and anxiety for both the patient and family.
- Control movement to optimize imaging studies and to improve safety for invasive procedures.
- Develop systems that are efficient and cost effective for the patient and for the health care system.

ANESTHESIA VERSUS SEDATION

The decision to deliver a general anesthetic with a secured airway versus deep sedation for most procedures outside the OR is based on special requirements for the procedure (breath holding), the pain of the procedure, the child's comorbidities, and the experience and comfort of the anesthesiologist with deep sedation techniques. Even though strong evidence supporting a particular technique is lacking, anesthesiologists should consider the advantages of providing sedation for many procedures and not simply use general endotracheal anesthesia for every patient. The anesthesia provider should choose a technique that best meets the goals, as stated earlier. For example, the laryngeal mask airway (LMA) can be used to maintain a patent airway with spontaneous ventilation and requires a lower dose of anesthesia, and, therefore, there is a more rapid emergence from anesthesia. Patients with upper respiratory tract infections, and those with asthma, may have fewer respiratory complications when an LMA is used.[10] Patients undergoing imaging studies who do not have a history of airway compromise can be managed with a natural airway and a shoulder roll with slight head extension to maintain pharyngeal patency during deep sedation. Propofol is one of the shortest-acting anesthetics and has been used as an antiemetic; therefore, this technique may be optimal in terms of recovery characteristics. A propofol infusion for these procedures with routine noninvasive monitors and nasal cannula CO_2 monitoring can provide a safe and efficient method of providing a motionless examination. If the child develops some degree of airway obstruction not relieved by improved positioning and an oral airway, an LMA can be used. The anesthesiologist has the means of providing immediate tracheal intubation to safely complete the imaging study. It is challenging to clearly distinguish deep sedation versus general anesthesia in a spontaneously breathing patient receiving a propofol infusion for imaging studies. Therefore, in our institution, we differentiate deep sedation from general anesthesia by the need for an invasive airway device (LMA or endotracheal tube [ETT]). Patients managed with a nasal cannula and propofol infusions are classified as undergoing deep sedation, no matter the dose of propofol.

PATIENT PREPARATION

A complete evaluation of the patient is paramount to conducting a safe procedure. This strategy is essential for every patient managed in the OR but is absolutely required in a procedure outside the OR, where limitation of space and challenging access to ancillary services (blood bank, pharmacy) and emergency personnel may exist.

A thorough evaluation of the patient's clinical history must include:

- Current medical or surgical diagnosis requiring the scheduled diagnostic or therapeutic procedure
- Current clinical condition of the patient with respect to hydration, airway compromise, respiratory symptoms, cardiac hemodynamics, hematologic status, infectious disease, mental status, and immunologic risk
- Review of past medical history
- Review of previous procedures requiring anesthesia or sedation and noted complications
- Current and recent medications, including other sedative/analgesic drugs; in a study analysis of 264 preventable and potential adverse drug events,[11] lack of patient information accounted for 18% of errors
- Review of allergies to medicines, latex, and foods
- Review of laboratory data and imaging studies
- Plan for additional laboratory analysis, imaging studies, or other diagnostic tests to reduce risk

A physical examination, with focus on the airway, lungs, heart, and neurologic status, must be performed. The specific procedure determines additional aspects of the physical examination, which must be assessed.

Careful attention to fasting status must be made. Except for emergency procedures, the standard American Society of Anesthesiologists (ASA) nil-by-mouth guidelines should be followed to avoid the risk of aspiration. An exception to these guidelines should be considered for patients undergoing computed tomography (CT) scanning of the abdomen with oral contrast. In our institution, we proceed with sedation/anesthesia 1 hour after ingestion of oral contrast. Although it is controversial, suboptimal CT images are commonly obtained from a prolonged delay after contrast ingestion, requiring a repeat of the CT scan, with the associated radiation exposure. We have used this shortened fasting guideline in CT for the past 7 years without a single incidence contrast aspiration.

Informed consent should include detailed information about planned management, concerns, potential risks, and benefits. The anesthesiologist should also include an explanation of the potential need for deepening sedation, inducing general anesthesia and placing an airway device, should the need arise.

To reduce the risk of postprocedure adverse behavior, the administration of anxiolytic or analgesic medications should be considered. A variety of distraction techniques that alleviate the stress of separation may also be used. Although the opportunity to induce deep sedation or general anesthesia with parental presence may be limited in many OR settings, the remote anesthesia site can commonly accommodate parental presence.

The Universal Protocol (preprocedure verification, site marking, and time-out) mandated by the Joint Commission and performed in the OR environment must be adopted in sites outside the OR.

SPECIFIC EXTRAMURAL SITES AND BEST PRACTICES

Essentially, every medical system that manages pediatric patients undergoing invasive procedures has developed unique processes to provide sedation for children. Sedation is commonly provided in clinics, such as oncology, orthopedics, and dental; on inpatient wards; in the emergency center; in burn centers; intensive care units; in postanesthesia care units; in radiology areas and procedure suites. In order to provide a safe environment for children undergoing deep sedation or anesthesia, these out of OR areas should be set up to provide[12]:

- Equipment and monitoring similar to the OR environment
  - Backup airway equipment such as oral and nasal airways, LMA, laryngoscopes and ETTs, and adequate suction
  - Standard ASA monitors including end-tidal CO_2 (ETCO$_2$) monitoring
  - Difficult airway cart
  - Malignant hyperthermia cart
  - Scavenging system
- Anesthesia providers who are familiar with the environment and assistants, such as nurse anesthetists, anesthesia technicians, sedation nurses, or respiratory therapists to assist with patient management when needed
- Effective communication system in order to obtain immediate skilled assistance from the OR when needed

Radiology

The radiology suite is commonly the busiest remote anesthesia site. Providing anesthesia and sedation in this site creates many unique issues and challenges. Some of the anesthesia equipment used in these locations must be modified or specially ordered for the specific environment, and any practitioner providing sedation or anesthesia must be familiar with the specific constraints of each site. However, regardless of the location, minimum standards for equipment, monitors, and conditions of anesthetic delivery set by the ASA must be in place. Specifically, the ASA requires off-site locations to have 2 sources of oxygen, suction, a self-inflating hand resuscitator bag, anesthesia machine with scavenging system for volatile agent administration, and standard-of-care monitors and equipment. Anesthesiologists should be involved in the development of these areas to ensure that standards are met as well as advocate for adequate space for the various equipment, monitors, and induction/emergence areas that are needed.

CT

CT uses ionizing radiation to differentiate between high-density and low-density structures.[13] The growth of CT use in children has been driven primarily by the decrease in the time needed to perform a scan (now <5 seconds, in some instances), largely eliminating the need for anesthesia to prevent the child from moving during image acquisition. Situations in which sedation or general anesthesia may be required include unstable respiratory or cardiovascular status, emergent situations (ie, head trauma), uncooperative children (young age or developmental delay), unstable airways, and the need for breath holding during imaging (ie, dynamic airway studies to evaluate tracheobronchomalacia).

In many cases, distraction techniques (colored lights and toys) and parental presence may obviate anesthesia. Varying levels of sedation (minimal to moderate to deep) can be accomplished using midazolam, propofol or dexmedetomidine.[14]

- CT uses ionizing radiation
- Procedures are short (uncommonly require sedation)
- Oral contrast administered for abdominal CT requires a deviation from ASA nil-by-mouth guidelines in order to obtain adequate imaging
- Breath holding may be required for chest CT, which typically requires sedation and assisted ventilation in younger patients

---

One area of controversy that anesthesiologists face in sedating children for CT is necessary violation of nil-by-mouth guidelines with oral contrast administration. Gastrografin (Bristol-Meyers Squibb, Princeton, NJ), 3% concentration at full strength, is hyperosmolar and hypertonic. If aspirated, it can cause pulmonary edema, pneumonitis, and death. For this reason, it is diluted to an isotonic 1.5% solution before ingestion. Even so, to be effective, images must be taken between 30 and 90 minutes after administration, falling outside usual nil-by-mouth guidelines of 2 hours for clear liquids. In addition, the volume of contrast required can be large (60–90 mL in neonates and 250–350 mL in children aged 1–5 years). In these cases, there are no data to suggest optimal sedation technique to account for theoretic aspiration risk. Care for these patients includes intravenous (IV) sedation with spontaneous ventilation and natural airway; inhaled induction and LMA placement; and rapid sequence induction and endotracheal intubation.[15]

For CT scans of the chest or abdomen that require breath holding for optimal image quality, anesthetic techniques include general anesthesia with volatile agents, mask ventilation with intermittent hyperventilation, apnea breath holding, and general endotracheal intubation with muscle relaxation. Because atelectasis is more frequent and severe in children undergoing general anesthesia compared with IV pentobarbital sedation, consideration should be given to the use of forced inspiration in children anesthetized for CT scan of the chest.[16]

Magnetic resonance imaging

Magnetic resonance imaging (MRI), including magnetic resonance angiography and magnetic resonance venography, is rapidly becoming one of the most frequently used diagnostic tools since its introduction in 1990. It is used in the diagnosis of neoplasms and vascular/cardiac malformations, evaluation of sleep apnea, developmental delay, seizures, stroke, behavioral disorders, autism, hypotonia, and metabolic/mitochondrial disorders, as well as infectious processes such as meningitis/encephalitis, osteomyelitis, and abscess formation.

- One of the most commonly used imaging tools
- Very strong magnetic field requires special safety precautions
  - Use of MRI-safe equipment
  - Screening of patient for potential implants
- Most younger children require sedation for immobility
- Persons inside the scanning room require auditory protection
- Children with comorbidities should be managed by an anesthesiologist

---

The MRI system is a superconducting magnet that creates a variety of safety issues not seen in other diagnostic/therapeutic areas. The strength of the magnetic field in the scanner is measured in Tesla (T) or the equivalent of 10,000 G. The earth's magnetic field is 0.5 G and the most common MRI machines are 1.5 to 3T. Thus, any ferromagnetic material brought near the machine becomes a major hazard, because it can become a projectile from the strong attractive force created by the scanner (and the magnet is always on). Additional patient injury can occur from implanted devices such as cardiac pacemakers, spinal cord or vagus nerve stimulators, and programmable insulin pumps or ventriculoperitoneal shunts, which may be affected by the magnet. Therefore, special MRI-compatible or MRI-safe equipment is frequently used in these areas, and special screening of patients and employees must be carried out before entering the scanner. The Web site http://www.mrisafety.com/ is a useful resource to identify potential hazards. Auditory hazards are created from the loud knocking sound produced by the scanner; therefore, any person remaining in the scanner while it is running should have earplugs or headphones in place. Burns or thermal injury can occur from coiled or frayed monitor cables (even if MRI safe), MRI-unsafe electrocardiography leads, and skin contact with the MRI bore or cables as they heat up during the scanning process.

MRI-compatible/MRI-safe equipment may not be available in every institution, and special care with alternative methods must be taken to deliver a safe anesthetic. Creating a hole in the console wall to thread necessary tubing (suction and medication infusion tubing, ventilator circuit for an MRI-unsafe machine, $ETCO_2$ monitoring tubing) from outside the scanner to the patient is one option. On average, 9.15 m (30 ft) of tubing is needed for each.[17–19]

Anesthetic care varies with practitioner preference, patient medical history, and physical status, as well as availability of support staff and equipment. With the advent of MRI-safe video goggles, many children are able to complete the examination without sedation. When sedation is required, infusions with dexmedetomidine or propofol with spontaneous ventilation, nasal cannula O_2 supplementation, and $ETCO_2$ are often used. General anesthesia with an LMA or ETT can be used, with careful taping of the pilot balloon to the circuit to prevent artifact on images of the head or neck. Bivona tracheostomy tubes may need to be replaced with MRI-safe tracheostomy tubes (ie, Shiley) or ETTs, because the Bivona tube is not considered MRI safe by the US Food and Drug Administration.

Interventional radiology
Interventional radiology (IR) procedures have definitely contributed to the expansion of the anesthesiologist's role in remote sites. With the recent advances in technology, increasing numbers of patients are coming to radiology for a minimally invasive alternative to larger procedures performed in the OR. In addition, some of these patients may be acutely ill, with a tenuous hemodynamic or respiratory status, and considered too high risk for the surgical alternative. A variety of procedures are performed in the IR suite, including peripherally inserted central catheter line placement, liver biopsies, abscess drain placements, nephrostomy and chest tube placements, lumbar punctures in morbidly obese patients, cerebral angiography and embolization, as well as sclerotherapy for vascular and lymphatic malformations. Unlike diagnostic radiologic procedures, IR procedures can pose significant procedural-related risks, similar to surgery performed in the OR. Preprocedural planning with the radiologist must occur. In our institution, all members of the interventional team, including the anesthesiologist, radiologist, nurses, and technicians, meet to discuss each case in a morning rounds session. Pertinent medical history and laboratory tests, planned procedure, including required equipment and special medications that are administered by either the radiologist or anesthesiologist, positioning, and any further testing or treatments required to optimize the patient before arrival are discussed. Depending on the patient status, planned procedure, need for absolute immobility or breath holding, anticipated procedure length, and postoperative disposition, patients may be managed using a range of techniques, from minimal IV sedation with spontaneous ventilation and natural airway to general anesthesia with LMA or ETT.

- Many procedures are performed on very high-risk patients, because IR is less invasive than surgery
- Sclerotherapeutic agents used for vascular and lympathic malformation have potential side effects
- Cerebral angiography and embolization of vascular malformations can produce profound hemodynamic changes

---

   With sclerotherapy and embolization of arteriovenous and lymphatic malformations, it is important to have an understanding of the various agents and their potential complications. Ethanol, polyvinyl alcohol foam, bleomycin, doxycycline, sodium tetradecyl sulfate, ethylene vinyl alcohol, cyanoacrylate glue, balloons, and coils have all been used. Polyvinyl alcohol foam causes direct mechanical obstruction and is often used for tumor embolization and preoperative devascularization of lesions but can break down over time, causing recanalization of vessel.[20] Coils need to be appropriately sized for the vessel or arteriovenous malformation (AVM) that is targeted. A small coil may embolize downstream; a large coil may herniate back into the parent vessel. Ethanol destroys the endothelial lining of the vessel, causing immediate thrombosis.

Systemic effects can include sedation or agitation, pulmonary hypertension, cardiac arrhythmias, and complete cardiovascular collapse.[21] Therefore, total dose should be limited to 1 mL/kg, and additional sedatives and narcotics must be cautiously administered. Hemolysis and subsequent hemoglobinuria are a concern, and careful attention to fluid management with aggressive hydration to flush the kidneys must occur to prevent renal injury or failure. Administering furosemide and sodium bicarbonate to alkalinize the urine may also be needed to reduce this risk. Bleomycin has been known to cause pulmonary fibrosis and skin hyperpigmentation. In our institution, a no-sting barrier is used before placement of any adhesive materials on the patient's skin. Special Velcro-based ETT holders are used, and eyes are protected with lubrication. Most sclerosing agents cause some degree of swelling. This swelling may cause airway compromise in patients with head or neck involvement, warranting extended intubation until resolution (**Fig. 1**).

Cerebral angiography is often used in the diagnosis and treatment evaluation for various medical conditions, including aneurysm, arteriovenous malformation, stroke, and vascular disease (such as moyamoya disease). It requires absolute patient immobility and controlled ventilation with intermittent breath holding and therefore is routinely performed under general endotracheal anesthesia. Consideration should be given to arterial line placement for blood pressure monitoring in these patients, especially when an intervention is anticipated. Maintaining normocarbia or even slightly hypercarbic ventilation aids in radiologic visualization by dilating the cerebral vasculature. Similarly, avoiding hyperventilation is important, especially in patients with a history of transient ischemic stroke or moyamoya disease, because these patients are at higher risk for perioperative neurologic complications.

Nuclear medicine

Nuclear medicine studies are used in the diagnosis of multiple disease states, including hematologic and oncologic processes and their response to treatment, localization of seizure foci in intractable epilepsy, and assessment of benign and malignant bone lesions, as well as assessing cardiac, renal, and thyroid function. Unlike other imaging modalities that focus on structures, nuclear medicine studies give functional information through the use of radioisotope medication uptake. About 90% of worldwide radioisotope use is for medical diagnoses. The most common radioisotope, used in about 80% of nuclear medicine studies, is technetium 99. With a half-life of 6 hours, it lasts long enough to examine metabolic activity but short enough to minimize radiation exposure to the patient. Even so, all radioisotopes produce waste products, which require special handling and storage until stabilized. These materials include medical waste such as syringes, paper, and cloth, as well as patient substances such as urine,

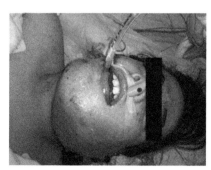 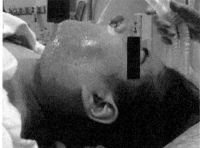

Fig. 1. Facial edema after sclerotherapy.

blood, and other bodily fluids. Therefore, all members of the patient care team should be cognizant of potential exposure to radioactive materials, and safety training should be instituted.[20,22,23]

- Radioactive agents are administered before scanning, and patients may need sedation in a warming room remote from the anesthesia provider
  - Requires remote monitoring setup
- Commonly require long periods of sedation

Anesthesia providers are challenged with increasingly longer studies requiring sedation or anesthesia and limited access to the patient during peak levels of potential radiation exposure. Hybrid imaging (single-photon emission CT, positron emission tomography [PET] CT; PET MRI) is becoming standard in nuclear medicine. These advanced imaging studies require longer time commitments (1–3 hours in some cases) and are very sensitive to patient movement. Often, patients need to be sedated for a warming phase, usually 30 minutes to 1 hour, after injection of the radioisotope before the start of the examination. During this period, risk of radiation exposure is high, and patients may be monitored from a remote location with closed circuit cameras. There is some concern that with the prolonged sedations required, patients are at higher risk of adverse outcomes. However, recent studies with propofol sedation for examinations lasting longer than 1 hour did not have any significant increase in adverse events compared with shorter studies.[21] Alternatively, providers may wish to use general anesthesia with an airway device (LMA or ETT) in place.

External beam radiation therapy
External beam radiation therapy (XRT) has become one of the cornerstone treatments in the management of malignant lesions. A linear accelerator machine is used to accelerate electrons to a very high energy state and then collide with material such as tungsten, which then releases energy in the form of radiographs, which are then focused at specific sites on the body to destroy tumor cells. The energy deposited into the tissues is measured in units of gray (Gy), and equal to 1 J/kg. A typical course of treatment involves 25 to 80 Gy divided into 30 equal portions, often once per day, over a 6-week period. Although the procedure itself is short and painless, it requires complete patient immobility to avoid damage to surrounding normal tissues. Initially, a planning or simulation session is undertaken, in which a plaster immobilization cast of the patient's head or torso is created to aid patient positioning for repeated treatments. This session also allows the radiation oncologist to plan the number and location of sites to be treated. Although this initial simulation can last from 20 to 90 minutes, the subsequent daily treatments usually last only 5 to 20 minutes and are therefore mainly performed under deep sedation with nasal cannula O_2. One exception is the treatment of retinoblastoma, because complete immobilization of the globe and extraocular muscles often requires muscle paralysis. Anxiolysis with midazolam or deep sedation with propofol infusion can be used to accomplish XRT.[24] Initial concerns for tachyphylaxis to propofol have not been substantiated.[25] Alternative medications used for XRT include dexmedetomidine and ketamine. However, the prolonged time required to bolus dexmedetomidine may inhibit its use for this brief procedure. The need for monitoring from a distance with telemetry and cameras makes this site uniquely challenging for the anesthesiologist. The typical configuration involves 2 cameras: one

directed at the patient to assess respiratory effort and patient motion and one directed at the monitors (and anesthesia machine, if general anesthesia is being used).

- Patients require complete immobility
- Daily treatments are common
- Remote monitoring is necessary
- Children commonly require monitored transport to a radiation center

---

Radiation therapy is also used in some operating arenas with either brachytherapy (intercavity implantation of radioactive material), intraoperative radiation therapy (IORT), and stereotactic radiosurgery.[26] In IORT, the procedure begins in the OR, where tumor debulking occurs. The patient is then transported to the XRT suite with the surgical site exposed for treatment. The patient is then returned to the OR for surgical closure. Stereotactic radiosurgery or Gamma Knife (Elekta Instruments, Stockholm, Sweden) surgery uses beams of γ radiation to treat various malignancies, arteriovenous malformations, and acoustic neuromas. The patient first has a stereotactic frame placed over the head and secured in place with screws. They are then transported to the MRI scanner, where three-dimensional reconstruction of the brain and plotting of coordinates are performed. The patient is then taken to the Gamma Knife unit for treatment. The head frame is removed, and the patient is taken to the recovery area. Although Gamma Knife surgery may occasionally be performed under deep sedation, general anesthesia is most commonly used, because these cases can last 9 to 12 hours. It is important to remember to transport the patient with equipment to rapidly remove the head frame should access to the airway be required. Both IORT and Gamma Knife procedures require a great deal of coordination among services to complete.

Procedure Suite

Procedure suites have been historically established for the individual medical specialists whose teams are charged with performing procedures and administering sedative medications to accomplish such procedures successfully. Although the volume of patients needing timely procedures and the advancement of technology persists, the complexity of patient clinical condition has resulted in the expansion of the anesthesiologist's role in these sites. A properly designed procedure suite functions similar to an OR. The design should take into account the need for patient admission and evaluation, the tools and room design needed for specific procedures, and an area for monitoring and observation during recovery. It is our opinion that procedure suites provide a significant advantage in safety and efficiency for patients who require moderate or deep sedation compared with a system in which the sedation practitioner travels to the bedside or clinic. Invasive procedures such as gastrointestinal endoscopy, bronchoscopy, bone marrow aspirations, lumbar punctures, dermatologic procedures, and kidney/liver biopsies are the types of procedures performed outside the OR in specialized procedure suites. These procedures produce strong noxious stimulation for children and therefore typically require deep sedation or general anesthesia. In our institution, the choice of sedation provider is dependent on the child's underlying medical condition, the associated risks, and the duration of the planned procedure. The ideal procedure suite provides the anesthesia practitioner with the option of using the same techniques and monitoring that are available in an OR, with backup equipment and support systems to treat procedural complications, such as the difficult airway, hemorrhage, anaphylaxis, and cardiac arrest. Considerations for some of these procedures are discussed.

Upper esophagogastroduodenoscopy

Upper esophagogastroduodenoscopy (EGD) in infants and small children is most commonly performed under general anesthesia with tracheal intubation to avoid airway compression caused by the endoscope pressing the trachealis muscle into the trachea. An LMA can be used; the cuff is deflated to allow passage of the endoscope and then reinflated once the scope has entered the esophagus. When the endoscopist passes the scope from the oropharynx into the esophagus, there is increased risk of dislodging the LMA or ETT, and we suggest that the anesthesiologist should hold on to the airway device during this portion of the procedure and when the endoscope is withdrawn.

- Many healthy children can be deeply sedated
- Most stimulation occurs during passage of the scope through the oropharynx into the esophagus
- Younger children (<10 years) and those with comorbidities should have an anesthesiologist providing care

---

The use of total IV anesthesia has been described for these procedures and is especially useful in endoscopy suites that do not have adequate scavenging and ventilation to allow the safe use of inhalational anesthetics.[27–29] Propofol can be used alone[30] but is more commonly combined with an opioid such as fentanyl or remifentanil[31,32] or with ketamine.[33] Outcomes after deep sedation with propofol versus inhalational anesthesia were similar.[28] The time to awakening was more rapid after the inhalational anesthetic, yet the time to hospital discharge was greater. In the propofol group, the incidence of agitation on emergence was less and the time to hospital discharge earlier.

Sedating a child for EGD is particularly challenging, because introducing the scope into the pharynx is stimulating and it must be removed in order to apply bag-valve-mask ventilation. Topical local anesthetic spray can be used to reduce stimulation, coughing, and gagging with introduction of the scope, and most patients require a deep level of sedation during this portion of the procedure. Once the scope is in the esophagus, the level of sedation can be reduced. These rapid adjustments in the level of sedation are most easily accomplished by using infusions or small boluses of short-acting sedatives and analgesics, such as propofol and remifentanil. Passing the scope through the pylorus is also stimulating and often requires deepening the level of sedation as well. Because the endoscope is passed through the oropharyngeal airway, there is a higher risk of apnea, laryngospasm, bronchospasm, and airway obstruction when these cases are performed without tracheal intubation. Early recognition and treatment by removal of the endoscope and bag mask ventilation are generally effective, although tracheal intubation may be required.[34] In addition to monitoring heart rate, blood pressure, and oxygen saturation, capnography helps the anesthesiologist recognize these airway-related problems and should be used routinely. At completion of the procedure, the endoscopist should aspirate the air that has been introduced into the gastrointestinal tract. Failure to do so may impair diaphragmatic excursion and compromise ventilation after the procedure.

In 2007, the PEDS-CORI (Pediatric Endoscopy Database System-Clinical Outcomes Research Initiative [the pediatric component of a national registry of endoscopic procedures]),[35] reported outcomes from data collected between 1999 and 2003. This report included data from 13 institutions involving 10,236 encounters. The study found an overall complication rate of 2.3%, and of these 80% were cardiopulmonary complications. Children with complications were younger and had a greater ASA physical status. There were fewer complications in patients who received general anesthesia (1.2%) compared with those who underwent sedation (3.7%). There are insufficient data to develop definitive guidelines, and many sedation practices use criteria to select patient for sedation that include ASA physical status 1 and 2, body mass index less than 95% for age, and weight more than 10 kg.

Bronchoscopy

Pediatric pulmonologists perform flexible bronchoscopy to evaluate a variety of respiratory diseases in children. In 2003, the American College of Chest Physicians published guidelines for interventional pulmonary procedures, leaving the choice of anesthesia versus sedation or topical anesthesia to the interventionalist. However, general anesthesia was recommended for pediatric bronchoscopic procedures.[36] Deep sedation or general anesthesia with topical anesthesia can be provided with the natural airway and nasal cannula for oxygen administration and CO_2 monitoring, or via facemask, LMA, or ETT. Many consider the LMA to provide ideal bronchoscopic conditions, because the large shaft more easily accommodates the bronchoscope, without significant compromise to gas flow, with ease of visualizing laryngeal function and the ability to administer positive pressure ventilation when needed.

Various agents can be used, including potent inhaled anesthetics or short-acting IV anesthetics, such as propofol, remifentanil, dexmedetomidine, fentanyl, and midazolam. The most stimulating portion of the procedure is the introduction of the bronchoscopy through the vocal cords, and the vocal cords are typically sprayed with lidocaine before passing the scope through the vocal cords. Lidocaine itself commonly causes coughing and may produce laryngospasm in lightly anesthetized patients. If the bronchoscopist touches the carina, a cough reflex is often produced, which is sometimes accompanied by bronchospasm. The anesthesiologist should be prepared to treat bronchospasm by increasing the depth of anesthesia or the administration of inhaled bronchodilators. In more severe cases, the procedure should be interrupted, the bronchoscope removed, and bronchodilators administered. Inhalational anesthetics have the added benefit of producing bronchodilation and ease of titration to alter the depth of anesthesia. However, when compared with sevoflurane, and when remifentanil was compared with propofol and remifentanil, the propofol group had less coughing and faster return of ciliary function.[37] Remifentanil, like all opioids, blunts airway reflexes and, because patients generally do not have pain after the procedure, some consider this the ideal opioid to use as an adjunct for these procedures.

BONE MARROW/LUMBAR PUNCTURE

Children with oncologic conditions frequently undergo brief, painful procedures such as bone marrow aspiration and biopsy, and lumbar puncture. A single frightful or painful experience may have long-term effects, in which every subsequent procedure is associated with fear and anxiety by the patient and family. Therefore, it is important to develop a process that minimizes pain and distress for the child and family. Some patients can be effectively managed with local anesthetics, distraction, and minimal sedation or anxiolytic medications; others require a brief general anesthetic in a procedure suite; and patients with underlying high-risk medical conditions are managed in an OR. At Texas Children's Hospital, we have developed and published a clinical algorithm to assist the decision-making process regarding the type of sedation and the optimal environment. We use an isolation room in our postanesthesia care unit as a deep sedation suite, where propofol or remifentanil are generally administered by an anesthesiologist (**Fig. 2**).[38]

Anesthesia providers should practice nonpharmacologic interventions that decrease anxiety and distress, such as nonprocedural distracting talk (eg, talk about friends, toys), humor, and medical reinterpretation (eg, reframing medical procedures and equipment as something fun and positive). They should be trained to provide developmentally appropriate procedural information. Undesired behaviors from the health care team include reassuring statements, empathizing, and apologizing.[39]

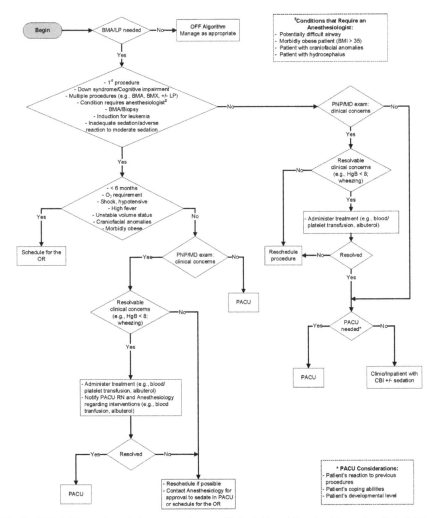

Fig. 2. TCH Evidence-Based Outcomes Center Clinical Algorithm for Managing Painful Procedures in the Cancer Center. BMA, Bone marrow aspiration; BMI, body mass index; BMX, Bone marrow biopsy; CBI, Cognitive-behavioral interventions; HgB, hemoglobin; LP; MD, medical doctor/physician; OFF, is off; PACU, postanesthesia care unit; PNP, Pediatric Nurse Practitioner; RN, registered nurse.

When sedation or anesthesia is required, the choice of pharmacologic agents and airway management is dependent on the individual patient and the environment. Rapid emergence from sedation-analgesia is desirable, significant respiratory depression should be avoided, and postoperative complications, such as nausea and vomiting as well as emergence agitation, should be minimized. Because of the rapid onset and offset of actions with minimal postoperative side effects, propofol is frequently used, often combined with other analgesics, such as fentanyl, remifentanil, and ketamine. Combining ketamine with propofol reduces respiratory depression and better maintains pharyngeal tone. Therefore, this combination is commonly used by nonanesthesiologists, because the need for airway interventions is reduced.

MOBILE SEDATION

Tasked with the challenge of providing procedural sedation for patients in outpatient clinics or inpatient floors because of advanced ASA classification, lack of skilled sedation providers, and limited additional space to perform procedures safely, our institution established a mobile sedation service. The team travels with all required equipment, supplies, and medications for safe administration of agents and resuscitation. The anesthesiologist can manage patients in the audiology, dental, hematology-oncology clinics. In our institution, the physical medicine and rehabilitation whirlpool suite is indeed 18 floors away from the OR, with limited access, and is probably the most remote anesthesia site.

SPECIFIC ISSUES

Nitrous oxide (N_2O) is an inhalation analgesic, which can be used for mild to moderately painful procedures in children, including laceration repair, fracture reduction, and peripheral venous catheter insertion. It has a very rapid onset of action (minutes) and a rapid return to baseline after discontinuation. It is sometimes delivered in a premixed tank at 50% with oxygen, or through flow meters that allow up to 70% N_2O administration with oxygen. According to American Academy of Pediatrics guidelines, N_2O delivery equipment must have the capacity of delivering 100% and never less than 25% oxygen concentration. A delivery system that covers the mouth and nose must be used in conjunction with a calibrated and functional oxygen analyzer.[7] N_2O generally produces minimal sedation in concentrations of 50% or less.[40–42] The child should be able to maintain verbal communication throughout the procedure. If N_2O is combined with other sedatives or hypnotic agents, a deeper level of sedation may develop, requiring an increased level of monitoring. The most common use of N_2O is in pediatric dentistry; however, some pediatric institutions report excellent success with the use of N_2O and rare side effects. Because N_2O is more soluble than nitrogen, it expands air-containing spaces in the body. Therefore, it is contraindicated for patients who have bowel obstruction or pneumothorax. In remote anesthesia sites, where the availability of anesthesia machines might be limited, a portable N_2O delivery system managed by a trained, highly skilled nursing team or respiratory therapist team can be used to sedate children for peripheral IV catheters in preparation for deep sedation or general anesthesia with IV sedative medications.

DIFFICULT AIRWAY

Patients with recognized syndromes associated with difficult intubation or a craniofacial abnormality on physical examination suggestive of difficult intubation are difficult to manage outside the OR. These locations that are remote from the OR typically do not have the full selection of tools to manage the airway in the OR such as video laryngoscopes and fiber-optic bronchoscopes. All sedating and anesthetizing locations must be equipped with standard laryngoscopes, with varying sizes and shape of blades to care for children. In addition, LMAs of all sizes must be available. The sedating physician/anesthesiologist must decide on the optimal technique of sedation or anesthesia and be prepared to intubate the trachea if airway obstruction or respiratory depression develops. If the difficult airway is recognized before the procedure, the anesthesiologist should consider starting the anesthetic in the OR, where additional personnel and equipment are more readily available. If difficult intubation was not anticipated beforehand, the LMA can be lifesaving.[43] There must also be a mechanism and protocol to call for immediate assistance (see later discussion).

CARDIOPULMONARY RESUSCITATION

The anesthesia provider directing cardiopulmonary resuscitation (CPR) in locations other than the OR must be prepared to potentially deal with a team that is less prepared and less practiced in these skills compared with OR personnel. Simulation has shown these weaknesses in 1 hospital. Before undertaking sedation/anesthesia of a child in a new location, the anesthesia provider should familiarize themselves with the location of the closest code cart and the contents of that cart if it is not standardized in the institution. In 2009, the ASA published a practice advisory for MRI that advises initiation of CPR in the MRI when an emergency situation develops and quickly removing the patient from the MRI scanner. The patient should be transferred to a previously designated location near the MRI that has monitoring and resuscitation equipment.[17,44]

POSTPROCEDURE CARE

Like procedures in the OR, careful observation and monitoring of the patient after sedation/anesthesia should continue into the recovery phase in remote sites. Emergence agitation, pain, respiratory events, and unstable hemodynamics should be managed in a safe environment and under the vigilance of skilled personnel. Close attention should be made to the patient's medical condition, which may pose a risk after sedation/anesthesia. Anticipated time of recovery (extended stay for patients with obstructive sleep apnea), possible hospitalization (premature infant at risk for postanesthesia apnea) or upgrade of inpatient care environment (unstable hemodynamics or acute respiratory event requiring intubation) must be communicated to the recovery phase nursing team, responsible medical or surgical team, and the parents. Children scheduled for outpatient procedures should meet strict discharge criteria to eliminate risk.

RISKS AND COMPLICATIONS

Risk related to sedation and anesthesia outside the OR can be broken down into inadequate sedation, oversedation/adverse response to sedatives, and failure to rescue. There is a theoretic risk of neurotoxicity from sedative exposure to the developing brain, and this is discussed in the article elsewhere in this issue.

In a study of 1140 sedations administered by nonanesthesiologists,[45] the most frequent complication was inadequate sedation, which was reported in 13.2% of patients. Even although outcomes from inadequate sedation have not been studied, they can be inferred from evidence regarding stress and anxiety in children having surgery. The incidence of negative behaviors 2 weeks after surgery is significantly greater in children who are anxious and have a stressful inhalation induction.

In 2000, Dr Charles Coté published a landmark article on the risk of oversedation and failure to rescue children after sedation.[46] This was a retrospective review of 95 cases reported over a 20-year period. Even though an incidence of severe adverse effects could not be determined, the findings from this article remain applicable. The incidence of death or severe neurologic injury was high (60 of 95 patients), and most of these events could have been prevented. Thirty-four of the patients received an overdose, and when 3 medications were used in combination, the risk of oversedation was significantly greater. The most frequent complications began as a respiratory event (80%), and most of these events progressed to cardiac arrest, which indicates an inability to rescue the child.

The Pediatric Sedation Research Consortium (PSRC) has established a large database of sedation procedures, outcomes, and complications. There are more than 35 institutions, which share prospective data on pediatric sedation, and several reports have been published from this database. In 2006, the PSRC reported an analysis of the first 30,037 records.[3] They found no deaths and only 1 cardiac arrest; unanticipated admission occurred in 1 per 1500 sedations; vomiting in 1 per 200, including 1 aspiration; stridor, laryngospasm, wheezing, and apnea in 1 per 400; and airway or ventilatory manipulations occurred in 1 per 200. Failed sedations were rare, at 8.9 per 1000. In 2009, the PSRC reported the analysis of 49,386 procedures in which propofol sedation/anesthesia was used outside the OR.[4] Propofol was administered by anesthesiologists, intensivists, emergency medicine specialists, pediatricians, and radiologists. No deaths were recorded; however, CPR was required in 2 children (anesthesiologists were not involved in their care), and aspiration occurred in 4 children. Desaturation of less than 90% for more than 30 seconds developed 154 times per 10,000 sedations/anesthetics, and 1 in 70 children required airway rescue. Unexpected admissions occurred 7.1 times per 10,000 sedations. No difference in major pulmonary complications was found for anesthesiologists versus other providers. Another report of the PSRC published in 2011[47] analyzed 131,751 procedural sedations and found no difference in the rates of major complications among different pediatric specialists administering procedural sedation. The study did not track whether high-risk patients were referred to the anesthesia service.

QUALITY IMPROVEMENT AND OUTCOME

In the 1990s, the Centers for Medicare and Medicaid Services and the Joint Commission mandated uniform standards for all sedated patients throughout an institution, which include standardized documentation, fasting guidelines, and informed consent procedures. These standards hold regardless of the location of the procedure and regardless of practitioner. The sedation personnel, monitoring equipment, and recovery facilities must be uniform within an institution, as well as a quality improvement process.[8] In 2010, the Joint Commission mandated that anesthesia departments provide the leadership and responsibilities for the delivery of deep sedation in addition to anesthesia.[9] Minimal and moderate sedation are not subject to anesthesia administration requirements. However, hospitals are required to develop protocols for patients receiving all levels of sedation. A quality improvement program for the department of anesthesiology should review anesthetic and sedation outcomes of patient both in the OR and outside the OR. The types of complications that are commonly assessed include:

- Aspiration events
- Unscheduled admissions to the hospital, or unplanned admission to an intensive care unit as a direct result of the sedation or anesthesia (ie, because of protracted emesis, prolonged sedation, or respiratory or cardiac complication)

- Failed procedures resulting from inadequate or problematic anesthesia or sedation
- Medication errors
- Airway injury
- Hypothermia
- Awareness
- Position injuries
- Respiratory arrest and hypoxemic events
- Cardiovascular compromise
- Anaphylaxis
- Cardiac arrest

Hospital systems have benefited from anesthesiology participation and leadership of a sedation committee, whose charter is the oversight of effective, efficient, and safe sedation throughout the institution. A sedation committee membership is made up of physicians, nurses, pharmacists, and quality specialists. Physicians who are common users of sedation, such as gastroenterologists, pulmonologists, emergency medicine specialists, intensivists, and oncologists should be represented on the committee. This committee should produce education programs and credentialing processes for sedating patients as well as policies on needed equipment, medications, monitoring, assessment, and recovery from sedation.

REFERENCES

1. Coté CJ, Cravero JP. Brave new world: do we need it, do we want it, can we afford it? Pediatr Anesth 2011;21:919–23.
2. Lalwani K, Michel M. Pediatric sedation in North American children's hospitals: a survey of anesthesia providers. Paediatr Anaesth 2005;15:209–13.
3. Cravero JP, Blike GT, Beach M, et al. Incidence and nature of adverse events during pediatric sedation/anesthesia for procedures outside the operating room: report from the Pediatric Sedation Research Consortium. Pediatrics 2006;118: 1087–96.
4. Cravero JP, Beach ML, Blike GT, et al. The incidence and nature of adverse events during pediatric sedation/anesthesia with propofol for procedures outside the operating room: a report from the Pediatric Sedation Research Consortium. Anesth Analg 2009;108:795–804.
5. Coté CJ. Round and round we go: sedation–what is it, who does it, and have we made things safer for children? Paediatr Anaesth 2008;18:3–8.
6. Scottish Intercollegiate Guidelines Network. SIGN Guideline 58: safe sedation of children undergoing diagnostic and therapeutic procedures. Paediatr Anaesth 2008;18:11–2.
7. Coté CJ, Wilson S. Guidelines for monitoring and management of pediatric patients during and after sedation for diagnostic and therapeutic procedures: an update. Pediatrics 2006;118:2587–602.
8. The Joint Commission. Anesthesia and sedation: the Joint Commission resources. Oakbrook Terrace (IL): The Joint Commission; 2001.
9. Joint Commission Resources Staff. The Joint Commission comprehensive creditation manual. E-ed. 2011. Available at: http://www.jointcommision.org/.
10. Tait AR, Pandit UA. Use of the laryngeal mask airway in children with upper respiratory tract infections: a comparison with endotracheal intubation. Anesth Analg 1998;86:706–11.

11. Leape LL, Bates DW, Cullen DJ, et al. Systems analysis of adverse drug events. JAMA 1995;274:35–43.
12. Cravero JP. Anesthesia outside the operating room. In: Cote CJ, Lerman J, Anderson BJ, editors. A practice of anesthesia for infants and children. 5th edition. Elsevier; 2013.
13. Brenner DJ, Hall EJ. Computed tomography–an increasing source of radiation exposure. N Engl J Med 2007;357:2277–84.
14. Mason KP, Zgleszewski SE, Dearden JL, et al. Dexmedetomidine for pediatric sedation for computed tomography imaging studies. Not Found In Database 2006;103:57–62.
15. Ziegler MA, Fricke BL, Donnelly LF. Is administration of enteric contrast material safe before abdominal CT in children who require sedation? Experience with chloral hydrate and pentobarbital. AJR Am J Roentgenol 2003;180:13–5.
16. Sargent MA, McEachern AM, Jamieson DH, et al. Atelectasis on pediatric chest CT: comparison of sedation techniques. Pediatr Radiol 1999;29:509–13.
17. Practice advisory on anesthetic care for magnetic resonance imaging: a report by the American Society of Anesthesiologists Task Force on Anesthetic Care for Magnetic Resonance Imaging. Anesthesiology 2009;110(3):459–79.
18. Lawson GR. Sedation of children for magnetic resonance imaging. Arch Dis Child 2000;82:150–3.
19. Sury MR. Paediatric sedation. Cont Educ Anaesth Crit Care Pain 2004;4:118–22.
20. Guistino A, Kondo KL. Pharmacology of sclerotherapy. Semin Intervent Radiol 2010;27(4):391–9.
21. Mason KP, Michna E, Zurakowski D, et al. Serum ethanol levels in children and adults after ethanol embolization or sclerotherapy for vascular anomalies. Radiology 2000;217:127–32.
22. Roca-Bielsa I, Vlajković M. Pediatric nuclear medicine and pediatric radiology: modalities, image quality, dosimetry and correlative imaging: new strategies. Pediatr Radiol 2013;43(4):391–2.
23. Nadel HR. Radiation safety summit: nuclear medicine and PET/CT justification and optimization. Pediatr Radiol 2011.
24. Griffiths M, Kamat P, McCracken CE, et al. Is procedural sedation with propofol acceptable for complex imaging? A comparison of short vs prolonged sedation in children. Pediatr Radiol 2013;43(10):1273–8.
25. Mettler F, Bhargavan M, Faulkner K, et al. Nuclear medicine studies in the United States and worldwide: frequency, radiation dose, and comparison with other radiation sources. Radiology 2009;253:520–31.
26. Harris E. Sedation and anesthesia options for pediatric patients in the radiation oncology suite. Int J Pediatr 2010;2010:870921.
27. Gilger MA. Sedation for pediatric GI endoscopy. Gastrointest Endosc 2007;65:211–2.
28. Kaddu R, Bhattacharya D, Metriyakool K, et al. Propofol compared with general anesthesia for pediatric GI endoscopy: is propofol better? Gastrointest Endosc 2002;55:27–32.
29. Schwarz SM, Lightdale JR, Liacouras CA. Sedation and anesthesia in pediatric endoscopy: one size does not fit all. J Pediatr Gastroenterol Nutr 2007;44:295–7.
30. Barbi E, Petaros P, Badina L, et al. Deep sedation with propofol for upper gastrointestinal endoscopy in children, administered by specially trained pediatricians: a prospective case series with emphasis on side effects. Endoscopy 2006;38:368–75.

31. Abu-Shahwan I, Mack D. Propofol and remifentanil for deep sedation in children undergoing gastrointestinal endoscopy. Paediatr Anaesth 2007;17:460–3.
32. Michaud L. Sedation for diagnostic upper gastrointestinal endoscopy: a survey of the Francophone Pediatric Hepatology, Gastroenterology, and Nutrition Group. Endoscopy 2005;37:167–70.
33. Tosun Z, Aksu R, Guler G, et al. Propofol-ketamine vs. propofol fentanyl for sedation during pediatric upper gastrointestinal endoscopy. Paediatr Anaesth 2007; 10:983–8.
34. Amournyotin S, Aanpreung P, Prakarnrattana U, et al. Experience of intravenous sedation for pediatric gastrointestinal endoscopy in a large tertiary referral center in a developing country. Paediatr Anaesth 2009;19:784–91.
35. Thakkar K, El-Serag HB, Mattek N, et al. Complications of pediatric EGD: a 4 year experience in PEDS-CORI. Gastrointest Endosc 2007;65(2):213–21.
36. Ernst A, Silvestri GA, Johnstone D. Interventional pulmonary procedures: guidelines from the American College of Chest Physicians. Chest 2003;123:1693–717.
37. Ledowski T, Paech MJ, Patel B, et al. Bronchial mucus transport velocity in patients receiving propofol and remifentanil versus sevoflurane and remifentanil anesthesia. Anesth Analg 2006;102:1427–30, 8.
38. Hockenberry MJ, McCarthy K, Taylor O, et al. Managing painful procedures in children with cancer. J Pediatr Hematol Oncol 2011;33(2):110–27.
39. Martin SR, Chorney JM, Tan ET, et al. Changing healthcare providers' behavior during pediatric inductions with an empirically based intervention. Anesthesiology 2011;115:18–27.
40. Zier JL, Tarrago R, Liu M. Level of sedation with nitrous oxide for pediatric medical procedures. Anesth Analg 2010;110:1399–405.
41. Zier JL, Liu M. Safety of high-concentration nitrous oxide by nasal mask for pediatric procedural sedation: experience with 7802 cases. Pediatr Emerg Care 2011; 27:1107–12.
42. Babl FE, Oakley E, Seaman C, et al. High-concentration nitrous oxide for procedural sedation in children: adverse events and depth of sedation. Pediatrics 2008;121:e528–32.
43. Schmidt U, Eikermann M. Organizational aspects of difficult airway management: think globally act locally. Anesthesiology 2011;114(1):3–6.
44. Blike GT, Christoffersen K, Cravero JP, et al. A method for measuring system safety and latent errors associated with pediatric procedural sedation. Anesth Analg 2005;101:48–58.
45. Kain ZN, Mayes LC, Wang SM, et al. Parental presence during induction of anesthesia versus sedative premedication: which intervention is more effective? Anesthesiology 1998;89:1147–56.
46. Coté CJ, Karl HW, Notterman DA, et al. Adverse sedation events in pediatrics: analysis of medications used for sedation. Pediatrics 2000;106:633–44.
47. Couloures KG, Beach M, Cravero JP, et al. Impact of provider specialty on pediatric procedural sedation complication rates. Pediatrics 2011;127:e1154–60.

Respiratory Complications in the Pediatric Postanesthesia Care Unit

Britta S. von Ungern-Sternberg, MD, PhD, DEAA, FANZCA[a,b,]*

KEYWORDS

- Pediatric anesthesia • Respiratory complications • Risk factors
- Postanesthesia care unit • Recovery room

KEY POINTS

- Despite a good safety record, respiratory complications are a major cause of morbidity and mortality in pediatric anesthesia.
- 1 in 10 children present with 1 or more respiratory complications during their stay in the PACU.
- The risk factors can be divided into patient factors, surgical factors, and factors caused by anesthesia management.
- Rapid recognition of respiratory complications in the PACU and appropriate treatment strategies are essential to avoid hypoxia.

INTRODUCTION

Although pediatric anesthesia is relatively safe, perioperative respiratory adverse events (PRAE) are one of the major causes of morbidity and mortality.[1–6] A large audit in an academic center in Singapore showed that PRAE accounted for more than three-quarters of all critical incidents in pediatric anesthesia.[1] In addition, one-third of all perioperative cardiac arrests are caused by respiratory complications.[2] One-fifth of all perioperative cardiac arrests occur during emergence from anesthesia and in the postanesthesia care unit (PACU), with half of these the PACU arrests being caused by respiratory problems.[7] Furthermore, when comparing pediatric and adult closed-claim legal cases with respect to the mechanisms of injury and outcome, PRAE are more common and the rate is greater in pediatric claims that resulted in death

Funding: B.S. von Ungern-Sternberg is partly funded by the Princess Margaret Hospital Foundation and Woolworths Australia.
a Department of Anesthesia and Pain Management, Princess Margaret Hospital for Children, Roberts Road, Subiaco, Western Australia 6008, Australia; b School of Medicine and Pharmacology, The University of Western Australia, 35 Stirling Highway, Crawley, Perth, Western Australia 6009, Australia
* Department of Anesthesia and Pain Management, Princess Margaret Hospital for Children, Roberts Road, Subiaco, Western Australia 6008, Australia.
E-mail address: britta.regli-vonungern@health.wa.gov.au

Anesthesiology Clin 32 (2014) 45–61
http://dx.doi.org/10.1016/j.anclin.2013.10.004

(70%) or brain damage (30%) in previously healthy children compared with adult claims.[8,9]

A study by our group of more than 9000 children showed that 15% of all children suffered from 1 or more PRAE with oxygen desaturation; pulse oximeter saturation (SpO_2) less than 95% (10%), coughing (7%), airway obstruction (4%), and laryngospasm (4%) were the most common, whereas bronchospasm (2%) and postoperative stridor (<1%) were less common.[3]

Although PRAE may occur at any time in the perioperative period, they are most frequently observed during the induction of anesthesia and the recovery period.[3] Besides pain, emergence delirium, and postoperative nausea and vomiting, PRAE are the most common problems encountered in the PACU; however, above all, the most common reason for an emergency call from the PACU is the occurrence of PRAE.

Our goal should therefore be to predict (even before the induction of anesthesia) which children are at a particularly high risk for PRAE in the perioperative period, to then adjust our anesthesia management for the individual patient in order to minimize the occurrence and severity of PRAE during the entire perioperative period, including the stay in the PACU. Most respiratory complications, if treated immediately and effectively, are not associated with any long-term negative effects for the patient.

DEFINITIONS AND SIGNS OF PRAE

PRAE in the PACU include apnea, bronchospasm, laryngospasm, severe persistent coughing, oxygen desaturation, and stridor/postextubation croup, with the following definitions[10]:

1. Laryngospasm: complete airway obstruction associated with muscle rigidity of the abdominal and chest walls. Warning signs for the occurrence of laryngospasm are cough, breath holding, and straining in inspiration and expiration.
2. Bronchospasm: increased respiratory effort, particularly during expiration, and wheeze on auscultation; in extreme cases, a silent chest can occur, making the diagnosis more challenging.
3. Severe persistent coughing: a series of pronounced, persistent severe coughs lasting more than 10 seconds.
4. Partial and complete airway obstruction: erratic respiratory efforts in combination with stridor or a snoring noise or with paradoxic movement of the abdomen in the presence of partial and complete airway obstruction, respectively.
5. Apnea: cessation of gas flow for more than 10 to 15 seconds (varying definitions) or less if associated with bradycardia, cyanosis, or pallor. Apnea can be of either central (no gas flow because of lack of respiratory effort), obstructive (no gas flow despite respiratory effort), or mixed (central and obstructive) origin.
6. Oxygen desaturations: definitions vary between SpO_2 of lower than 90% and 95%. Desaturations can be the consequence of any of these signs and can lead to hypoxia and cardiac arrest.
7. Stridor: a high-pitched wheezing sound, resulting from turbulent airflow in the upper airway.

INCIDENCE OF PRAE

Recent data in our institution have shown that 1 in 10 children in the PACU present with 1 or more PRAE.[3] Although the incidence of bronchospasm and laryngospasm is low in the PACU ($\leq$1%), 5% of children suffer from severe persistent coughing or desaturation (SpO$_2$ <95%).[3] Airway obstruction, which could be relived by simple airway maneuvers, was found in 1% of children in our institution independent of the presence of respiratory risk factors, whereas stridor was found mainly in high-risk children (for risk factors, see later discussion).[3]

Other groups have reported desaturation rates as high as 50% on arrival in the PACU.[11,12] High desaturation rates are commonly linked with the lack of oxygen administration on transfer to the recovery area.[11–13]

SEVERITY AND OUTCOME OF RESPIRATORY COMPLICATIONS

Potential complications of PRAE in the PACU are negative pressure pulmonary edema, prolonged oxygen requirements, prolonged hospital stay, behavioral problems, need for reintubation, need for admission to the intensive care unit (ICU)/neonatal ICU (NICU), cardiac arrest, permanent brain damage, and death. Most reintubations and nearly half of all the unplanned postoperative admissions to ICU are related to PRAE, the remaining mainly for surgical reasons.[14,15] Most PRAE resulting in permanent brain damage are caused by inadequate ventilation. Half of all cardiac arrests in the PACU are caused by PRAE.[2,7] Children cared for by pediatric anesthesiologists or in pediatric only centers had better outcomes after PRAE and cardiac arrest compared with children cared for by general anesthesiologists or in mixed population centers.[3,7,16]

General Risk Factors for Respiratory Complications

Although cardiac complications are mostly easy to predict in children because they mainly occur in children with known cardiac disease, respiratory complications are more commonly seen in previously healthy children or those with only minor comorbidities such as asthma or eczema. To determine who is at risk for respiratory complications, it is easiest to distinguish between factors related to the patient, the surgical procedure, and the anesthesia management (**Box 1**).[3,17–19]

The difficulty in studying and reporting risk factors of PRAE is that most PRAE and their risk factors are not independent from each other (eg, both bronchospasm or laryngospasm can lead to oxygen desaturations, and asthma is a risk factor for the occurrence of laryngospasm, bronchospasm, persistent coughing, and desaturation).[3]

Patient factors and pathophysiology: why are children at such a high risk for desaturations?

The main causes of postoperative hypoxemia in children are atelectasis and depression of respiratory drive by opioids and hypnotic agents, as well as decrease in muscle tone because of the muscle relaxing properties of anesthetics and residual neuromuscular blockade. In general, the resting volume of the lung is determined by the balance between the chest and lung recoil pressures. Because of the increased chest wall compliance, the functional residual capacity (FRC) is lower in younger children compared with older children or adults.[20,21] Chest wall compliance decreases rapidly during childhood, particularly in the first year of life.[20] Nearly all anesthetic agents induce a dose-dependent relaxation of respiratory muscles, which also reduces airway muscle activity.[22–25] This induced muscle relaxation interferes with the balance between the chest wall compliance, elastic lung recoil, and tension of the diaphragm, leading to a decrease in lung volumes and unequal distribution of ventilation.[24–28] In small children, this anesthesia-induced muscle relaxation in addition impairs the natural dynamic increase of FRC in the expiratory phase, leading to

Box 1
Factors increasing the risk of respiratory complications in the PACU
Patient
Young age, particularly (ex-) premature babies
Current or recent upper respiratory tract infection
Passive/active smoking
Recurrent wheezing
Current/past asthma
Nocturnal dry cough
Wheezing during exercise
Allergic rhinitis
Current/past eczema
Family history of asthma, eczema, or allergic rhinitis
Obstructive sleep apnea
Obesity
Unfasted patient
Bronchopulmonary dysplasia
Cystic fibrosis
Other respiratory illnesses
Surgical Procedure
Blood or secretions in the upper airway
Procedures with shared airway (eg, ear, nose, and throat, dental, respiratory medicine)
Sudden surgical stimulation
Emergency procedure
Anesthesia/Recovery Management
Invasive airway management
Repeated attempts at airway management
Desflurane as maintenance agent
Less experienced anesthesiologist
Less experienced PACU staff
Patient ratio in PACU
Opioid management
Administration of neuromuscular blocking agents
Timing of the removal of airway device
Topical lidocaine
Premedication with midazolam
Emergence (vs induction of anesthesia)
Mixed population hospital (vs solely pediatric)

an increased tendency for small peripheral airway collapse, even during normal tidal breathing.[29]

Children have lower oxygen reserves because of an increased tendency to airway collapse (increased compliance), leading to a decrease in FRC that makes them prone for hypoxemia.[21] This situation can be counteracted by the administration of positive end-expiratory pressure in the immediate postoperative period to prevent alveolar collapse by increasing FRC and dynamic lung compliance and decreasing total airway resistance.[28,30–33]

Age The age of the patient has a significant impact on the occurrence of PRAE, with neonates and young infants having the highest risk.[3] For example, the relative risk for laryngospasm decreases by 11% for each yearly increase in age.[3,34]

Clinical studies have shown that oxygen desaturation occurs faster, to deeper levels and with a slower recovery in infants compared with older children and adults.[35] Up to half of normally healthy infants and young children present with desaturations during the transport from operating room to the PACU or on arrival in the PACU.[11–13]

Prematurity Prematurity also increases the risk for PRAE, mainly because of the associated higher risk for apnea and bronchopulmonary dysplasia.

Bronchopulmonary dysplasia in (ex-) premature patients
Bronchopulmonary dysplasia occurs in a relatively high percentage of ex-premature preterm babies (birth weight <1500 g).[36] Even though many children are symptom-free in everyday life by 2 years of age, they still have a higher rate of bronchial hyperre-activity (BHR) compared with the normal population.[37] Many parents are unaware of the bronchopulmonary dysplasia that their child has, and history taking can therefore be deceiving.[37] A high index of suspicion should be used if a child was born prema-turely, especially if ventilated in the neonatal period.[38] The lack of surfactant and under-developed lungs, artificial ventilation, and other factors of the early neonatal period can result in inflammation and fibrosis of the alveoli and small airways.[36] These children display a hypersensitive pulmonary capillary network, which is prone to vasocon-striction after hypothermia, pain, or acidosis, for example. The BHR in these children with bronchopulmonary dysplasia has been shown from as early as 26 weeks after conception and 12 days of age and decreases slowly over the years, depending on the severity.[39]

Apnea in neonatal patients
Because respiratory control in neonates is not yet fully developed and needs weeks to months to mature,[10] the breathing pattern of preterm as well as term infants is often irregular and periodic and can be associated with severe apnea.[40] Brainstem respira-tory rhythmogenesis, peripheral and central chemoreceptor responses, and other parts of the respiratory control network are immature in premature babies, leading to an impaired response to hypercapnia and hypoxia.[10] In older children and adults, hypercarbia leads to an increase in tidal volume and respiratory rate. These responses are impaired in premature babies.[41] Hypoxia in preterm infants shows a biphasic response; at first, ventilation increases for approximately 1 minute and then de-creases, with the potential for apnea.[42] In the PACU, after emergence from anesthesia, any residual anesthetic drugs decrease the respiratory control to both hypoxia and hypercapnia.[43] Risk factors for postoperative apnea are given in **Box 2**.

BHR BHR is defined as a tendency of the smooth muscle of the tracheobronchial tree to contract more intensely in response to a given stimulus than it does in the response seen in normal individuals and is commonly caused by airway inflammation.

Box 2
Risk factors for postoperative apnea

- Inversely correlated to gestational age
- Inversely correlated to postconceptual age
- Associated with previous history of apnea
- Not associated with small-for-gestational-age infants (protective)
- Anemia, hematocrit level less than 30%, regardless of gestational age or postconceptual age
- Preventative treatment: caffeine 10 mg/kg

Asthma, BHR, upper respiratory tract infection (URTI), or passive smoking are all recognized risk factors for PRAE.[3,44–46] The incidence of asthma and BHR is high among children, with up to 40% of 6-year-old children having wheezing and around 20% having asthma requiring regular medication.[47,48] In addition, the incidence of URTI in children, particularly preschool children, presenting for anesthesia is high.[3,49] Although a recent URTI increases the risk of PRAE,[3,34] general anesthesia is often performed under these circumstances for several reasons: (1) URTI occurs frequently, especially in young children and children undergoing ear, nose, and throat (ENT) procedures, and there is clinical uncertainty for how long to postpone the procedure after an URTI[3]; (2) there are adverse economic and emotional impacts to canceling surgery.[50]

In general, all factors that are commonly associated with an increase in BHR lead to an increase in PRAE (**Box 3**). Children with BHR have an aggravated response to airway stimulations (eg, suctioning, removal of airway device in the PACU, which can lead to an increased risk for bronchospasm and desaturation in particular). In young children, symptoms of BHR might not yet have been noted by the parents, or the child might be to young to report them. Because eczema and to a lesser extent allergic rhinitis are often seen in children who later in life develop recurrent wheeze, asthma, and BHR, the presence of these early symptoms should alert the anesthesiologist as significant risk factors for respiratory complications.

BHR after an acute asthmatic/wheezing episode persists for several weeks beyond the presence of asthmatic symptoms.[51,52] Warning signs for significant BHR are a recent increase in asthma symptoms or treatment requirements or even

---

Box 3
Factors commonly associated with an increase in BHR

- Lung disease with airway inflammation (eg, asthma, cystic fibrosis)
- Current/recent (within 2 weeks) upper respiratory tract infections, particularly when associated with moist cough/green runny nose
- Dry nocturnal cough
- Wheezing with exercise
- Passive/active smoking
- Atopy
- Possible increase in children with eczema, allergic rhinitis, or family history of asthma, eczema, or allergic rhinitis

---

hospitalization. BHR is mainly caused by underlying airway inflammation, which should be treated and lung function optimized before surgery whenever possible.[53] Children with these warning signs should receive intensified therapy for their asthma/wheezing before elective surgery, preferably in a respiratory clinic, and surgery should be postponed. In addition, if surgery has to go ahead or even after the intensified therapy, these children can further benefit from a premedication with salbutamol 10 to 30 minutes before the induction of anesthesia, which significantly decreases the incidence of PRAE in these high-risk children.[19]

Obesity The incidence of childhood obesity, a risk factor for PRAE, is steadily increasing; in Australia, 25% of children are overweight (body mass index [BMI], calculated as weight in kilograms divided by the square of height in meters >85th centile) or obese (BMI >95th centile).[44,54–57] Obese children not only have a reduced lung function via a loss in lung volume and impaired respiratory mechanics[58] but also have a higher rate of asthma and other comorbidities (eg, obstructive sleep apnea, habitual snoring), further increasing the risk for PRAE.[17,44,55,57] Furthermore, many components of anesthesia (eg, supine positioning, anesthetic agents, and surgery) lead to an additional decrease in lung volumes, and the changes in lung function are expected to be greater in the obese patient.[28,33,59–66] Together, these factors increase the incidence of all PRAE, in particular, postoperative desaturations.

Surgical procedure
Procedures with a shared upper airway during the procedure (eg, ENT, dental, respiratory medicine) are more prone to lead to airway lesions, swelling, bleeding, or increased secretions postoperatively. Blood or increased secretions in the upper airway lead to an increased risk for PRAE.

ADENOTONSILLECTOMY

Children undergoing ENT surgery, particularly adenotonsillectomy, have an increased incidence of PRAE,[3,4,67] in particular oxygen desaturations and airway obstruction.[68,69]

Not only does the operation on the upper airway cause postoperative swelling, but these children also have a high incidence of obstructive sleep apnea syndrome, which is often the primary reason for surgery. It is therefore common practice in many institutions to monitor these children, particularly if they also show symptoms of obstructive sleep apnea, with continuous pulse oximetry for 24 hours after surgery.

Anesthesia Management

Airway device
Noninvasive airway management (supraglottic airway device or face mask) actively reduces PRAE (tracheal tube vs face mask relative risk [RR] [95% confidence interval] 5.1 [2.3–11.6], $P<.0001$).[3] The optimal timing of removal of any airway device is a topic of debate among pediatric anesthesiologists. However, there seem to be only minor differences between both techniques, regardless whether a laryngeal mask or an endotracheal tube is used.[70–72] Removal of a laryngeal mask airway in the awake state marginally increases the risk of PRAE compared with removal during deep anesthesia (RR 1.3 [1.1–1.5], $P = .001$).[3] A recent study from our group reported that awake extubation in high-risk children after adenotonsillectomy was associated with a higher incidence of severe persistent coughing (60% vs 36%) and hoarse voice (48% vs 26%), as well as more and longer episodes of oxygen desaturations.[70–72] Although persistent coughing is often seen as a minor problem, it can affect surgical hemostasis, with an

increased risk of postoperative bleeding, and can increase postoperative pain. On the other side, extubation while deeply anesthetized moderately increased rates of airway obstruction without increasing oxygen desaturations, because airway obstructions were easily removed by simple airway maneuvers.[72] Although deep extubation is less likely to stimulate the airway, and may increase efficiency and operating room turnover times, the setup of the PACU must enable close supervision by well-trained PACU nurses of the children extubated deep and must incorporate staff who are fully trained in performing simple airway maneuvers in case of airway obstruction.[72] With such a setup, it is not surprising that against common belief, the level of wakefulness in the PACU after pediatric anesthesia does not correlate with the occurrence of oxygen desaturation.[73]

In recent years, cuffed endotracheal tubes have increasingly been used also in younger children, including term neonates.[74] Cuffed endotracheal tubes are associated with lower rates of PRAE, even after correction for age, particularly if cuff pressure has been continuously monitored.[3,75] An increased cuff pressure correlates with negative outcome, particularly with the incidence of sore throat.[3,75]

DRUGS

Most anesthetic drug-related PRAE are caused by the mechanisms of reduced respiratory drive or impaired respiratory muscle function, leading to hypoventilation, atelectasis, and hypoxia. Rarely, anesthetic drugs can lead to allergic or nonallergic bronchoconstriction.

Neuromuscular Blocking Agents

Residual neuromuscular blockade has been found in nearly half of the patients who received intraoperative neuromuscular blocking agents, even though the patient was deemed appropriately reversed by the attending anesthesiologist.[76–80] This is not surprising, because neuromuscular monitoring is not standard in all institutions; it is particularly rarely used in many private institutions.[81] In addition, neuromuscular monitoring in children is technically challenging and cannot completely exclude residual paralysis. For example, a tetanic stimulation in an awake premature baby leads to a fade at 20 Hz; term neonates show fade on stimulation from 50 Hz onwards.[82] Residual neuromuscular blockade is even found after a single intubation dose.[83] Residual neuromuscular blockade often leads to hypoventilation, respiratory fatigue, and consequent hypoxia. Furthermore, infants show a fade without the administration of muscle relaxants under nitrous oxide and methohexital anesthesia.[84] To avoid residual neuromuscular blockade, reversal agents are given in many cases. However, reversal given too early is associated with the danger of recurarization, which can occur in the PACU or on the ward. The incidence of hypoxia in the PACU is nearly doubled in children who received neuromuscular blocking agents compared with those who did not.[3] Against more traditional anesthetic teaching routinely using neuromuscular blockade, it has been shown that endotracheal intubation can be performed equally well in most children without neuromuscular blockade.[85] Therefore, it is advisable not to use neuromuscular blocking agents in children unless they are necessary for procedural reasons.

Opioids

Most children admitted to the PACU have received opioids within their anesthesia regimen. Children with obstructive sleep apnea as well as neonates and young infants (<6 months) are particularly sensitive to opioids.[86] The highest-risk groups for patients after opioid administration are listed in **Box 4**. Particularly after major surgery, it is

> **Box 4**
> **Risk factors for respiratory complications with opioid administration**
>
> - Age younger than 6 months, particularly neonates
> - Cardiac disease
> - Underlying respiratory disease
> - Central/obstructive sleep apnea
> - Syndromes associated with airway obstruction
> - Hepatic/renal insufficiency
> - Neurodevelopmental disorders, global developmental delay
> - Concurrent administration of other sedative drugs (eg, benzodiazepines, clonidine, gabapentin)

often a fine balance to have the children pain free but not oversedated with opioids. It has been shown that reducing the dose of intraoperative morphine decreases the incidence of PRAE after tonsillectomy, particularly apneas, airway obstruction, and oxygen desaturations.[87] It is important that postoperative agitation is not misdiagnosed as pain, because this can falsely trigger further administration of opioids. If naloxone is given, it is important to consider the potential for resedation once naloxone has worn off. Therefore, the patients should remain in the PACU until the time naloxone is known to have lost effect.

Accidental drug injection

A further source for complications in the PACU is the accidental postoperative injection of an anesthetic drug (neuromuscular blocking agents, opioids, or hypnotics). Even small volumes of an anesthetic drug (particularly neuromuscular blocking agents) in an insufficiently flushed drip can cause muscle relaxation or neuromuscular blockade and can consequently lead to hypopnea or apnea or even cardiac arrest in infants because of a potentially high dose per body weight. Strict departmental guidelines about postoperative flushing of line with sufficient fluid are therefore crucial in the pediatric setting. In our institution, flushing of the line is part of the World Health Organization checklist at the end of surgery in the operating room. In addition, we routinely also mention the flushing of the line as part of our standardized handover in the PACU, which has decreased the number of incident reports filled out on the wards of white (propofol) residues in the line.

PREVENTION AND TREATMENT OF RESPIRATORY COMPLICATIONS
Infrastructure and Organization

Because children have high oxygen demands, they are particularly vulnerable to hypoxemia should a PRAE occur. However, many pediatric PACUs are solely staffed by nurses, without an attending anesthesiologist in the unit. The availability of medical backup in the PACU as well as the nurse/patient ratio varies between centers. Therefore, in anticipation of potential PRAE, regular training of the staff in rapid recognition and knowledge of the cause and treatment of PRAE in the PACU is vital.[21] For example, in our institution, we retrain our PACU nurses on a regular basis with hands-on airway management (eg, airway maneuvers, holding the face mask) in the operating room under the direct supervision of pediatric anesthesia consultants.

Furthermore, the PACU should be close to the operating rooms to allow for rapid and safe patient transport and fast response rates of the attending anesthesiologist when their immediate presence is required in the PACU because of a complication. Furthermore, an alarm system is of great benefit to allow for rapid backup in case of an emergency in the PACU. Given the small hypoxia tolerance in young children, time is vital. Each patient bed space should be well equipped, including compatible patient monitoring (SpO_2, CO_2, heart rate, blood pressure), oxygen supply, and suction. An emergency drug and airway cart should be readily available within the PACU. A thorough, preferably standardized, handoff report from the anesthesia team to the PACU team is of vital importance to make the PACU team aware of potential risk factors for complications. This handoff should include a check whether or not the intravenous (IV) line of the patient was appropriately flushed and whether the patient had received any drugs which could resedate or remuscle relax them. A nurse/patient care ratio of 1:1 is the goal in the immediate postoperative period. PACU staff must be well trained and competent in recognizing and treating respiratory complications in children.

Bronchospasm

As soon as bronchospasm is suspected in the PACU, 100% oxygen should be delivered, and repeated doses of salbutamol or levalbuterol should be given, preferably via mask and spacer, using a metered dose inhaler. If salbutamol/levalbuterol is insufficient to relieve the bronchospasm, IV ketamine, epinephrine, or magnesium should be considered.

Laryngospasm

The key point in the treatment of laryngospasm is to start therapy as early as possible once laryngospasm is suspected, before the development of hypoxia. Initial therapy includes jaw thrust and continuous positive airway pressure (CPAP) with 100% oxygen via a face mask. If this procedure is unsuccessful, 1 to 3 mg/kg of IV propofol is administered; if oxygen saturation begins to decrease and other treatment has failed, IV succinylcholine 1 to 2 mg/kg is the drug of choice to relieve laryngospasm. If succinylcholine is contraindicated, atracurium or rocuronium are safe alternatives. Most children recover from laryngospasm without any sequelae. However, some children are oxygen dependent for some time, particularly if they have underlying lung disease (eg, respiratory tract infection, cystic fibrosis). Laryngospasm can lead to atelectasis, loss of FRC, and retention of secretion, causing V/Q mismatch, which resolves once the child is sufficiently awake to cough and by doing so reexpand atelectatic lung segments.[88] Strong inspiratory efforts against a closed glottis can generate large negative intrapleural pressures, which can cause large fluid shifts from the vascular system into the interstitium by causing a sudden increase in left ventricular preload and afterload and consequently into the alveoli, leading to a negative pressure pulmonary edema.[89,90] Negative pressure pulmonary edema usually resolves quickly but may require the administration of high-flow oxygen, CPAP, and even admission to the ICU/NICU.

Desaturation

All patients should receive supplemental oxygen in the immediate postoperative period. This treatment also includes oxygen administration as a standard for all patient transfers. In our institution, we provide all patients with oxygen either via a facemask or via a laryngeal mask airway connected to a T-piece, allowing for manual ventilation or the administration of CPAP if required. Other supplemental oxygen administration options in the PACU include nasal cannula, simple face mask, or blow-by humidified oxygen via 22-mm corrugated tubing. The exact method is determined by supplemental oxygen requirement and tolerance of the child for device chosen.

Anesthesia decreases pulmonary gas exchange, mainly because of FRC loss, consequent airway closure, and atelectasis.[27] This situation can be minimized by performing a recruitment maneuver before removal of the airway device. Oxygen supplementation can be ceased entirely when pulse oximetry readings are normal and stable at or higher than preoperative levels with the patient breathing room air. Because of their higher susceptibility to oxygen toxicity, the level of oxygen supplementation necessary for appropriate oxygenation should be reviewed regularly in neonates, particularly if born premature. An air oxygen blender is useful particularly in this vulnerable population. For all patients, wakefulness does not correlate with the risk for oxygen desaturations.[73]

Severe persistent coughing and airway obstruction
Severe persistent coughing normally is self-limiting once the stimulus is removed and secretions have been mobilized. Airway obstruction in the PACU can easily be overcome in most children with simple airway maneuvers such as jaw thrust and chin lift and CPAP.[72] If these maneuvers are not sufficient, oral or rarely nasal airways can be used. In addition, it is advisable to recover all children in the lateral position, because this improves airway patency compared with the supine position.[91]

Stridor
Stridor and postintubation croup used to have an incidence of around 1% in intubated children,[92] but this has been decreasing over time with the increasing use of noninvasive airway devices and the introduction of cuffed endotracheal tubes, which are associated with lower rates of stridor compared with uncuffed endotracheal tubes.[3] Treatment, if at all, may consist of cool humidified mist or nebulized racemic epinephrine, which results in vasoconstriction of the swollen airway mucosa. Clinicians need to be aware of a potential rebound effect after nebulized racemic epinephrine, which necessitates an observation for 4 hours after nebulizer treatment in order to avoid an unobserved worsening of the respiratory symptoms. Furthermore, dexamethasone has been described to be useful in patients after longer-term ventilation (>48 hours),[93] whereas it has been controversial for postintubation croup after shorter intubation periods.[94,95]

Perioperative improvement of patients at risk of PRAE
To improve patient management and minimize respiratory complications in the PACU, it is crucial to start preventative measures as early as possible, even before the patient's admission. Prevention strategies are summarized in **Box 5**.

Therapy for asthma and BHR in general should be optimized by the treating physician with intensified inhaler therapy or in severe cases with oral corticosteroids before elective procedures.[38]

Performing a procedure at a purely pediatric hospital compared with a mixed population hospital is associated with significantly lower morbidity and mortality.[3,7,16] Furthermore, during anesthesia, preventative measures should be taken (eg, consultant anesthesiologist, noninvasive airway management, and premedication with salbutamol/levalbuterol).[3,18,19]

Anesthesia induction for patients at risk of PRAE, particularly bronchospasm, should include premedication with salbutamol/levalbuterol, IV induction, and maintenance with propofol.[3,18,19] In the PACU, close observation by staff trained to recognize and immediately treat respiratory complications in children is vital to assure a safe recovery.

Box 5
Prevention strategies for respiratory complications in the PACU

Patient

  Preoperative optimization of children with BHR (if possible)

  Age-appropriate fasting

Anesthesia

  Premedication with salbutamol in children with BHR

  Avoidance of premedication with midazolam; if needed, use clonidine

  Noninvasive airway management

  Prefer cuffed over uncuffed endotracheal tube

  Propofol anesthesia

  Regional anesthesia

  Avoidance of desflurane

  Appropriate opioid dosing

  Careful flushing of lines

  Monitoring of neuromuscular function after neuromuscular blocking agents

  Consultant pediatric anesthesiologist

  Pediatric hospital

PACU management

  Oxygen administration during transport

  Patient/nurse ratio in PACU 1:1

  Continuous Sao_2 monitoring

  CO_2 monitoring if possible

  Careful flushing of lines

ACKNOWLEDGMENTS

I thank Professor Adrian Regli, Intensive Care Unit, Fremantle Hospital, Perth, Australia for his valuable input into this article.

REFERENCES

1. Tay CL, Tan GM, Ng SB. Critical incidents in paediatric anaesthesia: an audit of 10 000 anaesthetics in Singapore. Paediatr Anaesth 2001;11:711–8.
2. Bhananker SM, Ramamoorthy C, Geiduschek JM, et al. Anesthesia-related cardiac arrest in children: update from the pediatric perioperative cardiac arrest registry. Anesth Analg 2007;105:344–50.
3. von Ungern-Sternberg BS, Boda K, Chambers NA, et al. Risk assessment for respiratory complications in paediatric anaesthesia: a prospective cohort study. Lancet 2010;376:773–83.
4. Mamie C, Habre W, Delhumeau C, et al. Incidence and risk factors of perioperative respiratory adverse events in children undergoing elective surgery. Paediatr Anaesth 2004;14:218–24.

5. Rosenstock C, Moller J, Hauberg A. Complaints related to respiratory events in anaesthesia and intensive care medicine from 1994 to 1998 in Denmark. Acta Anaesthesiol Scand 2001;45:53–8.
6. Cohen MM, Cameron CB, Duncan PG. Pediatric anesthesia morbidity and mortality in the perioperative period. Anesth Analg 1990;70:160–7.
7. Christensen R, Voepel-Lewis T, Lewis I, et al. Pediatric cardiopulmonary arrest in the postanesthesia care unit: analysis of data from the American Heart Association Get With The Guidelines-Resuscitation registry. Paediatr Anaesth 2013;23:517–23.
8. Morray JP, Geiduschek JM, Caplan RA, et al. A comparison of pediatric and adult anesthesia closed malpractice claims. Anesthesiology 1993;78:461–7.
9. Thach BT. Sleep apnea in infancy and childhood. Med Clin North Am 1985;69:1289–315.
10. Carroll JL, Agarwal A. Development of ventilatory control in infants. Paediatr Respir Rev 2010;11:199–207.
11. Laycock GJ, McNicol LR. Hypoxaemia during recovery from anaesthesia–an audit of children after general anaesthesia for routine elective surgery. Anaesthesia 1988;43:985–7.
12. Motoyama EK, Glazener CH. Hypoxemia after general anesthesia in children. Anesth Analg 1986;65:267–72.
13. Pullerits J, Burrows FA, Roy WL. Arterial desaturation in healthy children during transfer to the recovery room. Can J Anaesth 1987;34:470–3.
14. Kurowski I, Sims C. Unplanned anesthesia-related admissions to pediatric intensive care–a 6-year audit. Paediatr Anaesth 2007;17:575–80.
15. Ing C, Chui I, Ohkawa S, et al. Incidence and causes of perioperative endotracheal reintubation in children: a review of 28,208 anesthetics. Paediatr Anaesth 2013;23:621–6.
16. Keenan RL, Shapiro JH, Dawson K. Frequency of anesthetic cardiac arrests in infants: effect of pediatric anesthesiologists. J Clin Anesth 1991;3:433–7.
17. Nafiu OO, Burke CC, Chimbira WT, et al. Prevalence of habitual snoring in children and occurrence of peri-operative adverse events. Eur J Anaesthesiol 2011;28:340–5.
18. von Ungern-Sternberg BS, Saudan S, Petak F, et al. Desflurane but not sevoflurane impairs airway and respiratory tissue mechanics in children with susceptible airways. Anesthesiology 2008;108:216–24.
19. von Ungern-Sternberg BS, Habre W, Erb TO, et al. Salbutamol premedication in children with a recent respiratory tract infection. Paediatr Anaesth 2009;19:1064–9.
20. Papastemelos C, Panitch HB, England SE, et al. Developmental changes in chest wall compliance in infancy and early childhood. J Appl Physiol 1995;78:179–84.
21. Bancalari E, Clausen J. Pathophysiology of changes in absolute lung volumes. Eur Respir J 1998;12:248–58.
22. Drummond GB. Influence of thiopentone on upper airway muscles. Br J Anaesth 1989;63:12–21.
23. Grounds RM, Maxwell DL, Taylor MB, et al. Acute ventilatory changes during i.v. induction of anaesthesia with thiopentone or propofol in man. Br J Anaesth 1987;59:1098–102.
24. Dueck MH, Oberthuer A, Wedekind C, et al. Propofol impairs the central but not the peripheral part of the motor system. Anesth Analg 2003;96:449–55.

25. Haeseler G, Stormer M, Bufler J, et al. Propofol blocks human skeletal muscle sodium channels in a voltage-dependent manner. Anesth Analg 2001;92: 1192–8.
26. Macklem PT, Murphy B. The forces applied to the lung in health and disease. Am J Med 1974;57:371–7.
27. von Ungern-Sternberg BS, Hammer J, Schibler A, et al. Decrease of functional residual capacity and ventilation homogeneity after neuromuscular blockade in anesthetized young infants and preschool children. Anesthesiology 2006;105: 670–5.
28. von Ungern-Sternberg BS, Frei FJ, Hammer J, et al. Impact of depth of propofol anaesthesia on functional residual capacity and ventilation distribution in healthy preschool children. Br J Anaesth 2007;98:503–8.
29. Stocks J. Respiratory physiology during early life. Monaldi Arch Chest Dis 1999; 54:358–64.
30. Duggan M, Kavanagh BP. Pulmonary atelectasis: a pathogenetic perioperative entity. Anesthesiology 2005;2005:838–54.
31. von Ungern-Sternberg BS, Regli A, Frei FJ, et al. A deeper level of ketamine anesthesia does not affect functional residual capacity and ventilation distribution in healthy preschool children. Paediatr Anaesth 2007;17:1150–5.
32. von Ungern-Sternberg BS, Regli A, Frei FJ, et al. Decrease in functional residual capacity and ventilation homogeneity after neuromuscular blockade in anesthetized preschool children in the lateral position. Paediatr Anaesth 2007;17:841–5.
33. von Ungern-Sternberg BS, Regli A, Schibler A, et al. The impact of positive end-expiratory pressure on functional residual capacity and ventilation homogeneity impairment in anesthetized children exposed to high levels of inspired oxygen. Anesth Analg 2007;104:1364–8.
34. von Ungern-Sternberg BS, Boda K, Schwab C, et al. Laryngeal mask airway is associated with an increased incidence of adverse respiratory events in children with recent upper respiratory tract infections. Anesthesiology 2007;107: 714–9.
35. Xue FS, Huang YG, Tong SY, et al. A comparative study of early postoperative hypoxemia in infants, children, and adults undergoing elective plastic surgery. Anesth Analg 1996;83:709–15.
36. Bancalari E, Claure N, Sosenko IR. Bronchopulmonary dysplasia: changes in pathogenesis, epidemiology and definition. Semin Neonatol 2003;8:63–71.
37. Maxwell LG. Age-associated issues in preoperative evaluation, testing, and planning: pediatrics. Anesthesiol Clin North America 2004;22:27–43.
38. Von Ungern-Sternberg BS, Habre W. Pediatric anesthesia–potential risks and their assessment: part I. Paediatr Anaesth 2007;17:206–15.
39. Motoyama EK, Fort MD, Klesh KW, et al. Early onset of airway reactivity in premature infants with bronchopulmonary dysplasia. Am Rev Respir Dis 1987; 136:50–7.
40. Mathew OP. Apnea of prematurity: pathogenesis and management strategies. J Perinatol 2011;31:302–10.
41. Gerhardt T, Bancalari E. Apnea of prematurity: II. Respiratory reflexes. Pediatrics 1984;74:63–6.
42. Rigatto H, Kalapesi Z, Leahy FN, et al. Ventilatory response to 100% and 15% O_2 during wakefulness and sleep in preterm infants. Early Hum Dev 1982;7:1–10.
43. Kurth CD, Spitzer AR, Broennle AM, et al. Postoperative apnea in preterm infants. Anesthesiology 1987;66:483–8.

44. Tait AR, Voepel-Lewis T, Burke C, et al. Incidence and risk factors for perioperative adverse respiratory events in children who are obese. Anesthesiology 2008;108:375–80.
45. Olsson GL, Hallen B. Laryngospasm during anaesthesia. A computer-aided incidence study in 136,929 patients. Acta Anaesthesiol Scand 1984;28:567–75.
46. Olsson GL. Bronchospasm during anaesthesia. A computer-aided incidence study of 136,929 patients. Acta Anaesthesiol Scand 1987;31:244–52.
47. Oddy WH, Holt PG, Sly PD, et al. Association between breast feeding and asthma in 6 year old children: findings of a prospective birth cohort study. BMJ 1999;319:815–9.
48. Joseph-Bowen J, de Klerk NH, Firth MJ, et al. Lung function, bronchial responsiveness, and asthma in a community cohort of 6-year-old children. Am J Respir Crit Care Med 2004;169:850–4.
49. Tait AR, Malviya S, Voepel-Lewis T, et al. Risk factors for perioperative adverse respiratory events in children with upper respiratory tract infections. Anesthesiology 2001;95:299–306.
50. Tait AR, Voepel-Lewis T, Munro HM, et al. Cancellation of pediatric outpatient surgery: economic and emotional implications for patients and their families. J Clin Anesth 1997;9:213–9.
51. Whyte MK, Choudry NB, Ind PW. Bronchial hyperresponsiveness in patients recovering from acute severe asthma. Respir Med 1993;87:29–35.
52. Warner DO, Warner MA, Barnes RD, et al. Perioperative respiratory complications in patients with asthma. Anesthesiology 1996;85:460–7.
53. Parker SD, Brown RH, Hirshman CA. Differential effect of glucocorticoids on pulmonary responses and eosinophils. Respir Physiol 1991;83:323–31.
54. Fuiano N, Luciano A, Pilotto L, et al. Overweight and hypertension: longitudinal study in school-aged children. Minerva Pediatr 2006;58:451–9.
55. Setzer N, Saade E. Childhood obesity and anesthetic morbidity. Paediatr Anaesth 2007;17:321–6.
56. Nafiu OO, Reynolds PI, Bamgbade OA, et al. Childhood body mass index and perioperative complications. Paediatr Anaesth 2007;17:426–30.
57. Nafiu OO, Burke CC, Gupta R, et al. Association of neck circumference with perioperative adverse respiratory events in children. Pediatrics 2011;127: e1198–205.
58. Luce JM. Respiratory complications of obesity. Chest 1980;78:626–31.
59. von Ungern-Sternberg BS, Regli A, Schneider MC, et al. Effect of obesity and site of surgery on perioperative lung volumes. Br J Anaesth 2004;92:202–7.
60. von Ungern-Sternberg BS, Regli A, Bucher E, et al. Impact of spinal anaesthesia and obesity on maternal respiratory function during elective Caesarean section. Anaesthesia 2004;59:743–9.
61. von Ungern-Sternberg BS, Regli A, Reber A, et al. Comparison of perioperative spirometric data following spinal or general anaesthesia in normal-weight and overweight gynaecological patients. Acta Anaesthesiol Scand 2005;49:940–8.
62. von Ungern-Sternberg BS, Regli A, Reber A, et al. Effect of obesity and thoracic epidural analgesia on perioperative spirometry. Br J Anaesth 2005;94:121–7.
63. von Ungern-Sternberg BS, Hammer J, Frei FJ, et al. Prone equals prone? Impact of positioning techniques on respiratory function in anesthetized and paralyzed healthy children. Intensive Care Med 2007;33:1771–7.
64. von Ungern-Sternberg BS, Erb TO, Habre W, et al. The impact of oral premedication with midazolam on respiratory function in children. Anesth Analg 2009; 108:1771–6.

65. Regli A, Habre W, Saudan S, et al. Impact of Trendelenburg positioning on functional residual capacity and ventilation homogeneity in anaesthetised children. Anaesthesia 2007;62:451–5.
66. Von Ungern-Sternberg BS, Saudan S, Regli A, et al. Should the use of modified Jackson Rees T-piece breathing system be abandoned in preschool children? Paediatr Anaesth 2007;17:654–60.
67. Murat I, Constant I, Maud'huy H. Perioperative anaesthetic morbidity in children: a database of 24,165 anaesthetics over a 30-month period. Paediatr Anaesth 2004;14:158–66.
68. Ye J, Liu H, Zhang G, et al. Postoperative respiratory complications of adenotonsillectomy for obstructive sleep apnea syndrome in older children: prevalence, risk factors, and impact on clinical outcome. J Otolaryngol Head Neck Surg 2009;38:49–58.
69. Nixon GM, Kermack AS, McGregor CD, et al. Sleep and breathing on the first night after adenotonsillectomy for obstructive sleep apnea. Pediatr Pulmonol 2005;39:332–8.
70. Pounder DR, Blackstock D, Steward DJ. Tracheal extubation in children: halothane versus isoflurane, anesthetized versus awake. Anesthesiology 1991;74:653–5.
71. Patel RI, Hannallah RS, Norden J, et al. Emergence airway complications in children: a comparison of tracheal extubation in awake and deeply anesthetized patients. Anesth Analg 1991;73:266–70.
72. von Ungern-Sternberg BS, Davies K, Hegarty M, et al. The effect of deep vs. awake extubation on respiratory complications in high-risk children undergoing adenotonsillectomy: a prospective, randomised, controlled trial. Eur J Anaesthesiol 2013;30:529–36.
73. Soliman IE, Patel RI, Ehrenpreis MB, et al. Recovery scores do not correlate with postoperative hypoxemia in children. Anesth Analg 1988;67:53–6.
74. Weber T, Salvi N, Orliaguet G, et al. Cuffed vs non-cuffed endotracheal tubes for pediatric anesthesia. Paediatr Anaesth 2009;19(Suppl 1):46–54.
75. Ong M, Chambers NA, Hullet B, et al. Laryngeal mask airway and tracheal tube cuff pressures in children: are clinical endpoints valuable for guiding inflation? Anaesthesia 2008;63:738–44.
76. Cammu G, De Witte J, De Veylder J, et al. Postoperative residual paralysis in outpatients versus inpatients. Anesth Analg 2006;102:426–9.
77. Beemer GH, Rozental P. Postoperative neuromuscular function. Anaesth Intensive Care 1986;14:41–5.
78. Bevan DR, Smith CE, Donati F. Postoperative neuromuscular blockade: a comparison between atracurium, vecuronium, and pancuronium. Anesthesiology 1988;69:272–6.
79. Bevan DR, Kahwaji R, Ansermino JM, et al. Residual block after mivacurium with or without edrophonium reversal in adults and children. Anesthesiology 1996; 84:362–7.
80. Baillard C, Gehan G, Reboul-Marty J, et al. Residual curarization in the recovery room after vecuronium. Br J Anaesth 2000;84:394–5.
81. Fuchs-Buder T, Fink H, Hofmockel R, et al. Application of neuromuscular monitoring in Germany. Anaesthesist 2008;57:908–14.
82. Crumrine RS, Yodlowski EH. Assessment of neuromuscular function in infants. Anesthesiology 1981;54:29–32.
83. Debaene B, Plaud B, Dilly MP, et al. Residual paralysis in the PACU after a single intubating dose of nondepolarizing muscle relaxant with an intermediate duration of action. Anesthesiology 2003;98:1042–8.

84. Fisher DM. Neuromuscular blocking agents in paediatric anaesthesia. Br J Anaesth 1999;83:58–64.
85. von Ungern-Sternberg BS. Muscle relaxants are obligatory for pediatric intubation: con. Anaesthesist 2011;60:476–8.
86. Brown KA, Laferriere A, Lakheeram I, et al. Recurrent hypoxemia in children is associated with increased analgesic sensitivity to opiates. Anesthesiology 2006; 105:665–9.
87. Raghavendran S, Bagry H, Detheux G, et al. An anesthetic management protocol to decrease respiratory complications after adenotonsillectomy in children with severe sleep apnea. Anesth Analg 2010;110:1093–101.
88. Keating M, Johnson J, Erb TO, et al. Computed tomography changes of alveoli and airway collapse after laryngospasm. Anaesth Intensive Care 2011;39: 958–60.
89. Krodel DJ, Bittner EA, Abdulnour R, et al. Case scenario: acute postoperative negative pressure pulmonary edema. Anesthesiology 2010;113:200–7.
90. Halter JM, Steinberg JM, Schiller HJ, et al. Positive end-expiratory pressure after a recruitment maneuver prevents both alveolar collapse and recruitment/derecruitment. Am J Respir Crit Care Med 2003;167:1620–6.
91. von Ungern-Sternberg BS, Erb TO, Reber A, et al. Opening the upper airway-airway maneuvers in pediatric anesthesia. Paediatr Anaesth 2005;15:181–9.
92. Koka BV, Jeon IS, Andre JM, et al. Postintubation croup in children. Anesth Analg 1977;56:501–5.
93. Anene O, Meert KL, Uy H, et al. Dexamethasone for the prevention of postextubation airway obstruction: a prospective, randomized, double-blind, placebo-controlled trial. Crit Care Med 1996;24:1666–9.
94. Koren G, Frand M, Barzilay Z, et al. Corticosteroid treatment of laryngotracheitis v spasmodic croup in children. Am J Dis Child 1983;137:941–4.
95. Kuusela AL, Vesikari T. A randomized double-blind, placebo-controlled trial of dexamethasone and racemic epinephrine in the treatment of croup. Acta Paediatr Scand 1988;77:99–104.

Major Surgical Procedures in Children with Cerebral Palsy

Mary C. Theroux, MD[a,b],*, Sabina DiCindio, DO[a,b]

KEYWORDS

- Cerebral palsy • Spine fusion • Varus osteotomy • Pelvic osteotomy
- Baclofen pump • Spasticity • Coagulopathy

KEY POINTS

- Cerebral palsy is the most common and most debilitating neurological disease in children. Pediatric Anesthesiologist may expect to care for this population at an increasing frequency.
- Children with cerebral palsy have many co-morbid conditions which may result in increased morbidity and even mortality in the peri-operative period.
- This chapter describes the three most common major procedures that these children undergo and discusses the anesthetic care in detail.

INTRODUCTION

There are 3 surgical procedures that patients with cerebral palsy (CP) undergo that may be considered major procedures: femoral osteotomies combined with pelvic osteotomies, spine fusion, and intrathecal baclofen pump implant for the treatment of spasticity. Most patients with CP who undergo these procedures have spastic quadriplegic CP, and they are often developmentally delayed.

Many complications are known to occur at a higher rate in this population, and some may be avoided with prior awareness of the preoperative pathophysiology of the patient with CP. For example, awareness of suboptimal levels of clotting factors help plan for major surgeries with large blood loss by optimizing factor levels in a timely manner. Using information from trauma literature regarding transfusion and fluid resuscitation and adapting it to major surgeries in patients with CP in whom massive

Funding Sources: None.

Conflict of Interest: None.

[a] Department of Anesthesiology and Critical Care Medicine, Nemours/Alfred I. duPont Hospital for Children, Post Office Box 269, Wilmington, DE 19899, USA; [b] Department of Pediatrics, Jefferson Medical College, Thomas Jefferson University, Philadelphia, 111 S 11th Street, PA 19107, USA

* Corresponding author. Department of Anesthesiology and Critical Care Medicine, Nemours/Alfred I. duPont Hospital for Children, Post Office Box 269, Wilmington, DE 19899.

E-mail address: mtheroux@nemours.org

Anesthesiology Clin 32 (2014) 63–81

http://dx.doi.org/10.1016/j.anclin.2013.10.014

bleeding occurs will help decrease dilutional coagulopathy. Extubating patients earlier, such as the day of surgery, may have beneficial effects, and may result in decreased intensive care unit (ICU) and hospital days. Measures to decrease blood loss, such as use of tranexamic acid (TXA), are increasingly employed to help with an earlier extubation. Extensive lower extremity surgical procedures are often performed in this patient population because of the nature of their frequent bilateral disease and the need to decrease multiple hospitalizations and expenses. In order to provide optimal pain relief, the use of epidurals or caudal catheters using fluoroscopic aid is warranted. Treating spasticity postoperatively is important and controls pain more easily by preventing the cycle of pain leading to spasm and vice versa.

This article is organized into 2 major sections: (1) description of general risk associated with anesthesia and CP and (2) the 3 major surgical procedures and their specific risks (derotational femoral osteotomies and reconstructive acetabular surgeries, scoliosis correction, and baclofen catheter and pump placement).

GENERAL RISK OF ANESTHESIA AND SURGERY

The general risk of anesthesia is complicated by CP[1] and may be largely attributed to abnormal muscle tone and nutritional status. **Fig. 1** lists complications from a retrospective study examining 517 patients who underwent surgery and anesthesia at Mayo Clinic and the percentage of patients who had each complication. Some complications may be considered minor, but some may lead to major morbidity and mortality if left unattended.

Hypothermia

Hypothermia, the etiology of which is poorly understood, is the most prevalent complication (55.1%) observed in children with CP under anesthesia.[1] The global ischemic injury sustained by the patient that led to the development of CP in early childhood

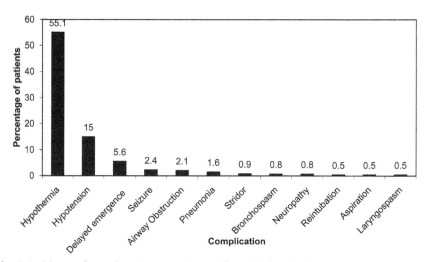

Fig. 1. Incidence of complications in patients with cerebral palsy. (*From* Wass CT, Warner ME, Worrell GA, et al. Effect of general anesthesia in patients with cerebral palsy at the turn of the new millennium: a population-based study evaluating perioperative outcome and brief overview of anesthetic implications of this coexisting disease. Child Neurol 2012;27(7):861; with permission.)

likely may have injured the hypothalamus, resulting in poor thermal regulation. A relative lack of adipose tissue protecting the body may also be a contributory factor to hypothermia complications. Unless special attention is paid to prevent it, a patient with spastic quadriplegic will likely sustain hypothermia in the operating room. At the authors' pediatric hospital, patients with CP scheduled for major surgeries are warmed using a forced air warming gown (Arizant Healthcare, St. Paul, Minnesota) system in the preoperative holding area, not only to minimize temperature decrease associated with the relatively sparse hospital clothing, but also to create a more favorable baseline temperature. When active warming, it is important to monitor temperature, because patients with CP may easily sustain temperatures greater than normal due to the inability to maintain normothermia when swings in ambient temperatures occur. When patients arrive for the 2 most common major surgical procedures, spine fusion for scoliosis and acetabulum/femur surgery for dislocated and subluxed hip joints, it is important to prevent them from plunging into a deep hypothermia, which is frequently sustained shortly after induction of anesthesia. Prewarming the patients while they are in the preoperative area not only allows a better baseline temperature but also facilitates line placement.

Hypotension

Hypotension that occurs in association with anesthesia and surgery in patients with CP may be attributed to different etiologic factors: (1) increased sensitivity to anesthetic agents, (2) chronic underhydration, and (3) volume of blood loss of great magnitude in relation to estimated blood volume. Among volatile anesthetics, halothane and sevoflurane have been studied in children with CP. Minimum alveolar concentration for halothane is decreased (0.7) in children with CP and severe mental retardation, and a further decrease (0.6) manifests in patients with CP who are on anticonvulsant medications, with normal children acquiring 0.9 in the same study.[2] There is evidence for a greater drop in bispectral (BIS) values in children with spastic quadriplegic CP with sevoflurane when compared with neurologically normal children.[3] Similarly, increased respiratory depression and greater obtundation are observed with narcotic analgesics in clinical practice, and greater titration of such medications is imperative in CP patients.

Most patients with spastic quadriplegic CP who are in need of major surgical procedures are nonambulatory and are fed via gastrostomy tube or are given pureed food by their caretaker. Children are given a prescribed amount of free water, typically via their gastrostomy feeding tube, and do not follow normal physiologic feedback initiated by thirst. Expect such children to be chronically underhydrated with higher than expected hemoglobin due to relative hemoconcentraion. It is important not to misjudge the degree of their underhydration and lack of clear, or any, urine upon Foley catheter placement. Repeating hemoglobin and clotting studies after hydrating the patient until free flow of urine is observed will provide values more representative of their actual baseline.

Patients with CP thus may sustain hypotension more easily than otherwise normal patients if induction of anesthesia is not given due consideration and special care. Other contributing factors to perioperative hypotension in CP, especially quadriplegic CP, include a propensity to greater blood loss during surgery, the etiology of which includes a subnormal level of clotting factors. A detailed description of increased bleeding and inadequate hemostatic ability in patients with CP follows later in this article.

Excessive salivation caused by a disturbed coordination of orofacial and palatolingual muscles is common and can be managed both pharmacologically, using anticholinergic medication, and mechanically, with sufficient anticipation and suctioning in the perioperative arena.[4] Oropharyngeal aspiration and silent aspiration in children with CP are not only prevalent but also have significant association with neurologic impairment, developmental delay, and aspiration-related lung disease.[5] Salivary aspiration may contribute to, and often aggravate, preexisting chronic lung disease and reactive airway disease in such patients.

A greater amount of blood loss has been recognized in patients with CP during spine fusion surgery when compared with idiopathic scoliosis patients.[6] A pilot study examining the etiology of increased bleeding in patients with CP showed clotting factor levels[7] (**Table 1**) that were lower than normal. Further study by the same investigators comparing the thromboelastography findings during spine fusions in children with CP and in children with idiopathic scoliosis found maximum amplitude of the thromboelastograph significantly lower in patients with CP at early blood loss. The results from this study provide insight into why patients with CP appear to lose a greater amount of blood during surgery. Additionally, subnormal calcium and magnesium levels were observed in patients with CP with early blood loss, which could further explain increased bleeding, as calcium is an essential component of the hemostatic mechanism.

Neuromuscular blocking agents are known to have altered sensitivity in patients with spastic quadriplegic CP. A dose response study showed patients with CP have an increased sensitivity to succinylcholine.[8] Further scrutiny of the neuromuscular junctions of the spastic quadriplegic CP patients has revealed an abnormal spread of acetylcholine receptors in approximately 30% of patients studied (**Fig. 2**).[9] Specifically, the abnormality occurred in the spread of acetylcholine receptors, which extended beyond the boundary of the neuromuscular junctions. Nonambulatory patients with CP were found to have significantly greater numbers of abnormal neuromuscular junctions, as well as greater abnormality in the spread of acetylcholine receptors.[10]

These abnormalities are further validated indirectly by the study of vecuronium, a nondepolarizing neuromuscular blocking agent, which showed a decreased potency of vecuronium in patients with CP.[11] This study did not enroll patients who were on seizure medications in order to avoid the confounding effect of anticonvulsants on the results.[12] Implications of these abnormalities may be twofold:

1. The paralytic effects of succinylcholine may not be clinically significant because of the differences in the potency of the drug in patients with CP, while decreased potency of vecuronium may be more clinically apparent.
2. Caution may need to be exercised if succinylcholine is used in patients with CP, because some patients may harbor enough neuromuscular junctions with abnormal acetylcholine receptors to lead to complications, such as hyperkalemia, upon receiving succinylcholine.

To follow up on the findings of increased sensitivity to succinylcholine by CP patients, the investigative team embarked on research examining neuromuscular junctions in this population. The incident was thought to be the result of succinylcholine administration. Neuromuscular junctions are known to be up-regulated in patients who are in a state of immobility; patients with CP, particularly those who have spastic quadriplegic CP, are often bedridden and immobile.[13–18]

Topiramate is a relatively new anticonvulsant drug commonly used in patients with CP. Other indications for the use of this drug are migraine and bipolar disease. An adverse effect of topiramate is the development of closed angle glaucoma, which, when it occurs, typically presents within the first year of treatment.[19,20] Delayed onset

Table 1
Conventional clotting studies (PT/PTT) and factors II, VII, IX, X in 5 consecutive patients performed prior to induction of anesthesia and repeated at an estimated blood loss of approximately 20% (of their estimated blood volume)

Patient	Base PT	BL_{25} PT	Base PTT	BL_{25} PTT	Base II	BL_{25} II	Base VII	BL_{25} VII	Base IX	BL_{25} IX	Base X	BL_{25} X
1	10	12	29	38	90	68	43	49	70	74	58	45
2	10	15	34	67	100	46	110	30	100	37	100	57
3	12	15	28	43	85	48	64	12	100	52	100	22
4	13	14	39	48	90	55	70	70	37	52	60	39
5	13	16	30	46	100	46	80	64	74	29	57	57

Normal range for PT = 9–11 min, normal range for PTT = 23–38 min, and normal range for factor levels = 50%–150% of normal.
No blood or blood products had been given during this period.

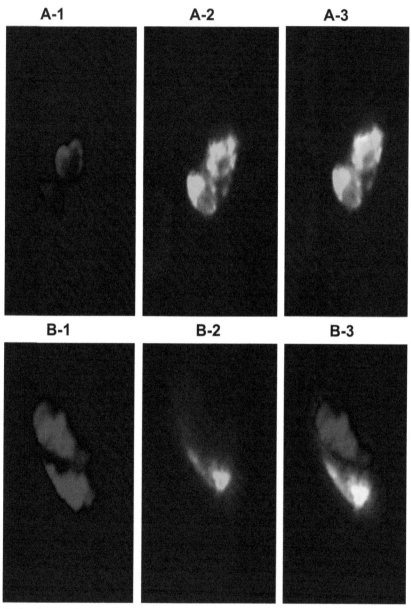

Fig. 2. (*A-1*) Normal neuromuscular junction first stained with α-bungarotoxin (*red*) to show the spread of acetylcholine receptors (AchRs). (*A-2*) The same neuromuscular junction stained with acetyl cholinesterase (*green*) to define the limits of the junction. (*A-3*) The superimposed neuromuscular junction with both α-bungarotoxin and acetyl cholinesterase staining. Red staining outside of the green indicates spread of AchRs outside the limits of the neuromuscular junction. (*B-1–B-3*) The same staining methods of a neuromuscular junction from a patient with CP. Significant spread of AchRs outside of the limits of the neuromuscular junction is seen.

has also been reported.[21] The proposed mechanism of closed angle glaucoma is choroidal effusion and forward rotation of the iris–lens diaphragm.[22] The effusion places pressure on the vitreous body and causes anterior displacement and closure of the angle. Conditions of surgery and anesthesia, especially those requiring prone positioning with large shifts in fluid status, may predispose patients on topiramate to developing acute closed angle glaucoma. The authors have seen such an incidence of acute closed angle glaucoma in a patient with CP who had been on topiramate for more than 1 year. After revision of her spine fusion, which lasted 4 hours, she developed closed angle glaucoma within the first 48 to 72 hours of recovery. Medical management, and, finally, surgical intervention were necessary to adequately treat her condition. Awareness, recognition, and treatment of closed angle glaucoma in patients who are on topiramate are necessary.

No discussion of CP is complete without a thorough review of spasticity, which is the most functionally debilitating feature of CP.[23] Cerebral palsy is associated with spasticity in 75% to 85% of the patient population.[24] Clinically, spasticity can present as hyperactive reflexes, clonus, weakness, and discoordination. Some patients benefit from their spasticity, as their stiffness aids with upright positioning and ambulation.[25–27] Other patients with spasticity have decreased range of motion, functional impairment, pain, and deformities. For patients who do not benefit from their increased muscle tone, the goals of spasticity therapy are to increase mobility and independence, to prevent or slow the development of contractures, to improve positioning, and to increase ease of care in those severely affected.[26,27]

Considering that environmental factors can aggravate spasms, it is important to address any or all pertinent afflictions. These can include pain, fatigue, excitement, cold, illness, sleep disturbance, immobility, and/or hormonal fluctuation.[27,28] Physical therapy and occupational therapy aim to maximize patient function and optimize results of surgery. Therapy directed toward focal spasticity can be achieved with denervation of neuronal input with phenol or Botulinum toxin injections. Orthopedic procedures improve limb mobility and provide long-term efficacy. Selective dorsal rhizotomy (SDR) is used to treat lower extremity spasms. In conjunction with postoperative rehabilitation, SDR has a favorable outcome; however, pediatric patients having SDR often sustain lower extremity weakness. Increased spasticity because of pain often escalates during postoperative care and pain management. Different modalities of treatment of spasticity are discussed in the baclofen pump insertion section of this article.

SURGERY FOR SCOLIOSIS AND KYPHOSIS CORRECTION

The most commonly performed surgery for scoliosis and kyphosis correction in children with CP involves primary instrumentation that fuses the spine from T1 to sacrum. An occasional patient with mild CP may undergo a segmental spine fusion similar to an idiopathic scoliosis correction. The discussion of scoliosis correction in this article refers to the commonly performed spine fusion (T1 to sacrum) and instrumentation. There are currently 2 instrumentations being used: (1) a precontoured rod known as unit rod, which uses sublaminar wires to fix along the vertebral segments,[29] and (2) a modular system, or custom rod, which is contoured by the surgeon and employs a double-rod system using screws with or without sublaminar wires to fix the rod at vertebral segments (**Fig. 3**).

The quality of curve correction is different between the 2 systems. The unit rod provides superior correction, especially of pelvic obliquity, which has an impact on the patient's ability to sit (**Fig. 4**). However, unit rod instrumentation leads to greater blood loss and longer ICU and hospital stay.[30]

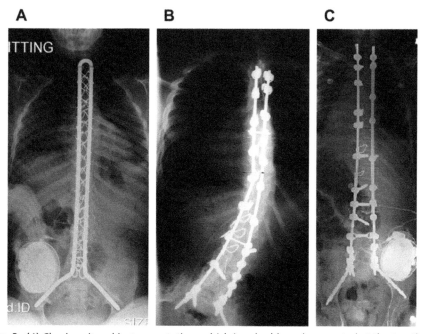

Fig. 3. (A) Classic unit rod instrumentation, which is a double rod connected at the top that has 2 pelvic legs drilled into the iliac bones. (B, C) Modular or custom rods, which may use screws and or sublaminar wires (B) and may use the pelvic legs (C) or may not use the pelvic legs (B).

A subpopulation of children with CP needs anterior spine release prior to posterior spine fusion. For children with spastic quadriplegic CP who are severely developmentally delayed, the anterior release is performed approximately 1 week prior to posterior spine fusion.[31] Occasionally, a child who is clinically judged to be healthier than the average CP patient will have both anterior release and posterior spine fusion performed on the same day. Flexibility is increased by anterior disc excision, allowing greater correction with posterior instrumentation. Some surgeons prefer a thoracoscopic approach, particularly when the number of discs released is not large. This approach requires one-lung ventilation, facilitating approach to the disc through the scope, which otherwise can be difficult because of the movement of the lung. There are studies, intended to benefit pediatric population, in piglets that examine one-lung ventilation and interventions to reduce injury from one-lung ventilation.[32–34]

Indications for anterior spine release include scoliosis curve approaching 90° in a growing child, a stiff curve where side bending to midline is difficult, or a kyphotic curve that is stiff or is a significant impairment to sitting.

Anesthetic Management for Spine Fusion in Patients with CP

Spine fusion is the most extensive of the elective surgical procedures that patients with CP undergo. A multidisciplinary approach is best when caring for these patients, as most who need posterior spine fusion have the most debilitating kind of spastic quadriplegic CP, with severe developmental delay and multisystem involvement. Preoperative workup should include neurology, pulmonology, and, less commonly cardiac consultations. At our Institution we have, in the past, routinely performed cardiac evaluations including an echocardiogram in patients with a scoliotic curve

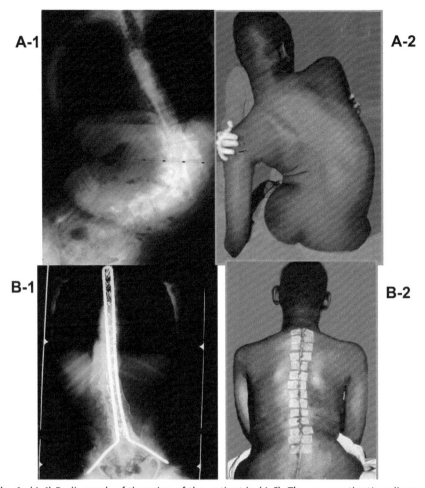

Fig. 4. (*A-1*) Radiograph of the spine of the patient in (*A-2*). The same patient's radiograph of the spine is shown in (*B-1*), with the patient in a sitting position postoperatively following spine fusion with unit rod instrumentation in (*B-2*). The obvious correction of the patient's pelvic obliquity is evident in the postoperative film. (*Courtesy of* Freeman Miller, MD, Wilmington, DE.)

>900. However, a recent examination of our data has yielded little or no helpful findings (manuscript in preparation). Therefore we no longer recommend cardiac evaluation based on the degree of the scoliotic curve alone in our CP population. Note that history of activity at school or ability to play sports is not of value, as most or all of such patients are either physically inactive or only minimally active. Neurology consultation is necessary for the consideration of seizure medications prior to and immediately following spine fusion, during which the levels of seizure medications fall precipitously and are often undetectable. A team dedicated to medically complex patients is ideal and should be involved in care prior to surgery. Care should be continued postoperatively until the patient is discharged from the hospital.

Besides the general risk discussed earlier, spine fusion will require 2 large intravenous lines, a central line, and an arterial line due to the anticipated blood loss.

Anesthetic agents used will largely be dictated by whether somatosensory and motor-evoked potentials are being monitored during the spine fusion.[35] Most patients with CP will have neuromonitoring employed (**Table 2**), with the exception of an occasional patient who will have such poorly recordable evoked potentials that monitoring may be abandoned; in this case, a combination of volatile anesthetics, muscle relaxants, and narcotics is used. History of seizures, which was considered a relative contraindication for neuromonitoring because of the possibility of provoking an episode of seizure, is no longer considered a contraindication. In such situations, the neurophysiology team often uses reduced-strength stimuli. When neuromonitoring is planned, several anesthetics are recommended as part of the total intravenous technique (note that a total intravenous technique is not practiced at all institutions, and opinions vary among the neurophysiology teams as to the optimal anesthetic techniques for neuromonitoring. It is not the intent of this article to cover this controversial subject).

Recommended intravenous anesthetics for planned neuromonitoring include

- Fentanyl, preferably continuous infusion or intermittent boluses; sufentanil, which is often an ideal agent for idiopathic patients, might be too potent for the patient with severe CP
- Remifentanil infusion, which helps to decrease the amount of propofol
- Ketamine infusion
- Low-dose dexmedetomidine, no higher than 0.2 µg/kg/min (this dose has the least influence on neuromonitoring)

Other considerations include

- Optimizing the patient status by treating any preoperative treatable conditions, such as reactive airway disease
- Considering a prophylactic dose of methylprednisolone, 2 mg/kg up to 40 mg, especially for anterior spine release and patients with reactive airway disease[32,36]
- Using simple measures, such as suctioning via endotracheal tube, before turning the patient
- Using procoagulants to reduce blood loss

Among procoagulants studied thus far, TXA has been shown to be more efficacious in decreasing blood loss during spine surgery in patients with CP.[37–41] TXA both reduces firbinolysis and reduces platelet aggregation.[42] The dosage regime that the authors currently use is a bolus of 50 mg/kg followed by 10 mg/kg/h infusion until skin

Table 2
Number and percentage of patients with CP- and non-CP-related neuromuscular scoliosis (NMS) for whom monitorable somatosensory-evoked potentials (SSEP) and/or transcranial electric motor·evoked potentials (TceMEP) could be recorded at baseline

Type of NMS	SSEP	TceMEP
Mild CP	4/4 (100%)	3/3(100%)
Moderate CP	12/12 (100%)	7/7(100%)
Severe CP	16/23 (70%)	9/10(90%)
No CP scoliosis	25/29 (86%)	25/29(86%)

From DiCindio S, Theroux M, Shah S, et al. Multimodality monitoring of transcranial electric motor and somatosensory-evoked potentials during surgical correction of spinal deformity in patients with cerebral palsy and other neuromuscular disorders. Spine 2003;28(16):1852; with permission.

closure.[43] Fluid management during spine fusion needs to take into consideration the suboptimal factor levels in patients with CP. Early use of fresh frozen plasma, cryoprecipitate, platelets, and red cells is most logical, or severe coagulopathy may result. Given the expected blood loss of a one-to-three blood volume (sometimes more), patients may benefit from a management similar to patients undergoing major trauma. Limiting crystalloids and transfusing plasma, platelets, and red cells have improved patient outcomes in the trauma literature.[44–49] the authors have found that patients with CP undergoing spine surgery may benefit from a similar strategy of intraoperative fluid management. The authors' data from an ongoing study is indicative of greater physiologic patient stability during both the intraoperative and postoperative periods with this regime of fluid management. For institutions in which blood loss from spine fusion is not of the same magnitude, it is logical to modify such trauma protocol-based transfusion guidelines.

Postoperative management of these patients may frequently require mechanical ventilation and ongoing fluid management including use of vasopressors. Patients frequently undergo a systemic inflammatory response, which may be associated with hypotension requiring use of vasopressors. Length of stay in the ICU is expected to be 3 to 10 days, and the authors are currently examining factors that influence this duration.[30]

DEROTATIONAL FEMORAL OSTEOTOMIES AND RECONSTRUCTIVE ACETABULAR SURGERIES

Indications include subluxation and dislocation of the hip joints.

Pathophysiology

There is a high incidence of subluxation and dislocation of hip joints in patients with spastic CP, especially in nonambulatory patients. Spasticity in these children allows flexion and adduction to overpower extension and abduction, which, over a period of time, results in subluxation or dislocation of the hip joints.[50] These conditions are painful, may cause decubitus ulcers, may interfere with perineal hygiene, and may lead to imbalance while sitting. Operative treatment of these conditions is varus derotational osteotomy (VDRO) and pelvic osteotomy, and this may be combined with soft tissue release as necessary. Revisions of such procedures may be necessary if timing of the procedure is inaccurate, or insufficient attention is paid to the contributing factors, including spasticity of adductor muscles.[51] Bilateral hip procedures are almost always performed in this patient population.[52,53] Given that each hip would be subjected to a pelvic osteotomy as well as a femoral osteotomy, significant surgical trauma, blood loss, and postoperative pain should be expected. Emphasis is placed on adequate treatment of pain, which, unless treated optimally, will trigger spasms, resulting in a vicious cycle of pain, spasm, pain. Detailed treatment of pain is discussed later in this article.

Surgical Procedure

Proximal femoral osteotomy and peri-ileal pelvic osteotomies are the most common osteotomies performed for spastic disease of the hip joints in patients with CP. Proximal shortening is performed to correct varus, derotation, or flexion extension. Blade plates are inserted into the lateral aspect of the femoral shaft using screws (**Fig. 5**), and the wound is packed. The peri-ileal pelvic osteotomy (referred to as pelvic osteotomy from here on) is performed next, the indication for which is correction of posterior superior acetabular dysplasia, the most common spastic hip disease. A second incision

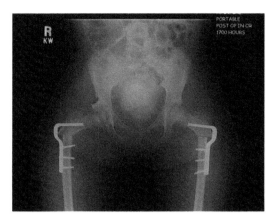

Fig. 5. Radiograph of the pelvis showing the blade plates in the proximal femur, which are fixed using screws. Acetabular osteotomy does not use instrumentation and therefore is not distinguishable by radiograph. (*Courtesy of* Freeman Miller, MD, Wilmington, DE.)

is necessary and starts medial to the anterior superior iliac spine and extends laterally. Reshaping of the acetabulum by wedge osteotomy is the main goal of this aspect of the surgery.

Anesthetic Management of Bilateral Femur/Pelvic Procedures

Besides general risk, blood loss is often underestimated in pelvic osteotomies. A significant amount of blood is lost on the drapes during drilling, and unlike spine fusion, the surgical site is not as well suited for suctioning of blood. Expect hemoglobin to drop 1 to 2 g postoperatively; consider this in deciding the need for transfusion during the surgery. A good general rule is to consider transfusion if acetabular osteotomies have been performed in addition to varus femoral osteotomies due to greater post operative drop in their hemoglobin levels.

Factors important in postoperative pain management include

- Spasticity and pain need to be treated simultaneously
- For lower extremity osteotomies, consider a regional technique, which reduces postoperative spasm[54]
- When performing epidural anesthetics, use of fluoroscopy or ultrasound may be necessary to aid in identifying midline structures due to kyphosis/scoliosis of the spine
- Documenting catheter tip position using iohexol (Omnipaque) is recommended
- Benzodiazepines have remained the mainstay of treatment of spasticity in the immediate postoperative period
- Use of dexmedetomidine 0.5 to 1 μg/kg is useful as an adjuvant and is increasingly employed intraoperatively or in the postoperative recovery period
- Postoperative pain management of a spine fusion patient is largely determined by whether the patient remains intubated
- Use of agents such as fentanyl infusion will not be tolerated by a patient with CP who has a natural airway
- Minimizing opioids and taking advantage of adjuvant medications is recommended
- Adjuvants are intravenous acetaminophen, dexmedetomidine, and clonidine patch (when patient is stable hemodynamically); ketorolac may be used after

discussion with the surgeon (unlike idiopathic spine fusion, where ketorolac is commonly used for postoperative pain management, greater caution is exercised when using ketorolac in CP patients for postoperative pain management; due to the extensive nature of the surgical dissection, the surgeons are often reluctant to the use of ketorolac in the immediate postoperative period for fear of increased postoperative bleeding and may elect to wait till the first postoperative day)

- Patients who may have had prior spine fusion (T1 sacrum) may still be able to have an epidural placed caudally (**Fig. 6**)

INTRATHECAL BACLOFEN PUMP INSERTION

Although treatment for spasm is initiated using oral medications with the goal to inhibit excitatory or augment inhibitory neurotransmitters at the spinal cord,[55,56] these drugs have limited use because of adverse effects (**Table 3**). Another option for the treatment of generalized spasticity is intrathecal baclofen (ITB), which requires a surgical procedure.

Indications for ITB include when spasticity does not respond to oral medication or is associated with adverse effects. ITB for cerebral spasticity was approved in 1996 by the US Food and Drug Administration (FDA) for patients older than 4 years. It is associated with fewer adverse effects than oral medications at same dosage.[56] Lumbar administration of baclofen results in one-fourth the concentration in the craniocervical region.[57] Tolerance to baclofen is not documented.[58,59] Half-life of baclofen administered intrathecally is 4 to 5 hours. Baclofen, 4-amine-3-(4-chlorphenyl)-butanoic acid, is a muscle relaxant and antispasmodic drug. It is structurally similar to

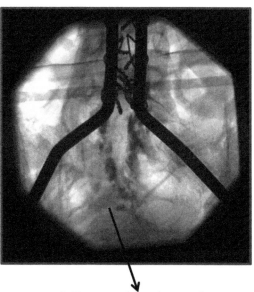

Epidurogram shows the spread
of Omnipaque in the epidural space

Fig. 6. Caudal catheter and epidurogram using iohexol in a patient with CP who had a prior spine fusion from T1 to sacrum using a unit rod. Patients with CP often lack adipose tissue around the sacrococcygeal area, and bony landmarks are often felt more easily. However, in the presence of a spine fusion, an epidurogram is recommended.

Table 3		
Mechanism of action and adverse effects of commonly used oral agents		
Oral Pharmacotherapy for Spasticity		
Medication	Mechanism of Action	Adverse Effects
Benzodiazepine	Binds GABA-a receptor and increases GABA activity	Sedation, ataxia, physical dependence, impaired memory
Alpha-2 adrenergic agonist	Binds alpha-2 receptors and hyperpolarizes neurons, decreases excitatory neurotransmitter release	Sedation, hypotension, nausea, vomiting, hepatitis
Dantrolene	Inhibits release of calcium at sarcoplasmic reticulum	Weakness, nausea, vomiting, hepatitis
Baclofen	Binds GABA-b receptors, inhibits release of excitatory neurotransmitters in spinal cord	Sedation, ataxia, weakness, hypotension

gamma-aminobutyric acid (GABA) and selective for GABAb receptors. GABAb receptors are superficially located in the spinal cord in laminae 1 through 4. Binding of the GABAb receptors inhibits monosynaptic and polysynaptic spinal reflexes by inhibiting release of excitatory neurotransmitters presynaptically. Implanted pumps are used to deliver continuous ITB. The pump weight, diameter, and size vary based on the model. Reservoirs of different sizes can hold 10, 18, 20, or 40 mL of baclofen. Within the implant, there is a peristaltic pump with a battery, which has a 3- to 7-year life span and a telemetric control that allows for adjustments in dosing. Despite manufacturer's recommendations for use in patients over 4 years old, patient size is considered to be a greater limitation to placement than age.[60] The patient has to have enough distance from the lowest rib superiorly, the iliac crest inferiorly, and the umbilicus medially to fit the pump (**Fig. 7**). Prior to pump placement, a test dose of 25 to 100 μg of baclofen is given by lumbar puncture. If bolus dosing results in a reduction by 1° of the Ashworth score, a scale used for assessing spasticity, the patient is a candidate for pump placement.[28,60]

Surgery for Baclofen Pump Insertion

The pump is placed with the patient under general anesthesia. The procedure itself takes 1 to 1.5 hours. The surgeon creates a pocket in the anterior abdomen. This pocket can be subfascial or subcutaneous. The intrathecal catheter is introduced through a Touhy needle into the intrathecal space, tunneled around the flank, either subcutaneously or under the fascia, and connected to the pump. The position of the catheter is determined by the clinical goal. T8 to T10 levels allow for leg relaxation; T3 to T6 levels allow for lower extremity and some upper extremity relaxation. C5–T5 placement is chosen for patients with severe upper extremity spasticity or opisthotonic posturing.[61] A diaphragm located within the pump allows for reservoir refills every 2 to 3 months. Drug dose escalation occurs more frequently within the first 2 years, with fewer adjustments in dosing being required subsequently.[60]

Significant complications associated with the ITB pump include

- Drug delivery system (catheter breaks, dislodgements, and kinks with an incidence of 5%–15%)
- Infection, incidence of 5% to 46%[61–64]
- Cerebrospinal fluid leakage, incidence of 2% to 8%[62,65]
- Pocket seromas and/or hematoma

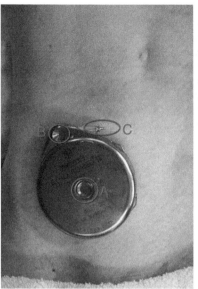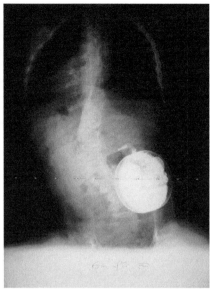

Fig. 7. Baclofen pump inserted into the right lower quadrant in a patient with cerebral palsy. Figure on the *left* shows the pump in the location of the abdomen where it will be inserted. (*Circled A-C*) indicates the reservoir, the connecting catheter exiting from the pump to attach with the catheter placed intrathecally. Figure on the *right* is the X-Ray of the pump after placement in the patient. (*Courtesy of* Freeman Miller, MD, Wilmington, DE.)

Medication-related adverse effects include

- Constipation, incidence of 19% to 38%[62]
- Nausea and vomiting, incidence of 11% to 14%
- Headache, incidence of 11% to 12%
- Increased oral secretions
- Lower extremity deep vein thrombosis
- Decubitus ulcers
- Hypotonia
- Somnolence

Drug titration alleviates most issues related to dosing.

Baclofen Overdose

There are many case reports related to baclofen overdose.[62] This can be due to pump malfunction, but it can also be associated with drug error. Mild overdoses can be treated with physostigmine or flumazenil.[66] Clinically, the authors have not seen much efficacy with the use of either of these 2 drugs to reverse baclofen-related obtunded state. A severe overdose of baclofen can lead to coma and flaccidity requiring mechanical ventilation. At the authors' institution, 3 episodes of overdose occurred with ITB pump placement. This was determined when the patient did not arouse from anesthesia, and careful review of the drugs suggested the most likely source was an overdose of baclofen. Subsequently, the patients were admitted to the ICU; one patient required assisted ventilation. All 3 patients had returned to baseline within 24 to 36 hours.

Withdrawal from baclofen is felt to have greater consequence. The adverse effects range from mild to severe. Mild withdrawal can present as increased spasticity, itching, and agitation. Severe withdrawal can present as psychosis, hyperthermia, dyskinesia, neuroleptic malignant syndrome, and, potentially, death.[60,67] Withdrawal can be treated with initiation of oral baclofen, benzodiazepines, supportive measures, and surgical correction of the system malfunction. In protracted cases, temporary placement of a subarachnoid catheter to administer intrathecal baclofen is warranted.

Many studies have demonstrated improvement in pain, comfort, and decreased worsening of deformities with ITB.[58,68] Functional and motor capabilities have also shown improvement with ITB.[69] Despite a significant risk of complications, ITB has a high (81%) rate of caregiver satisfaction, and 87% of caregivers are willing to recommend ITB therapy.[70]

REFERENCES

1. Wass CT, Warner ME, Worrell GA, et al. Effect of general anesthesia in patients with cerebral palsy at the turn of the new millennium: a population-based study evaluating perioperative outcome and brief overview of anesthetic implications of this coexisting disease. J Child Neurol 2012;27(7):859–66.
2. Frei FJ, Haemmerle MH, Brunner R, et al. Minimum alveolar concentration for halothane in children with cerebral palsy and severe mental retardation. Anaesthesia 1997;52(11):1056–60.
3. Choudhry DK, Brenn BR. Bispectral index monitoring: a comparison between normal children and children with quadriplegic cerebral palsy. Anesth Analg 2002;95(6):1582–5.
4. Wilken B, Aslami B, Backes H. Successful treatment of drooling in children with neurological disorders with botulinum toxin A or B. Neuropediatrics 2008;39(4):200–4.
5. Weir KA, McMahon S, Taylor S, et al. Oropharyngeal aspiration and silent aspiration in children. Chest 2011;140(3):589–97.
6. Kannan S, Meert KL, Mooney JF, et al. Bleeding and coagulation changes during spinal fusion surgery: a comparison of neuromuscular and idiopathic scoliosis patients. Pediatr Crit Care Med 2002;3(4):364–9.
7. Brenn BR, Theroux MC. Clotting factors in children with neuromuscular scoliosis undergoing posterior spinal fusion. Spine (Phila Pa 1976) 2004;29(15):E310–4.
8. Rose JB, Theroux MC, Katz MS. The potency of succinylcholine in obese adolescents. Anesth Analg 2000;90(3):576–8.
9. Theroux MC, Akins RE, Barone C, et al. Neuromuscular junctions in cerebral palsy: presence of extrajunctional acetylcholine receptors. Anesthesiology 2002;96(2):330–5.
10. Theroux MC, Oberman KG, Lahaye J, et al. Dysmorphic neuromuscular junctions associated with motor ability in cerebral palsy. Muscle Nerve 2005;32(5):626–32.
11. Hepaguslar H, Ozzeybek D, Elar Z. The effect of cerebral palsy on the action of vecuronium with or without anticonvulsants. Anaesthesia 1999;54(6):593–6.
12. Moorthy SS, Krishna G, Dierdorf SF. Resistance to vecuronium in patients with cerebral palsy. Anesth Analg 1991;73(3):275–7.
13. Martyn JA, White DA, Gronert GA, et al. Up-and-down regulation of skeletal muscle acetylcholine receptors. Effects on neuromuscular blockers. Anesthesiology 1992;76(5):822–43.

14. Gronert GA, Theye RA. Pathophysiology of hyperkalemia induced by succinyl-choline. Anesthesiology 1975;43(1):89–99.
15. Fung DL, White DA, Jones BR, et al. The onset of disuse-related potassium efflux to succinylcholine. Anesthesiology 1991;75(4):650–3.
16. Gronert GA. Succinylcholine-induced hyperkalemia and beyond. 1975. Anes-thesiology 2009;111(6):1372–7.
17. Gronert GA, Theye RA. Effect of succinylcholine on skeletal muscle with immo-bilization atrophy. Anesthesiology 1974;40(3):268–71.
18. Martyn JA, Richtsfeld M. Succinylcholine-induced hyperkalemia in acquired pathologic states: etiologic factors and molecular mechanisms. Anesthesiology 2006;104(1):158–69.
19. Ho JD, Keller JJ, Tsai CY, et al. Topiramate use and the risk of glaucoma devel-opment: a population-based follow-up study. Am J Ophthalmol 2013;155(2): 336–41.e1.
20. Chalam KV, Tillis T, Syed F, et al. Acute bilateral simultaneous angle closure glaucoma after topiramate administration: a case report. J Med Case Rep 2008;2:1.
21. Czyz CN, Clark CM, Justice JD, et al. Delayed topiramate-induced bilateral angle-closure glaucoma. J Glaucoma 2013. [Epub ahead of print].
22. Sankar PS, Pasquale LR, Grosskreutz CL. Uveal effusion and secondary angle-closure glaucoma associated with topiramate use. Arch Ophthalmol 2001; 119(8):1210–1.
23. Delgado MR, Hirtz D, Aisen M, et al. Practice parameter: pharmacologic treat-ment of spasticity in children and adolescents with cerebral palsy (an evidence-based review): report of the Quality Standards Subcommittee of the American Academy of Neurology and the Practice Committee of the Child Neurology So-ciety. Neurology 2010;74(4):336–43.
24. Brunstrom JE. Clinical considerations in cerebral palsy and spasticity. J Child Neurol 2001;16(1):10–5.
25. Murphy NA, Irwin MC, Hoff C. Intrathecal baclofen therapy in children with ce-rebral palsy: efficacy and complications. Arch Phys Med Rehabil 2002;83(12): 1721–5.
26. Butler C, Campbell S. Evidence of the effects of intrathecal baclofen for spastic and dystonic cerebral palsy. AACPDM Treatment Outcomes Committee Review Panel. Dev Med Child Neurol 2000;42(9):634–45.
27. Krach LE. Pharmacotherapy of spasticity: oral medications and intrathecal bac-lofen. J Child Neurol 2001;16(1):31–6.
28. Gilmartin R, Bruce D, Storrs BB, et al. Intrathecal baclofen for management of spastic cerebral palsy: multicenter trial. J Child Neurol 2000;15(2):71–7.
29. Dias RC, Miller F, Dabney K, et al. Surgical correction of spinal deformity using a unit rod in children with cerebral palsy. J Pediatr Orthop 1996; 16(6):734–40.
30. Sponseller PD, Shah SA, Abel MF, et al. Scoliosis surgery in cerebral palsy: differences between unit rod and custom rods. Spine (Phila Pa 1976) 2009; 34(8):840–4.
31. Tsirikos AI, Chang WN, Dabney KW, et al. Comparison of one-stage versus two-stage anteroposterior spinal fusion in pediatric patients with cerebral palsy and neuromuscular scoliosis. Spine (Phila Pa 1976) 2003;28(12):1300–5.
32. Theroux MC, Olivant A, Lim D, et al. Low dose methylprednisolone prophylaxis to reduce inflammation during one-lung ventilation. Paediatr Anaesth 2008; 18(9):857–64.

33. Theroux MC, Fisher AO, Horner LM, et al. Protective ventilation to reduce inflammatory injury from one lung ventilation in a piglet model. Paediatr Anaesth 2010; 20(4):356–64.

34. Olivant Fisher A, Husain K, Wolfson MR, et al. Hyperoxia during one lung ventilation: inflammatory and oxidative responses. Pediatr Pulmonol 2012;47(10): 979–86.

35. DiCindio S, Theroux M, Shah S, et al. Multimodality monitoring of transcranial electric motor and somatosensory-evoked potentials during surgical correction of spinal deformity in patients with cerebral palsy and other neuromuscular disorders. Spine (Phila Pa 1976) 2003;28(16):1851–5 [discussion: 1855–6].

36. Anderson PR, Puno MR, Lovell SL, et al. Postoperative respiratory complications in non-idiopathic scoliosis. Acta Anaesthesiol Scand 1985;29(2):186–92.

37. Thompson GH, Florentino-Pineda I, Poe-Kochert C, et al. Role of Amicar in surgery for neuromuscular scoliosis. Spine (Phila Pa 1976) 2008;33(24):2623–9.

38. Sethna NF, Zurakowski D, Brustowicz RM, et al. Tranexamic acid reduces intraoperative blood loss in pediatric patients undergoing scoliosis surgery. Anesthesiology 2005;102(4):727–32.

39. Shapiro F, Sethna N. Blood loss in pediatric spine surgery. Eur Spine J 2004; 13(Suppl 1):S6–17.

40. Shapiro F, Zurakowski D, Sethna NF. Tranexamic acid diminishes intraoperative blood loss and transfusion in spinal fusions for duchenne muscular dystrophy scoliosis. Spine (Phila Pa 1976) 2007;32(20):2278–83.

41. Theroux MC, Corddry DH, Tietz AE, et al. A study of desmopressin and blood loss during spinal fusion for neuromuscular scoliosis: a randomized, controlled, double-blinded study. Anesthesiology 1997;87(2):260–7.

42. Verma K, Errico TJ, Vaz KM, et al. A prospective, randomized, double-blinded single-site control study comparing blood loss prevention of tranexamic acid (TXA) to epsilon aminocaproic acid (EACA) for corrective spinal surgery. BMC Surg 2010;10:13.

43. Goobie SM, Meier PM, Sethna NF, et al. Population pharmacokinetics of tranexamic acid in paediatric patients undergoing craniosynostosis surgery. Clin Pharmacokinet 2013;52(4):267–76.

44. Dehmer JJ, Adamson WT. Massive transfusion and blood product use in the pediatric trauma patient. Semin Pediatr Surg 2010;19(4):286–91.

45. Ho AM, Dion PW, Yeung JH, et al. Fresh-frozen plasma transfusion strategy in trauma with massive and ongoing bleeding. Common (sense) and sensibility. Resuscitation 2010;81(9):1079–81.

46. Phan HH, Wisner DH. Should we increase the ratio of plasma/platelets to red blood cells in massive transfusion: what is the evidence? Vox Sang 2010;98(3 Pt 2):395–402.

47. Makley AT, Goodman MD, Friend LA, et al. Resuscitation with fresh whole blood ameliorates the inflammatory response after hemorrhagic shock. J Trauma 2010;68(2):305–11.

48. Griffee MJ, Deloughery TG, Thorborg PA. Coagulation management in massive bleeding. Curr Opin Anaesthesiol 2010;23(2):263–8.

49. Pidcoke HF, Aden JK, Mora AG, et al. Ten-year analysis of transfusion in Operation Iraqi Freedom and Operation Enduring Freedom: increased plasma and platelet use correlates with improved survival. J Trauma Acute Care Surg 2012;73(6 Suppl 5):S445–52.

50. Howard CB, McKibbin B, Williams LA, et al. Factors affecting the incidence of hip dislocation in cerebral palsy. J Bone Joint Surg Br 1985;67(4):530–2.

51. Dhawale AA, Karatas AF, Holmes L, et al. Long-term outcome of reconstruction of the hip in young children with cerebral palsy. Bone Joint J 2013;95-B(2): 259–65.
52. Miller F, Girardi H, Lipton G, et al. Reconstruction of the dysplastic spastic hip with peri-ilial pelvic and femoral osteotomy followed by immediate mobilization. J Pediatr Orthop 1997;17(5):592–602.
53. Oh CW, Presedo A, Dabney KW, et al. Factors affecting femoral varus osteotomy in cerebral palsy: a long-term result over 10 years. J Pediatr Orthop B 2007; 16(1):23–30.
54. Brenn BR, Brislin RP, Rose JB. Epidural analgesia in children with cerebral palsy. Can J Anaesth 1998;45(12):1156–61.
55. Gracies JM, Elovic E, McGuire J, et al. Traditional pharmacological treatments for spasticity. Part I: local treatments. Muscle Nerve Suppl 1997;6:S61–91.
56. Goldstein EM. Spasticity management: an overview. J Child Neurol 2001;16(1): 16–23.
57. Kroin JS, Ali A, York M, et al. The distribution of medication along the spinal canal after chronic intrathecal administration. Neurosurgery 1993;33(2):226–30 [discussion: 230].
58. Awaad Y, Tayem H, Munoz S, et al. Functional assessment following intrathecal baclofen therapy in children with spastic cerebral palsy. J Child Neurol 2003; 18(1):26–34.
59. Akman MN, Loubser PG, Donovan WH, et al. Intrathecal baclofen: does tolerance occur? Paraplegia 1993;31(8):516–20.
60. Albright AL. Neurosurgical treatment of spasticity and other pediatric movement disorders. J Child Neurol 2003;18(Suppl 1):S67–78.
61. Borowski A, Pruszczynski B, Grzegorzewski A, et al. Dega transiliac acetabular osteotomy in cerebral palsy hip joint. Chir Narzadow Ruchu Ortop Pol 2009; 74(1):13–7 [in Polish].
62. Kolaski K, Logan LR. A review of the complications of intrathecal baclofen in patients with cerebral palsy. NeuroRehabilitation 2007;22(5):383–95.
63. Dickey MP, Rice M, Kinnett DG, et al. Infectious complications of intrathecal baclofen pump devices in a pediatric population. Pediatr Infect Dis J 2013; 32(7):715–22.
64. Vender JR, Hester S, Waller JL, et al. Identification and management of intrathecal baclofen pump complications: a comparison of pediatric and adult patients. J Neurosurg 2006;104(Suppl 1):9–15.
65. Albright AL. Intraventricular baclofen infusion for dystonia. Report of two cases. J Neurosurg 2006;105(Suppl 1):71–4.
66. Saissy JM, Vitris M, Demaziere J, et al. Flumazenil counteracts intrathecal baclofen-induced central nervous system depression in tetanus. Anesthesiology 1992;76(6):1051–3.
67. Samson-Fang L, Gooch J, Norlin C. Intrathecal baclofen withdrawal simulating neuroleptic malignant syndrome in a child with cerebral palsy. Dev Med Child Neurol 2000;42(8):561–5.
68. Gooch JL, Oberg WA, Grams B, et al. Complications of intrathecal baclofen pumps in children. Pediatr Neurosurg 2003;39(1):1–6.
69. Motta F, Antonello CE, Stignani C. Intrathecal baclofen and motor function in cerebral palsy. Dev Med Child Neurol 2011;53(5):443–8.
70. Borowski A, Pruszczynski B, Miller F, et al. Quality of life in cerebral palsy children treated with intrathecal baclofen pump implantation in parents' opinion. Chir Narzadow Ruchu Ortop Pol 2010;75(5):318–22 [in Polish].

Challenges in Pediatric Neuroanesthesia

Awake Craniotomy, Intraoperative Magnetic Resonance Imaging, and Interventional Neuroradiology

Craig D. McClain, MD, MPH*, Mary Landrigan-Ossar, MD, PhD

KEYWORDS

- Pediatric • Intraoperative magnetic resonance imaging • Awake craniotomy
- Neurointerventional • Neuroendovascular • Pediatric neuroanesthesia

KEY POINTS

- There are many complexities to the care of children undergoing awake craniotomies.
- The anesthesiologist must be prepared to deal with a variety of urgent and emergent intra-operative scenarios.
- When the techniques of cortical mapping are combined with an awake, responsive patient, optimal outcomes can be realized.
- Intraoperative magnetic resonance imaging offers high-resolution intraoperative images that can assess the extent of resection in pseudoreal time.
- Angiography and embolization are frequent procedures performed in the neurointerventional suite to address a variety of pediatric neurovascular lesions.

INTRODUCTION

Anesthesiologists involved in caring for children undergoing neurosurgical procedures are required to have an intimate understanding of normal neurocognitive development, the effects of anesthetics on the developing nervous system, the fundamental differences between children and adults, and the implications of these surgical approaches to children. Several surgical approaches such as image-guided procedures and awake craniotomies add to the complex environment faced by the anesthesiologist. In addition, the neurointerventional suite has become increasingly used as

Disclosures: the authors have no disclosures to make.
Department of Anesthesiology, Perioperative and Pain Medicine, Boston Children's Hospital, Harvard Medical School, 300 Longwood Avenue, Bader 3, Boston, MA 02115, USA
* Corresponding author.
E-mail address: craig.mcclain@childrens.harvard.edu

children with a variety of neurovascular lesions present for often lengthy and complicated procedures for definitive diagnosis or treatment. Planning and executing safe, age-appropriate perioperative care in these environments is challenging. This article offers some insight into the complexities of care of children undergoing awake craniotomies as well as procedures in intraoperative magnetic resonance imaging (iMRI) suites and neurointerventional radiology.

AWAKE CRANIOTOMY
History of Awake Craniotomy

Evidence of craniotomy predates the invention of surgical anesthesia by several millennia. There is evidence of trepanation (creating a hole through the skull and dura) in human skulls unearthed in France from approximately 6500 BC.[1] In addition, it is clear that several pre-Columbian societies in Mesoamerica practiced trepanation, most notably, the Incas.[2,3] During the Middle Ages and Renaissance in western Europe, trepanation was performed to alleviate headaches and seizures.[4] Dutch painter Hieronymus Bosch famously captured this practice in his painting, *The Extraction of the Stone of Madness*, from the late fifteenth century.

The modern use of awake craniotomy (AC) began in the second half of the nineteenth century, when local anesthetics became widely available. With good local anesthesia, Horsley was able to perform ACs.[5] However, the modern understanding of the benefit of AC began in 1951, when Wilder Penfield, the first director of the famous Montreal Neurologic Institute, published his landmark monograph, *Epilepsy and the Functional Anatomy of the Human Brain*.[6] Penfield described the use of craniotomy performed under local anesthesia only to facilitate resection of epileptogenic foci. Before resection, Penfield stimulated various locations of the cortex and observed the responses in the awake patient. This practice allowed him to generate cortical maps of motor and sensory areas, which result in cortical homunculus.

The 1960s brought the advent of neuroleptic anesthetic techniques, which continued to provide a responsive patient but offered some degree of analgesia and sedation in order to tolerate prolonged awkward positions.[7] A combination of drugs such as droperidol and fentanyl were commonly used to facilitate a patient who was drowsy and comfortable, yet still able to arouse to stimulation and follow commands. The downside of prolonged use of dopaminergic drugs became apparent when the occurrence of side effects, including extrapyramidal effects and dysphoria, was noted.

AC as a method of treating seizure foci and tumors became popular again in the 1990s and early 2000s, with the widespread use of shorter-acting hypnotic agents and opioids, such as propofol and remifentanil.[8,9] Current anesthetic techniques use a wide range of agents. Dexmedetomidine, an α_2 agonist with sedating and analgesic properties, is a relatively newer drug that offers some distinct advantages over other techniques using sedative hypnotics and opioids.[10,11] One of the most advantageous aspects of dexmedetomidine is its ability to offer mild analgesia and good sedation without compromising the airway.

AC in Children

Equipment
No special equipment is needed for the performance of AC. The anesthesiologist should have the operating room (OR) prepared for the same problems that may be encountered during a craniotomy under general anesthesia. Invasive blood pressure monitoring is useful. The anesthesiologist should be prepared to convert to a general anesthetic if needed. Airway management while the patient is in head pins can be

particularly problematic. It can be lifesaving to have properly sized supraglottic airway devices within easy reach. More advanced airway tools may be necessary to provide definitive airway management.

The anesthesiologist must be prepared to deal with a variety of urgent and emergent intraoperative scenarios. This strategy applies to any surgical case, but may be more important for an AC. Seizures, which can occur during cortical mapping in an AC, must be quickly and effectively controlled to prevent patient injury. Seizures are more common in younger patients with frontal lobe lesions.[12] Generalized tonic clonic movements can be devastating to a patient who is fixed in head pins. Injuries that may result can range from scalp lacerations to skull fractures and even cervical spine injuries. Anesthesiologists should always have a heightened sense of concern with an unrelaxed patient fixed in head pins (awake or under general anesthesia).

Indications

The benefits of having a responsive patient during surgery performed near eloquent cortex are legion. Most commonly, AC is performed on patients with lesions located near, adjacent to, or even within eloquent cortex. Intraoperative cortical mapping can be used to identify areas that are dysfunctional as well as those cortical areas that control important functions such as speech and motor movements. When the techniques of cortical mapping are combined with an awake, responsive patient, optimal outcomes can be realized. A prospective comparison in 2011[13] of AC versus craniotomies performed under general anesthesia for resection of supratentorial lesions found a statistically significant improvement in resection quality and better neurologic outcome in the awake patients.

Certainly a useful technique in adults, AC in pediatric neurosurgical patients presents the anesthesiologist with a tremendous challenge, because of the differences in level of cognitive development of children. The youngest patient reported in the literature to have successfully undergone an AC is a 9-year-old boy, who underwent resection of a glioblastoma in the left frontotemporal region using propofol sedation.[14] Despite this reported success, it is unlikely that many children younger than 10 years are emotionally mature enough to tolerate such a procedure.

Contraindications

Proper patient selection is probably the single most important factor in achieving an optimal outcome for an AC. Relative contraindications include patient's age (<11 or 12 years old) and the patient's general level of emotional maturity. There may be 12-year-old patients who are candidates for an AC, whereas a particular 16-year-old may not be amenable to such an approach. It is crucial to have thorough discussions with both the patient and their parents before embarking on such an endeavor. Further, similar conversations should occur with the neurosurgeon and neurologists involved in order to determine the plan of cortical mapping and what the patient is required to do.

Patient preparation

As noted earlier, proper patient selection and preparation are paramount. During preoperative conversations with the parents and child, the keen pediatric anesthesiologist is able to get a good assessment of the child's emotional maturity and consequent ability to tolerate the proposed procedure. The patient must be able to calmly and coherently express their needs and concerns to the anesthesiologist, and there needs to be a certain degree of trust.

Technique best practice

A variety of anesthetic approaches are currently used. There is no single best approach. Each has its advantages and disadvantages. The individual anesthesiologist needs to have a clear understanding of what the surgical and neurophysiologic needs are. The specific anesthetic technique may be adopted to best facilitate the goals within the resource constraints (both human and physical) of the given environment.

Essentially, the differences in technique boil down to the degree of anesthesia/sedation used before and after cortical mapping. One approach is to perform the entire procedure with the patient completely awake.[15] This approach necessitates a mature, motivated, and cooperative child, because several tasks need to be accomplished with an awake or minimally sedated patient, including line placement, infiltration of local anesthetic, placement of head pins, positioning, skull and dural opening, and resection. This type of approach is well described in the adult literature. A variation on this technique uses short-acting sedatives and analgesics, such as propofol and fentanyl, titrated to induce unconsciousness but maintain spontaneous ventilation for instillation of local anesthetics, insertion of monitoring catheters, placement of head pins, and skull opening.[9,16] Subsequently, patients can be allowed to awaken to facilitate cortical mapping before definitive resection. After that, the patient may then have sedatives and opioids reinstituted for the closure.

Another approach is the asleep-awake-asleep technique.[17] This approach consists of inducing general anesthesia and maintaining airway control with a supraglottic device. General anesthesia is maintained for line placement, placement of head pins, positioning, and skull and dural opening. The patient is then awakened, the supraglottic airway is removed, and the surgeons then proceed with mapping and resection. At the conclusion of the resection, general anesthesia is once again induced and the supraglottic airway reinserted for closure of the dura, skull, and skin. Although this technique offers the patient a stress-free procedure up to the point of functional testing and cortical mapping, there are some disadvantages. Airway management during emergence and induction while the patient is in head pins presents a greater challenge. Should the patient cough or buck while immobilized, cervical spine injuries or scalp lacerations can occur. In addition, brain swelling is a real concern in a patient who is breathing spontaneously under general anesthesia with an inhalational anesthetic and possibly nitrous oxide.

Procedural steps

Line placement and placement of head pins in a child is the first challenge for the anesthesiologist. As noted earlier, short-acting, potent sedatives and analgesics such as propofol and remifentanil may be useful to ensure patient cooperation with placement of multiple intravenous (IV) lines, arterial lines, and a Foley catheter. These same agents may also be useful for placement of head pins. Another useful adjunct for scalp analgesia to facilitate placement of head pins is a scalp block.[18] Dosing adjustments of local anesthetic should be made to account for differing sizes of pediatric patients.

Positioning is best undertaken with an awake patient if at all possible. The advantage to having an awake patient at this juncture is that the patient can communicate what is most comfortable to them and give feedback as to how to optimize the position. A comfortable position is crucial, because the patient needs to remain there for several hours. It is common for patients to become anxious. Discomfort from awkward positions only exacerbates this problem. An important aspect of optimal patient positioning is the creation of a tent or drape tunnel so that the patient does not feel covered up and can see the anesthesiologist (**Fig. 1**).

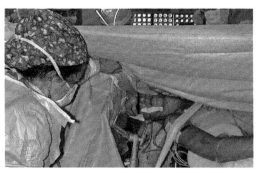

Fig. 1. Pediatric patient during an AC. Note creation of tunnel or tent so that patient can see anesthesiologist and communicate. Note also the head pins in place and the awkward position that the patient is required to maintain for several hours.

Regardless of the chosen technique, it is most important that the anesthesiologist themselves (or a trusted designee) remain in close visual contact and verbal communication with the patient at all times. Communication of every aspect of patient care in the OR suite must be clear and age appropriate for the patient. It is the anesthesiologist's job to decrease the patient's stress. In this setting, that responsibility involves letting the patient know who is in the room, what kinds of questions are being asked, explaining what they may feel, explaining noises, getting feedback about level of comfort, and distracting the patient to minimize anxiety. This is one of the most challenging aspects of an AC. It is useful to aggressively control traffic in the room, so that there is not a constant parade of people of various specialties coming in and out and inundating the room with multiple conversations. These things can be confusing and anxiety provoking to a patient who cannot see where the voices and noises are coming from and may feel like no one is talking to them.

If the patient is sedated during cranial and dural opening and initial exposure, it is important for them to be awake enough to engage in neurologic testing by the team. This testing may involve language skills, identifying pictures, memory tests, and so forth. This is the crucial moment for creating the cortical map to help facilitate resection of the lesion. If this part of the procedure cannot be accomplished effectively, the whole point of performing the procedure on an awake patient is rendered moot.

After mapping and resection, the remaining surgical steps involve closure and removing the head fixation device. This procedure can be performed using sedation as needed. It is often a welcome break for the patient to be sedated at this point, because they are often uncomfortable from awkward positions by this point of the procedure.

Postprocedure care

Caring for patients who have undergone ACs in the postoperative period should have little difference from postoperative care for pediatric patients who have had craniotomies performed under general anesthesia. Frequent neurologic assessments are the most sensitive indicator of postoperative problems. Control of pain and hemodynamic parameters is an important goal. The common complications after a craniotomy performed under general anesthesia are similar to those for ACs: bleeding, cerebrospinal fluid (CSF) leaks, electrolyte disturbances, and postoperative emesis. If the procedure is performed to resect seizure foci, caregivers must be keenly aware of the risk for postoperative seizures and have a plan for treatment.

Avoiding complications

Regardless of the technique chosen, it is important for the anesthesiologist to have an in-depth discussion with the patient with respect to intraoperative needs and expectations. The preoperative period is the time to decide whether the patient is a candidate for an AC. There are no randomized controlled trials comparing the safety or effectiveness of the techniques just described.

Common complications during ACs include seizures, failure of adequate communication with the patient, and hemodynamic derangements, including tachycardia and hypertension.[12,19,20] These problems have been noted in larger series of adult ACs. There are no such data for children. Despite this situation, anesthesiologists should be prepared to immediately address such concerns in pediatric patients.

iMRI
History of iMRI

The development of iMRI represents a significant leap in the continued effort to improve intraoperative navigation and the quality of resection of intracranial masses.[21] iMRI was first used in the mid-1990s for adult intracranial procedures.[22] However, its success was soon exported to pediatric neurosurgical procedures.[23] Coupled with a frameless navigation system, iMRI offers state-of-the-art ability to localize lesions as well as improve the quality and pseudoreal time assessment of resection during neurosurgical procedures. iMRI suites are common, with an increasing number of such suites being located in pediatric hospitals.[24,25] Thus, it is becoming increasingly important for pediatric anesthesiologists to be familiar with the unique considerations of working in an iMRI suite.

Before the advent of iMRI, frame-based or frameless navigation systems were used to aid in localization of intracranial lesions in children. Both types of navigation systems are predicated on layering a series of fixed points (often using either fiducials or a face recognition system) over previously obtained imaging. Although these systems were certainly advantageous, they had their limitations.

First, although these systems offer improved ability to localize lesions that may be difficult to differentiate with the naked eye (such as in deep brain structures or near eloquent cortex), they offer no opportunity to intraoperatively assess extent of resection. iMRI offers high-resolution intraoperative images, which can assess the extent of resection in pseudoreal time. This technique may lead to improved patient outcomes and decrease the need for unnecessary second operations in some situations.

Further, these types of navigation systems cannot account for the phenomenon of brain shift, which occurs naturally during intracranial surgery.[26] Brain shift describes the movement of intracranial structures throughout the procedure. Brain shift leads to decreased accuracy of navigation because of position changes, egress of CSF from the cranium, and mass resection. The degree of brain shift can vary with resected tissue type, patient position, CSF loss, size of craniotomy, hyperventilation, and amount of tissue resected. As the duration of the surgery increases, so does the degree of brain shift. This situation leads to the decreased accuracy of conventional intraoperative navigation systems. The advantage that iMRI offers is that images obtained intraoperatively can update the navigation systems and allow for continued precision.

Equipment

Much like any anesthetic performed to facilitate diagnostic MRI, anesthetics delivered during procedures that use iMRI require a significant investment in special equipment.[27,28] Special MRI-conditional physiologic monitors are required, as are MRI-conditional anesthesia machines and MRI-conditional infusion pumps. Depending on the particular configuration of a given iMRI suite, it may be possible to use normal surgical instruments, microscopes, drills, tables, and so forth (**Fig. 2**). However, in suites in which there is either a movable patient and stationary magnet or a movable magnet with a stationary patient, the patient still needs to have safe delivery of an anesthetic during imaging sequences. This procedure necessitates the MRI-safe anesthesia equipment during the maintenance phase of the anesthetic.

There are a limited number of manufacturers who produce such equipment. The equipment itself tends to be more expensive and more delicate than standard physiologic monitors, anesthesia machines, and infusion pumps. Also, there are certain limitations to such equipment. Pulse oximeters are often more sensitive to motion artifact and it can be difficult to obtain a consistent signal in a small child or cold digit. Electrocardiographic (ECG) interpretation can be challenging, especially during imaging, when the fluctuating magnetic fields can cause significant interference. ST analysis can be profoundly unreliable. Core temperature monitoring is not nearly as simple in an MRI environment. Some manufacturers have produced a temperature probe, which can be covered with a disposable condom.

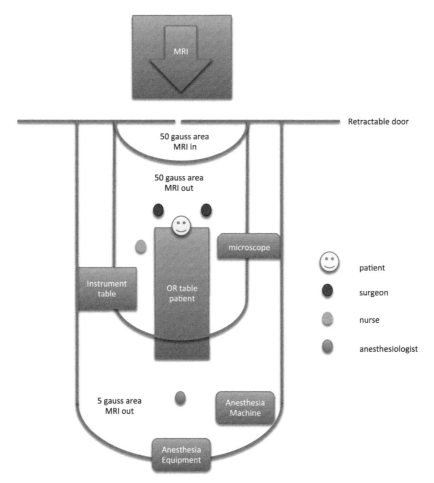

Fig. 2. A common iMRI setup. This system uses a movable magnet and stationary patient. This is the system used at our institution.

There are also several pieces of essential equipment that do not have an MRI-safe or conditional analogue. This equipment includes forced-air warming devices, nerve stimulators, precordial Doppler probes, and fluid warmers. The lack of availability of certain MRI-compatible equipment creates challenges in the iMRI environment. This situation results in the anesthesiologist being responsible for accounting for several items that must be removed from within the 5-Gauss line when magnet deployment and imaging occur. The existence of a movable magnetic field creates unique challenges to the care team. The modern iMRI environment is not analogous to diagnostic MRI, in which is a stationary field. Because of the movable field, iMRI is unlike any other environment within which the anesthesiologist works.

Indications
The indications for a pediatric neurosurgical procedure using iMRI can be diverse, depending on the capabilities of the magnet itself.[29] Most commonly, iMRI is used to help facilitate intracranial tumor resection. iMRI can be used to help localize small masses, improve precision of other intraoperative navigation systems, and assess extent of intraoperative resection in pseudoreal time. In addition, iMRI may be used to help delineate the extent of cortical disconnection in major seizure surgery, such as corpus callosotomy or functional hemispherectomy.

As imaging technology improves, the opportunities for iMRI to aid in pediatric neurosurgical procedures will expand. For example, there are new approaches to ablation of deep brain lesions using stereotactic MRI-guided laser-induced thermal ablation.[30,31] This technique requires multiple intraoperative images, with the ablation completed in real time while imaging.

Contraindications
A large volume of literature champions the safety of iMRI for many different tumor types and surgical approaches. However, there is little guidance for practitioners on exclusion criteria for patients being operated on in an iMRI suite. It may be easiest to break down the absolute and relative contraindications into some broad categories.

First, we can look at the patient characteristics that may prevent that child from even entering the iMRI suite. Children who have certain implantable devices may be absolutely excluded from a high-strength magnetic field environment. Examples of these devices may include implanted cardiac devices (ICDs) (pacemakers and defibrillators).[32,33] Although this remains generally the case, the prevalence of magnetic resonance (MR)-compatible ICDs and pacemakers is becoming more common. Other devices such as vagal nerve stimulators or certain types of programmable ventricular shunt valves may be acceptable, depending on the field strength of the magnet.[34] It is crucial to always consult with the MR technologist or radiologist when there is a question about the safety of implantable devices.

There are also some relative contraindications because of both the environment of the room and the size of the bore of the magnet. It can be difficult to perform lengthy surgical procedures on infants and small children in an iMRI suite for several reasons. First, the room itself must be kept cold to provide an optimal magnetic field for imaging. Thus, patients such as neonates under general anesthesia, who cannot effectively self-regulate temperature, are at particular risk for hypothermia and its consequences.[35] In our suite, we prefer to avoid having such patients in the iMRI room, unless there is some compelling reason to use the magnet and it aids in optimizing the child's outcome. In addition, the MRI-conditional equipment itself can be more difficult to use in small children, in our experience. Movement artifact is more common with pulse oximetry and ECG. Because of these issues with small children, we prefer not to care for children less than 10 kg or 1 year old, unless there is significant potential benefit that would alter the risk/benefit ratio in favor of accepting the risks.

Some patients may be too large to safely place in the magnet intraoperatively. Magnet bores vary in size, and practitioners must be aware of the limitations of their particular magnet. Once the patient is under anesthesia and under surgical drapes, they are not able to alert the care team to potential positioning problems within the magnet. In order to maintain sterility during intraoperative imaging, the patient remains draped and padded underneath. This situation further increases the footprint of the patient (**Fig. 3**). It is useful to have a template for sizing the patient preoperatively to determine if larger or obese patients are able to fit in the iMRI. Caregivers should take into account that the bulk from the drapes and padding is not accounted for in this situation.

Patient preparation
Specific patient preparation for procedures in an iMRI suite should be directed at screening to ensure the appropriateness of the patient for a high-strength magnetic field environment. Usually, the MR technician is considered the safety official.[36] Therefore, questions and concerns about the appropriateness of given implantable devices for a given MRI should be directed to the MR technician. All implanted devices, such as ventriculoperitoneal shunts, baclofen pumps, aneurysm clips, orthopedic hardware, and so forth, must be noted and cleared by the safety officer. In addition to the patient, all other people entering the room must also be cleared, including all medical personnel and parents if it is planned that a parent is to be present during the induction.

Aside from these considerations, the preparation of the patient for a procedure in an iMRI suite should proceed similar to the preparation of a patient for the same procedure in a conventional OR suite.

Technique best practice
Although the equipment that the anesthesiologist uses caring for the patient in an iMRI suite may be different from a conventional OR, the basic approach and anesthetic techniques should not be significantly different from similar procedures performed in a conventional OR suite. For craniotomies, common techniques such as total IV anesthesia or inhaled anesthesia and high-dose opioid are acceptable. No single best anesthetic technique has been identified for craniotomies.[37]

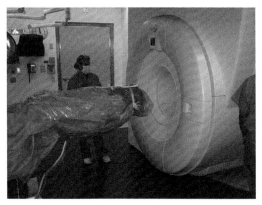

Fig. 3. Patient being placed into movable 1.5-T iMRI. Note the degree of draping to pad and protect the patient as well as maintain sterility.

Procedural steps

When caring for patients in an iMRI environment, practitioners must develop processes that account for the different risk profile resulting from the movable magnetic field presented to the patient and caregivers. These additional considerations include accounting for necessary MRI-incompatible equipment used before placing the patient in the high-strength magnetic field. Examples include IV needles, airway equipment, manometers, flashlights, scissors, and so forth. Inadvertently leaving MRI-incompatible equipment around the patient and subsequent placement in a high-strength magnetic field can result in serious injury or even death to the patient or caregivers if the object is ferromagnetic and becomes a missile. Even if the object is not ferromagnetic, it may still present danger to the patient by being a potential source of thermal injury. Some objects can also cause problems by interfering with image quality by introducing interference.

Other necessary MRI-incompatible devices include forced-air warming devices and nerve stimulators. These devices are certainly useful and necessary in modern practice, but no MRI-compatible version is commercially available. They can be used safely before placement of the patient in the high-strength magnetic field. Thus, the issue that arises has to do with the safe use of MRI-incompatible equipment in a movable magnetic field environment.

One solution is to create a series of checklists. We have used such a system in our practice with great success. When setting up our iMRI suite, we designed several different checklists to be implemented at critical steps in the surgical procedure to account for potential hazards and try to minimize adverse events. The first checklist occurs after induction but before draping the patient. This checklist is designed to ensure that, after induction, line placement, and positioning, there are no unaccounted for MRI-incompatible materials near the patient that would be hidden by the drapes when it comes time to image. After the initial checklist and ensuring appropriate counts of equipment and instruments, the surgical procedure occurs. Before deploying the movable magnet, another checklist is implemented. At this point, the nurses ensure accurate counts of all instruments and sutures. The same process occurs for the anesthesia provider. The anesthesiologist must ensure that the airway equipment, all IV lines and wires, nerve stimulator, forced-air warmer, fluid warmer, and precordial Doppler are moved outside the 5-Gauss line. Once all equipment is accounted for, the magnet is deployed and intraoperative imaging occurs. If repeat imaging is required after further resection, the process is repeated.

Postprocedure care

Postoperative care of children who have undergone neurosurgical procedures using iMRI is, in most ways, the same as for those undergoing similar procedures in a conventional OR suite. One caveat is that in suites that take advantage of a high field strength magnet (eg, 1.5 or 3 T), intraoperative images may obviate routine postoperative MRI. This has certainly been the case at our institution, where we have essentially eliminated the need for routine postoperative MRI evaluation of children who have undergone craniotomy with iMRI. There remain instances of requests for postoperative MRI, but these are universally because of some specific concern that would not be evident on intraoperative images obtained at the end of the case. iMRI has been shown to help in early diagnosis of some rare serious complications, such as intracranial bleeding, before significant patient compromise.[38] Avoidance of such routine postoperative imaging is advantageous, especially in young children. In addition to avoiding the logistic challenges of scheduling an MRI in busy centers, young children may avoid a second anesthetic and the attendant risks.

Avoiding complications

Proper training, patient selection, and establishment of strong lines of communication across disciplines optimize the environment to offer the safest, best possible outcome to the patient. We began the development of our suite by using a multidisciplinary approach involving all clinical departments involved in caring for patients in this environment: anesthesiology, neurosurgery, radiology, and nursing. We have continued to have regular meetings of a core group to ensure that this cross-disciplinary communication is maintained as this technology evolves. This strategy allows us a great deal of flexibility to address concerns as they arise. These concerns can include problems with or updates to the iMRI system itself, issues with the anesthesia equipment, advances in technology that affect the room, near misses, and the use of simulation approaches to address rare but serious concerns related to the suite.

The use of iMRI is becoming increasingly common. Practitioners must be aware of the unique considerations when caring for patients in this environment. Its proponents tout the purported benefits of iMRI. Practitioners must recognize that there are also some potential downsides as well. Delivering an anesthetic for a patient in diagnostic MRI is challenging enough. The additional concerns of performing a surgical procedure in a suite with a movable high-strength magnetic field demand a thoughtful approach from the anesthesiologist.

NEUROINTERVENTIONAL PROCEDURES

It is becoming increasingly common for children with a variety of intracranial diseases to require anesthesia for diagnostic imaging. In particular, children with some neurovascular lesions require either isolated diagnostic imaging or therapeutic interventions in the neurointerventional suite. Angiography and embolization are frequent procedures performed in the neurointerventional suite to address a variety of pediatric neurovascular lesions. This section describes the complex considerations of caring for children with significant neurovascular disease out of the OR.

DIAGNOSTIC CEREBRAL ANGIOGRAPHY
Equipment

Specialized anesthesia equipment is not generally necessary in the interventional radiology (IR) suite, unlike in MRI. Nonetheless, there are several considerations worthy of comment. It is generally accepted that older anesthesia equipment is relegated to the non-OR anesthesia (NORA) milieu.[39,40] Closed-claims data have shown that patients in the NORA environment are more likely to suffer more serious harm, and inadequate monitoring is cited as a contributor.[41] Anesthesia equipment in IR, in which lengthy complex cases are performed on sicker patients, should be standardized with that being used in the main OR. This strategy promotes safety not only by allowing the use of up-to-date technology for complex patients but also by reducing the chance of operator unfamiliarity with little-used devices.

Radiation safety in IR is another area of particular concern for anesthesiologists. As IR anesthesia services increase, anesthesiologists will have increased exposure to radiation. In the procedure room, anesthesiologists' exposure to radiation is 3-fold greater than that of radiologists on the opposite side of the procedure table, because of scatter radiation.[42] To reduce exposure, anesthesiologists should wear lead aprons, preferably wrap-around, and protective eyewear. Portable lead shields should be placed between the radiation source and the anesthesiologist. If feasible, the anesthesiologist should leave the room during angiography runs.[43] Portable dosimeters should be worn and monitored in compliance with local regulations. Because cerebral angiography is generally performed with biplane imaging, the dose to the anesthesiologist is increased, making these precautions even more necessary (**Fig. 4**).

Indications

Diagnostic cerebral angiography in pediatric patients is generally reserved for those cases in which computed tomographic angiography or MR angiography provides partial or questionable information and is the reference standard for diagnosis of neurovascular pathology.[44,45] This finding is borne out across several institutions, where the most common indications are stroke (including moyamoya disease), hemorrhage, and postoperative evaluation of cerebrovascular treatment.[46,47]

Patient Preparation

Because this procedure is often brief, little beyond routine preparation for general anesthesia is required. Preoperative blood pressures are helpful in establishing a baseline for comparison with intraoperative values. Parents may continue clear oral fluids until 2 hours before the procedure in the hope that euvolemia contributes to hemodynamic stability on induction of anesthesia. IV access should be sufficient for adequate hydration, because the likelihood of significant blood loss is low.

Technique Best Practices and Procedure Steps

Once arterial access is accomplished (usually via a femoral artery), a catheter is advanced over a guide wire with fluoroscopic guidance to the carotid or vertebral arteries. Angiography is performed with apnea for the 10-second to 15-second angiographic runs. Once imaging is complete, the arterial sheath is removed, and pressure is held until hemostasis is achieved (15–20 minutes). Patients are kept flat in the recovery area for several hours to assist with hemostasis.[47]

General endotracheal anesthesia is most commonly used in pediatric patients.[48] A more mature patient can successfully accomplish the procedure with anxiolysis. However, sedation beyond anxiolysis can be problematic, because the patient may become disinhibited and not be able to comply with breath holding.

Fluid management during cerebral angiography is aimed at preserving normotension by restoring euvolemia after fasting. Euvolemia to slight hypervolemia is preferable to reduce the chances of kidney damage in the setting of a contrast-induced osmotic diuresis.[49,50] Painful stimuli associated with this procedure are minimal

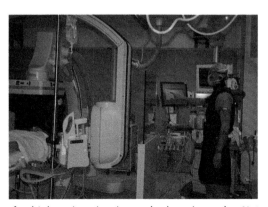

Fig. 4. Room setup for biplane imaging in cerebral angiography. Note radiation sources both below the procedure table and immediately adjacent to the anesthesiologist.

once arterial access is established, and the need for long-acting opioids is low. Muscle relaxation can be helpful in achieving apnea for angiography but is not mandatory.

Postprocedure Care

One challenge for pediatric patients is the need for flat bed rest for 2 to 6 hours after removal of the femoral sheath, to reduce the chances of postprocedural bleeding or hematoma.[51] Behavioral techniques such as reassurance and distraction can be useful, and chemical adjuncts can help for a younger or less compliant child. Deep extubation aided by longer-acting narcotics or an α_2 agonist, such as clonidine, can assist a child to sleep quietly in the recovery area.[48,52]

Avoiding Complications

Complication rates for cerebral angiography in the range of less than 0.4% have been found in large pediatric series with experienced neuroradiologists.[45,46,48] The most common problem seen is bleeding or hematoma at the femoral puncture, and even this is rare.[53] Neurologic or vascular complications of catheterization are extremely low in children, as are nephropathic consequences of contrast administration in patients with no preexisting renal dysfunction.

The risk of acute allergic-like reactions when low-osmolality contrast is used is less than 1%.[54,55] These reactions usually occur within 1 hour of administration and range from nausea, rash, and mild hemodynamic changes to severe reactions involving urticaria, bronchospasm, and hemodynamic collapse. Although similar to anaphylaxis, their nature is still a matter of debate. Mild reactions are treated symptomatically and are usually self-limited. Treatment of severe reactions is the same as the treatment of anaphylaxis, with hemodynamic and airway support, antihistamines, steroids, and epinephrine when indicated.[55] In patients at high risk for a reaction (history of previous reaction, asthma, or atopy), pretreatment with corticosteroids and antihistamines is standard.

NEUROENDOVASCULAR INTERVENTIONS
Equipment

Equipment requirements and safety considerations for neurointerventional procedures are similar to those required for diagnostic cerebral angiography.

Indications

Indications for neurointerventional procedures include embolization of intracerebral vascular anomalies, such as arteriovenous malformations, arteriovenous fistulae, and aneurysms, and targeted injection of intra-arterial chemotherapy for tumors (**Fig. 5**).[56–59]

Patient Preparation

Because of the often lengthy nature of these procedures, meticulous patient positioning and padding are crucial, because it may be impossible to reposition a patient once a procedure is under way. Good IV access should be obtained primarily for hydration and drug administration, because the chance of blood transfusion is small. An arterial line for blood pressure monitoring is usually required for close blood pressure monitoring as well as regular assessment of activated clotting times (ACTs) if heparin is administered.

A   **B**

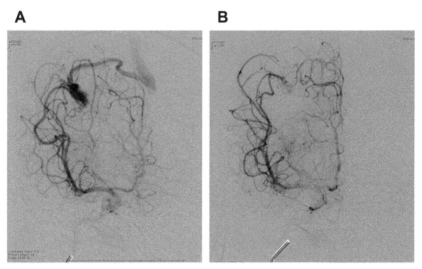

Fig. 5. Angiography before (*A*) and after (*B*) embolization of right frontal lobe arteriovenous malformation in a 9-month-old male.

Technique Best Practices and Procedure Steps

All endovascular work is performed via catheters guided fluoroscopically to the vessel of interest. Embolic agents such as coils or glue can be deployed or chemotherapeutic drugs can then be injected. Once the procedure is complete, arterial access is discontinued, and pressure is held at the puncture site. The patient must then lie flat for several hours to assist hemostasis.

These long procedures are performed almost exclusively under general anesthesia in pediatric patients. The requirements of an immobile patient and the need for frequent periods of apnea make this the safest choice. Consistent muscle relaxation is a necessity, because it would be catastrophic for a patient to move during a critical period.[60,61] These procedures are not particularly painful, and aggressive pain management may not be necessary. As in diagnostic angiography, euvolemia to slight hypervolemia should be maintained to offset the diuretic effect of contrast.[49] A continuous infusion of heparinized saline is used in the guide catheter to prevent microemboli; this can result in a significant amount of fluid being delivered to the patient via the femoral sheath, which may not be recognized by the anesthesiologist.[62] In addition to this infusion, patients are often heparinized to an ACT of 250 to 300 during the procedure.[56]

Blood pressure parameters are generally agreed between the anesthesiologist and neurointerventionalist, and close control of blood pressure is crucial when arteriovenous malformations and aneurysms are being treated. Deliberate hypotension has been described, as has induced asystole to facilitate injection of glue or coil placement into a high-flow lesion.[61] These procedures have not been well described in pediatric patients, and the technique of balloon-assisted glue embolization may make such radical measures unnecessary.[63]

Hemodynamic changes can occur during neurointerventional procedures and should be monitored closely to maintain stability. Intra-arterial embolization using Onyx (ev3, Irvine, CA), a popular type of glue, has been reported to induce bradycardia.[64] When a high-flow lesion, which has already affected a patient's hemodynamics, is closed, it is not uncommon to observe immediate positive changes in the patient's condition.[56]

Postprocedure Care

It can be challenging to keep a young child still for several hours after a procedure, and both chemical and behavioral assistance may be used as described earlier.

After embolization of an intracranial vascular malformation, close control of blood pressure may be required to reduce the risk of postprocedure hemorrhage.[65] This requirement is particularly true of partial embolization, such as before a surgical resection. There is evidence for close blood pressure control after the procedure, but there are few descriptions of how this is to be achieved.[66] Our group has had success with a low-dose dexmedetomidine infusion used after the embolization.

Avoiding Complications

The complications described for diagnostic angiography apply to interventional procedures as well. Although the most frightening complication for an anesthesiologist to contemplate is frank rupture of an intracranial vessel, its incidence is estimated at less than 0.5% of cases.[47] Treatment of this complication involves immediate occlusion of the perforated vessel and possible hematoma evacuation, with supportive treatment as necessary by the anesthesiologist. Migration of embolic agents has been described; both local flow into unintended vessels and distant glue embolization have been described. One series described a rate of migration of approximately 3%, with complications more likely to occur in more complex arteriovenous malformations or in those with deep draining veins.[67] A multispeciality team in the neurointerventional suite who know how to handle a crisis is an invaluable asset should a complication arise.[68]

REFERENCES

1. Walker AA. Neolithic surgery. Archaeology 1997;50(5):19.
2. Lumholtz C, Hrdlicka A. Trephining in Mexico. Am Anthropol 1897;10(12): 389–96.
3. Oakley K, Brooke MA, Akester A, et al. Contributions on trepanning or trepanation in ancient and modern times. Man 1959;59:92–6.
4. Piggott S. A trepanned skull of the beaker period from Dorset and the practice of trepanning in Prehistoric Europe. Proceedings of Prehistoric Society 1940;6(3): 112–32.
5. Girvin JP. Neurosurgical considerations and general methods for craniotomy under local anesthesia. Int Anesthesiol Clin 1986;24:89–114.
6. Jasper H, Penfield W. Epilepsy and the functional anatomy of the human brain. 1st edition. New York: Little, Brown; 1951.
7. Tasker RR, Marshall BM. Analgesia for surgical procedures performed on conscious patients. Can Anaesth Soc J 1965;12:29–33.
8. Olsen KS. The asleep-awake technique using propofol-remifentanil anaesthesia for awake craniotomy for cerebral tumours. Eur J Anaesthesiol 2008; 25:662–9.
9. Soriano SG, Eldredge EA, Wang FK, et al. The effect of propofol on intraoperative electrocorticography and cortical stimulation during awake craniotomies in children. Paediatr Anaesth 2000;10:29–34.
10. Ard J, Doyle W, Bekker A. Awake craniotomy with dexmedetomidine in pediatric patients. J Neurosurg Anesthesiol 2003;15:263–6.
11. Everett LL, Van Rooyen IF, Warner MH, et al. Use of dexmedetomidine in awake craniotomy in adolescents: report of two cases. Paediatr Anaesth 2006;16: 338–42.

12. Nossek E, Matot I, Shahr T, et al. Intraoperative seizures during awake craniotomy: incidence and consequences: analysis of 477 patients. Neurosurgery 2013;73(1):135–40.
13. Sacko O, Lauwers-Cances V, Brauge D, et al. Awake craniotomy vs surgery under general anesthesia for resection of supratentorial lesions. Neurosurgery 2011;68:1192–9.
14. Klimek M, Verbrugge SJ, Roubos S, et al. Awake craniotomy for glioblastoma in a 9-year-old child. Anaesthesia 2004;59:607–9.
15. Hansen E, Seemann M, Zech N, et al. Awake craniotomies without any sedation: the awake-awake-awake technique. Acta Neurochir 2013;155:1417–24.
16. Keifer JC, Dentchev D, Little K, et al. A retrospective analysis of a remifentanil/propofol general anesthetic for craniotomy before awake functional brain mapping. Anesth Analg 2005;101:502–8.
17. Hagberg CA, Gollas A, Berry JM. The laryngeal mask airway for awake craniotomy in the pediatric patient: report of three cases. J Clin Anesth 2004;16:43–7.
18. Pinosky ML, Fishman RL, Reeves ST, et al. The effect of bupivacaine skull block on the hemodynamic response to craniotomy. Anesth Analg 1996;83: 1256–61.
19. Skucas AP, Artu AA. Anesthetic complications of awake craniotomies for epilepsy surgery. Anesth Analg 2006;102:882–7.
20. Nossek E, Matot I, Shahar T, et al. Failed awake craniotomy: a retrospective analysis in 424 patients undergoing craniotomy for brain tumor. J Neurosurg 2013;118:243–9.
21. Manninen PH, Kucharczyk W. A new frontier: magnetic resonance imaging-operating room. J Neurosurg Anesthesiol 2000;12:141–8.
22. Black PM, Moriarty T, Alexander E, et al. Development and implementation of intraoperative magnetic resonance imaging and its neurosurgical applications. Neurosurgery 1997;41:831–42.
23. Nimsky C, Ganslandt O, Gralla J, et al. Intraoperative low-field magnetic resonance imaging in pediatric neurosurgery. Pediatr Neurosurg 2003;38:83–9.
24. Cox RG, Levy R, Hamilton MG, et al. Anesthesia can be safely provided for children in a high-field intraoperative magnetic resonance imaging environment. Paediatr Anaesth 2011;21:454–8.
25. McClain CD, Rockoff MA, Soriano SG. Anesthetic concerns for pediatric patients in an intraoperative MRI suite. Curr Opin Anaesthiol 2011;24:480–6.
26. Nimsky C, Ganslandt O, Cerny S, et al. Quantification of, visualization of, and compensation for brain shift using intraoperative magnetic resonance imaging. Neurosurgery 2000;47:1070–80.
27. Practice advisory on anesthetic care for magnetic resonance imaging: a report by the Society of Anesthesiologists Task Force on Anesthetic Care for magnetic resonance imaging. Anesthesiology 2009;110:459–79.
28. Patteson SK, Chesney JT. Anesthetic management for magnetic resonance imaging: problems and solutions. Anesth Analg 1992;74:121–8.
29. Levy R, Cox RG, Hader WJ, et al. Application of intraoperative high-field magnetic resonance imaging in pediatric neurosurgery. J Neurosurg Pediatr 2009; 4:467–74.
30. Curry DJ, Gowda A, McNichols RJ, et al. MR-guided stereotactic laser ablation of epileptogenic foci in children. Epilepsy Behav 2012;24:408–14.
31. Tovar-Spinoza Z, Carter D, Ferrone D, et al. The use of MRI-guided laser-induced thermal ablation for epilepsy. Childs Nervous System 2013;29(11): 2089–94.

32. Pavlicek W, Geisinger M, Castle L, et al. The effects of nuclear magnetic resonance on patients with cardiac pacemakers. Radiology 1983;147:149–53.
33. Erlebacher JA, Cahill PT, Pannizzo F, et al. Effect of magnetic resonance imaging on DDD pacemakers. Am J Cardiol 1986;57:437–40.
34. Crane BT, Gottschalk B, Kraut M, et al. Magnetic resonance imaging at 1.5T after cochlear implantation. Otol Neurotol 2010;31:1215–20.
35. Bissonnette B. Temperature monitoring in pediatric anesthesia. Int Anesthesiol Clin 1992;30:63–76.
36. Kanal E, Borgstede JP, Barkovich AJ, et al. American College of Radiology white paper on MR safety. AJR Am J Roentgenol 2002;178:1335–47.
37. Todd MM, Warner DS, Sokoll MD, et al. A prospective, comparative trial of three anesthetics for elective supratentorial craniotomy: propofol/fentanyl, isoflurane/nitrous oxide, and fentanyl/nitrous oxide. Anesthesiology 1993;78:1005–20.
38. McClain CD, Soriano SG, Goumnerova LC, et al. Detection of unanticipated intracranial hemorrhage during intraoperative magnetic resonance image-guided neurosurgery. Report of two cases. J Neurosurg 2007;106(Suppl 5): 398–400.
39. Frankel A. Patient safety: anesthesia in remote locations. Anesthesiol Clin 2009; 27:127–39.
40. Melloni C. Anesthesia and sedation outside the operating room: how to prevent risk and maintain good quality. Curr Opin Anaesthesiol 2007;20:513–9.
41. Metzner J, Posner KL, Domino KB. The risk and safety of anesthesia at remote locations: the US closed claims analysis. Curr Opin Anaesthesiol 2009;22: 502–8.
42. Anastasian ZH, Strozyk D, Meyers PM, et al. Radiation exposure of the anesthesiologist in the neurointerventional suite. Anesthesiology 2011;114:512–20.
43. Dagal A. Radiation safety for anesthesiologists. Curr Opin Anaesthesiol 2011; 24:445–50.
44. Kaufman TJ, Kallmes DF. Diagnostic cerebral angiography: archaic and complication-prone or here to stay for another 80 years? AJR Am J Roentgenol 2008;190:1435–7.
45. Burger IM, Murphy KJ, Jordan LC, et al. Safety of digital subtraction angiography in children: complication rate analysis in 241 consecutive diagnostic angiograms. Stroke 2006;37:2535–9.
46. Robertson RL, Chavali RV, Robson CD, et al. Neurologic complications of cerebral angiography in childhood moyamoya syndrome. Pediatr Radiol 1998;28: 824–9.
47. Alexander MJ, Spetzler RF. Pediatric neurovascular disease: surgical, endovascular and medical management. New York: Thieme; 2006.
48. Wolfe TJ, Hussain SI, Lynch JR, et al. Pediatric cerebral angiography: analysis of utilization and findings. Pediatr Neurol 2009;40:98–101.
49. Bush WH, Swanson DP. Acute reactions to intravascular contrast media: types, risk factors, recognition and specific treatments. AJR Am J Roentgenol 1991; 157:1153–61.
50. Mallinckrodt Optiray 240 Package Insert. 2011.
51. Logemann T, Luetmer P, Kaliebe J, et al. Two versus six hours of bed rest following left-sided cardiac catheterization and a meta-analysis of early ambulation trials. Am J Cardiol 1999;84:486–8.
52. Malviya S, Voepel-Lewis T, Ramamurthi RJ, et al. Clonidine for the prevention of emergence agitation in young children: efficacy and recovery profile. Paediatr Anaesth 2006;16:554–9.

53. Gross BA, Orbach DB. Addressing challenges in 4 F and 5 F arterial access for neurointerventional procedures in infants and young children. J Neurointerv Surg 2013;1–6.

54. Dillman JR, Strouse PJ, Ellis JH, et al. Incidence and severity of acute allergic-like reactions to IV nonionic iodinated contrast material in children. AJR Am J Roentgenol 2007;188:1643–7.

55. Pasternak JJ, Williamson EE. Clinical pharmacology, uses, and adverse reactions of iodinated contrast agents: a primer for the non-radiologist. Mayo Clin Proc 2012;87:390–402.

56. Theix R, Williams A, Smith E, et al. The use of onyx for embolization of central nervous system arteriovenous lesions in pediatric patients. AJNR Am J Neuroradiol 2010;31:112–20.

57. Walcott B, Smith ER, Scott RM, et al. Dural arteriovenous fistulae in pediatric patients: associated conditions and treatment outcomes. J Neurointerv Surg 2013; 5:6–9.

58. Saraf R, Shrivastava M, Siddhartha W, et al. Intracranial pediatric aneurysms: endovascular treatment and its outcome. J Neurosurg Pediatr 2012;10:230–40.

59. Shields C, Bianciotto C, Jabbour P, et al. Intra-arterial chemotherapy for retinoblastoma: report no. 1, control of retinal tumors, subretinal seeds, and vitreous seeds. Arch Ophthalmol 2011;129(11):1399–406.

60. Schulenburg E, Matta B. Anaesthesia for interventional neuroradiology. Curr Opin Anaesthesiol 2011;24:426–32.

61. Ogilvy C, Stieg P, Awad I, et al. Recommendations for the management of intracranial arteriovenous malformations. Stroke 2001;32:1458–71.

62. Blanc R, Deschamps F, Orozco-Vasquez J, et al. A 6F guide sheath for endovascular treatment of intracranial aneurysms. Neuroradiology 2007;49:563–6.

63. Andreou A, Ioannidis I, Nasis N. Transarterial balloon-assisted glue embolization of high-flow arteriovenous fistulas. Neuroradiology 2008;50:267–72.

64. Lv X, Li C, Jiang Z, et al. The incidence of trigeminocardiac reflex in endovascular treatment of dural arteriovenous fistula with onyx. Interv Neuroradiol 2010;16:59–63.

65. Lv X, Wu Z, Li Y, et al. Hemorrhage risk after partial endovascular NBCA and ONYX embolization for brain arteriovenous malformation. Neurol Res 2012;34: 552–6.

66. Natarajan S, Ghodke B, Britz G, et al. Multimodality treatment of brain arteriovenous malformations with microsurgery after embolization with onyx: single-center experience and technical nuances. Neurosurgery 2008;62:1213–26.

67. Ledezma C, Hoh B, Carter B, et al. Complications of cerebral arteriovenous malformation embolization: multivariate analysis of predictive factors. Neurosurgery 2006;58:602–11.

68. Miguel K, Hirsch J, Sheridan R. Team training: a safer future for neurointerventional practice. J Neurointerv Surg 2011;3:285–7.

Neuromonitoring for Scoliosis Surgery

Chris D. Glover, MD*, Nicholas P. Carling, MD

KEYWORDS

- Anesthesia • Pediatrics • Scoliosis • Evoked potentials • Electromyography • TIVA
- Propofol

KEY POINTS

- Somatosensory evoked potentials (SSEPs) are more sensitive to inhalation agents, with decreases in amplitude and increases in latency, compared with intravenous agents, such as propofol, ketamine, dexmedetomidine, and opioids.
- Ketamine and etomidate may be used to augment SSEPs.
- Motor evoked potentials (MEPs) are the modality of choice for monitoring motor tract function, are easily abolished by inhalational agents, and negate the use of full neuromuscular blockade.
- Patients with immature neural pathways or preexisting neuromuscular disease may have abnormal baseline SSEP recordings.
- Maintenance of adequate physiologic parameters for normal neuronal functioning is critical to intraoperative neuromonitoring (IONM) during scoliosis repair.

INTRODUCTION

The management of the pediatric patient presenting for scoliosis repair places many demands on pediatric anesthesiologists. These procedures are fraught with complications and require strict attention to acid-base status, hemodynamic fluctuations, coagulation, and temperature maintenance with constant neurologic monitoring to assess for neurologic injury to the spinal cord and nerve roots. Neurologic injury resulting in postoperative paralysis or sensory loss is an uncommon yet devastating and unpredictable complication of spine surgery.[1] The goal of IONM is to assess the integrity of neural pathways that may become compromised during a procedure from direct injury to the spinal cord or nerves during instrumentation, from excessive traction placed on the spinal cord, or from inadequate perfusion of the spinal cord. IONM facilitates the identification of neural irritation or injury along a time frame that allows

Disclosures: No relevant financial disclosures.
Department of Pediatrics and Anesthesiology, Texas Children's Hospital, Baylor College of Medicine, 6621 Fannin Street, Suite A3300, Houston, TX 77030, USA
* Corresponding author.
E-mail address: chris.glover@bcm.edu

Anesthesiology Clin 32 (2014) 101–114
http://dx.doi.org/10.1016/j.anclin.2013.10.001
1932-2275/14/$ – see front matter © 2014 Elsevier Inc. All rights reserved.

for corrective anesthetic and surgical interventions. IONM also aids in defining the nature of the injury so that the surgical procedure may be completed while minimizing the risk of further neurologic injury.[2] In order to fully understand how anesthetic choices and management influence IONM during scoliosis surgery and how this may affect neurologic outcomes, it is necessary to understand how the various types of neurophysiologic monitors (SSEPs, MEPs, and electromyography [EMG]) provide an assessment of neuronal functioning, how individual anesthetic agents can affect each type of neuromonitoring technique, and how physiologic parameters can alter normal neuronal function. In doing so, it becomes evident that the anesthetic principles and considerations are similar for providing anesthetic care to adult and pediatric patients for scoliosis repair and that the immature neural development of young pediatric patients or those with preexisting neurologic deficits may render neurophysiologic monitoring more unreliable and sensitive to anesthetic techniques.[3]

BACKGROUND

Scoliosis is a multidimensional deformity of the thoracolumbar spine resulting from a lateral and rotational deformity of the spine that occurs at an incidence of 1% to 2%.[4] The degree of scoliosis is quantified by the Cobb angle, which is measured by the intersection of perpendicular lines extending from lines along the vertebral body at the superior and inferior margins of the spine deformity.

Scoliosis can be categorized as idiopathic, congenital, or neuromuscular. Idiopathic scoliosis can be further subdivided based on age of onset (**Table 1**). Despite extensive research, the cause and pathogenesis remain unknown, although leading hypotheses center on a multifactorial origin.[5,6] Adolescent idiopathic scoliosis is the most common variant seen, with an incidence of 1% to 3% in children aged 10 to 16 years. The vast majority of these patients can be managed with conservative therapy. Congenital scoliosis, a defect noted at birth that occurs from vertebral or costal maldevelopment, occurs in approximately 1 of every 1000 live births.[7] Animal studies have postulated that congenital scoliosis may be linked to maternal toxin exposure during fetal development. The rate of disease progression is rapid in the first 5 years of life and again during puberty, coinciding with stages of rapid spine growth. Neuromuscular scoliosis is commonly associated with patient conditions listed in **Table 1**. Because severity of symptoms is associated with progression of this disease, surgical correction is usually undertaken when the Cobb angle is greater than 50° in those considered skeletally mature and greater than 40° in those with skeletal immaturity to arrest progression.

Table 1
Scoliosis classification and associated conditions

Scoliosis Classification	Associated Conditions
Idiopathic	Infantile (0–3 y)
	Juvenile (4–10 y)
	Adolescent (>10 y)
Congenital	Bony deformity
	Neural tube defects
Neuromuscular	Cerebral palsy
	Poliomyelitis
	Muscular dystrophy
	Spinal muscular atrophy
	Neurofibromatosis

ANATOMY OF THE SPINAL CORD AND PATTERNS OF INJURY

The blood supply of the spinal cord is organized segmentally both along the longitudinal axis of the spinal cord as well as cross-sectionally. Longitudinally, paired posterior spinal arteries supply the posterior third of the spinal cord whereas a single anterior spinal artery supplies the anterior two-thirds of the spinal cord.[8] Longitudinally, the paired posterior arteries and the collateral circulation that exists from the subclavian and intercostal arteries provide some redundancy in blood flow for the posterior third of the cord, making the dorsal columns less likely to suffer ischemic insult. Segmentally, sulcal arteries branch from the anterior spinal artery and penetrate into the spinal cord to supply the gray matter of the anterior horn.[9] The blood flow through the anterior spinal artery is not continuous because the collateral circulation from iliac and intercostal arteries is widely variable. Watershed areas along the thoracic spine can be attributed to this lack of collateral circulation. Because of this flow variability along the anterior spinal artery, segmental medullary and radicular arteries arising from the aorta facilitate perfusion for the lower thoracic and lumbar spinal cord. The most significant of these medullary arteries is the artery of Adamkiewicz, which usually anastomoses with the anterior spinal artery between T8 and L3, and is the primary source of blood supply for the lower two-thirds of the spinal cord. As a result of this vascular anatomy, the thoracic spinal cord receives less overall blood supply than the cervical and lumbosacral regions, placing the thoracolumbar area at increased risk for hypoperfusion when manipulation of the spinal column or aorta occurs.[10]

Cerebral and spinal cord blood flow follow the same principles of autoregulation and response to hypoxia, hypercarbia, and temperature. Spinal cord perfusion is dependent on the arterial blood pressure minus the central venous pressure or the cerebrospinal fluid pressure, whichever of the latter two is higher.

Neurologic injury during spine surgery can occur from a multitude of causes and is the most concerning complication associated with repair. Injury can involve nerve roots as well as the spinal cord with a permanent deficit, such as quadriplegia, as one catastrophic outcome. A previous combined analysis by the Scoliosis Research Society and the EuroSpine in 1991 reported on 51,000 surgical cases and noted an overall injury occurrence of 0.55%.[11] Distraction of the spine accounts for the highest risk of spinal cord injury. Direct trauma from surgical manipulation, damage to vasculature with surgical exploration, and positional issues can also lead to spinal cord ischemia. Patient conditions associated with a higher incidence of neurologic injury include combined anterior and posterior repair, neuromuscular scoliosis, and significant kyphosis.[12–14] Other studies point to neurologic injury occurring at an incidence of 0.5% to 1% of all cases. A 2011 analysis of data submitted to the Scoliosis. Research Society puts the incidence of new neurologic deficit (NND) associated with spine surgery at 1%, with revision cases having 40% higher incidence of neurologic injury when compared to primary cases. Pediatric cases versus adult cases reported an approximately 60% higher incidence of NND (1.32% vs 0.83%). Cases with implants doubled the chance of developing a neurologic deficit in the perioperative period. The cohort with the highest rate of NND's at 2.5' were pediatric patients undergoing revision with implants.[15]

Positioning injuries for scoliosis repair can range from isolated neuropathies along the extremities to quadriplegia, with one study reporting a prevalence of ulnar neuropathy at 6.2% with occurrence at a higher frequency related to prone positioning and in those whose arms were abducted greater than 90°.[16,17] The presentation of spinal cord injury can be varied given the separate blood supply (discussed previously).

Selective insult to the posterior blood supply can result in sensory deficits with intact motor function. Impaired anterior cord perfusion can result in flaccid paralysis with impairment in temperature and pain (spinothalamic tracts) but intact proprioception and sensation (dorsal columns) and is known as anterior spinal artery syndrome.[18]

Intraoperative neurophysiologic monitoring allows assessment of the integrity of the spine through the surgical period with real-time feedback to allow for interventions if needed, all with the goal of minimizing neurologic injury. All potentials are graded on their respective amplitudes, latencies, and shape. With respect to injury, expected neurophysiologic findings center on a decrease in amplitude potentials and increase in latency caused by decreased impulse transmission from damaged axons. Isolated latency changes are rare and are usually associated with hypothermia and/or hypercarbia. Significant findings requiring intervention include unilateral or bilateral amplitude changes of greater than 50%.

The quest for appropriate spinal cord monitoring techniques dates back to the early 1960s when Harrington[19] introduced instrumentation to allow for correction of spinal column deformities. A retrospective analysis performed by the Scoliosis Research Society in 1974 found that from 1965 to 1971, neurologic complications occurred at a rate of 0.72%, with partial or irreversible injury occurring in 0.65% in this patient cohort.[13] This discussion is an overview of the commonly used intraoperative monitoring techniques used today; readers are referred to several excellent reviews and studies cited in the References for more detailed information.[1–3,21,24,26,32]

WAKE-UP TEST

The wake-up test has historically been considered the first method to assess the functional integrity of the motor tracts during spine surgery and remains the standard for assessing global motor function. Developed by Stagnara and Vauzelle in 1973, anesthesia was reversed after implant placement and the patient was allowed to emerge intraoperatively from anesthesia with assessment of motor function in the lower extremities.[20,21] A major limitation of this form of testing is that although it can localize injury along the motor pathway, it can only do so for a single point in time.[22] An anesthetic technique tailored for rapid emergence should be a part of the anesthetic plan in those undergoing spinal fusion. A preoperative anesthetic consultation is imperative to decrease anxiety, to inform the patient and family about the details of the wake-up process, and to answer questions related to emergence, pain, and recall. Performance of the wake-up test first entails removing the anesthetic from the patient. The operating room environment should be made conducive to wake-up with minimized noise and activity. With indications of emergence, the anesthesiologist remains at the head of the bed asking the patient to follow a set of commands, such as "move your hands" or "move your feet," with operating room personnel assessing the upper and lower extremities. Once the patient has followed the indicated commands, the anesthetic is then reintroduced.

The wake-up test is still performed today, although it occurs more commonly in the face of changing neurophysiologic findings. There seems little debate that SSEP and MEP changes likely correlate with compromised spinal cord function with much higher sensitivity and specificity than the wake-up test.[23] Risks associated with the wake-up test include the potential for recall, increased surgical time, and potential for accidental tracheal extubation. Risks can be further compounded by delay in wake-up, resulting in a potential increase in time from diagnosis to treatment in those with actual injury. Practically, the wake-up test may offer therapeutic benefit in patients with potential spinal cord compromise because the hemodynamic changes associated with an intraoperative wake-up (increase in blood pressure) would have a positive affect on spinal cord perfusion.

SOMATOSENSORY EVOKED POTENTIALS

SSEP monitoring became widely adopted in the 1980s and is currently the mainstay for intraoperative monitoring during scoliosis repair (**Fig. 1**). Tamaki and Yamane[24] and Nash and colleagues[25] first reported its use in the late 1970s. SSEPs monitor the integrity of the dorsal column-medial lemniscus pathway, which mediates proprioception, vibration, and tactile discrimination. The dorsal column medial lemniscus pathway comprises afferent axons from the periphery, which ascend via the dorsal columns and synapse at the lower medulla, where they cross the midline and form the medial lemniscus. Second- and third-order neurons project from the thalamus to the primary sensory cortex. Pain and temperature are not mediated by this process and are instead mediated through the spinothalamic system. SSEPs involve

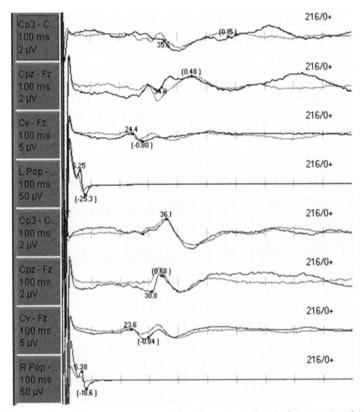

Fig. 1. SSEP recording. This recording was taken from the left side (blue tracings) and right side (red tracings) with control (green tracings). The total time of this trace is exhibited in the second line of each waveform and in this example is 100 ms. The abbreviations Cp3, Cpz, Cv, and L Pop refer to active electrode positions whereas C and Fz are the reference electrodes. 216/0 Refers to the average of 216 waveforms over the rejected waveforms during the time period measured (100 ms). The various voltages listed reference the sensitivity of the waveform. These numbers listed above are the latency associated with the examination whereas the numbers listed in parenthesis are the amplitudes.

stimulation of the peripheral nerve at fixed intervals distal to the surgical site, leading to signal propagation from the periphery to the primary sensory cortex. These cortical and subcortical signals are then recorded via scalp electrodes. The amplitude and latency of the responses are measured and then averaged with a comparison to base-line recordings to assess the potential for neurologic injury.[20] Changes are considered significant if the amplitude is decreased by more than 50% and/or the latency is increased by 10%.[26]

In addition, testing at the level of the brachial plexus can give insight into potential limb ischemia or nerve compression due to patient positioning, stretch injury to nerves, or during surgical manipulation. Any reduction of 50% in amplitude and/or a 10% increase in latency should cause personnel to investigate for potential neurologic defect.[20,26] Anesthetic agents have been noted to affect SSEPs (**Table 2**).[27,28]

Regarding safety and efficacy, a large multicenter study by Nuwer evaluated the efficacy of SSEP monitoring in diagnosing neurologic injury and found a statistically significant reduction in the total number of neurologic deficits (0.55% v 0.72%). He further pointed out that definite neurologic injury in the face of stable SSEPs occurred at a rate of just 0.063%. Although SSEP specificity in the detection of neurologic de-fects approaches 99%, a major limitation of SSEP monitoring is that this modality can only monitor the ascending dorsal columns. Specific patient conditions, such as neuromuscular scoliosis, cerebral palsy, and Down syndrome, have all been moni-tored reliably.

No information should be inferred on the integrity of the motor tracts or nerve roots from SSEP monitoring. Multiple reports of motor paresis after procedures with un-changed intraoperative SSEPs contributed to the search for other modalities to allow for improved intraoperative monitoring of the motor tracts of the spine.[23,29–32]

MOTOR EVOKED POTENTIALS

Mertin and Morton[33] revolutionized spinal cord monitoring in 1980 by demonstrating that single-pulse voltage applied transcranially could result in contralateral motor activity, marking the first time integrity of the corticospinal tract could be assessed. Translating these findings to the operating room was difficult given the

Table 2		
Anesthetic agents and somatosensory evoked potential effects		
Anesthetic Agents	**Amplitude**	**Latency**
Volatile agents • Isoflurane • Desflurane • Sevoflurane	↓↓	↑↑
Barbiturates	↓	↑
N₂O	↓	↔
Midazolam	↓	↔
Propofol	↔	↔
Dexmedetomidine	↔	↔
Opioids	↔	↔
Etomidate	↑	↔
Ketamine	↑↑	↔

Symbols: ↓, decrease; ↑, increase; ↔, no change.

exquisite sensitivity of this single-pulse technique to volatile anesthetics.[34] This difficulty remained until introduction of multiphase techniques in the mid-1990s. Incorporation of propofol into anesthesia practice was also occurring over this period.[35,36]

Currently, transcranial stimulation can occur via magnetic pulse or via electrical energy (**Fig. 2**). The multipulse technique relies on a train of 5 to 7 short successive electrical pulses applied over the scalp, causing pyramidal cell activation and summation at the anterior horn, resulting in alpha motor neuron firing of skeletal muscle.[36] Transcranial MEPs (TcMEPs) can be recorded at multiple levels. Direct (D) waves are recorded through epidural electrodes.[37] This recording of D waves is not routinely used because electrodes need to be placed into the epidural space. TcMEPs are recorded more commonly as compound muscle action potentials (cMAPs) via surface electrodes or subdermal needles placed in peripheral muscles.[38] Monitoring commonly occurs in adductor pollicis, adductor hallucis, and tibialis anterior. The control cMAP is taken in the upper extremity for comparison to the lower extremity cMAP. Determining which TcMEP changes are significant remains difficult because of the large variability seen in the response to stimulation under anesthesia.[39] The

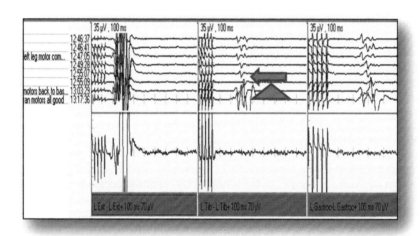

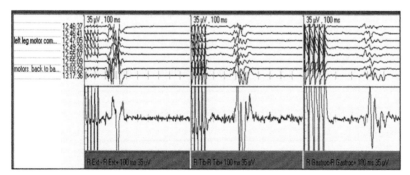

Fig. 2. TcMEP—exhibits a TcMEP tracing and associated change on the left tibial electrode (L tib) only signified by the arrow. Sensitivity of the waveform noted to be 35 μV over an examination time of 100 ms. The terminology, *R Ext – R ext*, refers to the active electrode versus the reference. TcMEP to baseline with intervention as noted by the triangle along the right side of the body. *Upper panel* is L side tracings, *Lower panel* is R side tracings.

most common methods for evaluation are using criteria similar to SSEP monitoring, where a threshold decrease signals potential injury, or evaluating TcMEP as all-or-none method.

Monitoring TcMEPs has several advantages. TcMEPs are exquisitely sensitive to spinal cord impairment and are able to detect spinal cord impairment an average of 5 minutes before SSEPs in a study by Schwartz.[23] TcMEPs are also sensitive to blood pressure changes given the blood supply to the anterior spinal cord. A major limitation with this monitoring modality is cMAPs' exquisite sensitivity to volatile anesthetics.[40] Other limitations include avoidance or limitation in the use of nondepolarizing muscle relaxants as well as the need for intermittent testing because patient movement makes operating conditions less than ideal.[41,42]

ELECTROMYOGRAPHY

Nerve root injuries are some of the most common neurologic deficits seen after scoliosis surgery, accounting for 65% of all NNDs.[11] SSEPs do not have the specificity or sensitivity to identify individual nerve root injury because they assess multiple nerve roots simultaneously. EMG assesses for potential nerve injury by electrical stimulation along the pedicle track or screw with placement of recording needle electrodes in specific muscles innervated by nerve roots (**Table 3**). A normal EMG has low-amplitude, high-frequency activity. EMG can be classified as free-running or triggered EMG.

Free-running and spontaneous EMGs are passive continuous EMGs and primarily used to map and assess nerve root function. Trauma to nerve roots causes depolarization with a subsequent muscle action potential in the muscles monitored. This sustained "burst" on the EMG is an asynchronous wave and can imply use of irrigation, contact of the nerve root, abrupt traction, and/or stretch injury. Long and sustained bursts imply nerve root irritation and potential risk for injury with the need for prompt action by the operative team (increasing blood pressure, release of distraction, and removal of hardware).[43]

Triggered EMG or stimulus-evoked EMG is primarily used to assess pedicle screw placement and cortical integrity of the vertebra. This is based on the principle that the conduction of an electrical stimulus between bone and soft tissue is relatively high. With cortical perforation, the resistance to the electrical stimulus drops significantly, resulting in cMAPs seen at very low voltage. Triggered cMAPS with unusually low voltage on EMG imply incorrect pedicle screw placement and the need for re-evaluation by a surgeon.[44,45] Pedicle screw malposition occurs in approximately 5% to 15% of cases.[46] In a large retrospective analysis of 1078 patients, Raynor and colleagues[47] found threshold levels less than 2.8 mA were 100% specific for cortical breech with sensitivity of 8.4%. Specificity decreased to 99% in those where the threshold was less than 4 mA but the sensitivity increased 4-fold. Current

Table 3	
Electromyography nerve roots and corresponding muscles monitored	
Nerve Root	**Muscles Monitored**
C8-T1	Adductor pollicis
T2-T6	Intercostals
T6-T12	Rectus abdominus
L3-L4	Vastus lateralis
L4-L5	Anterior tibialis
S1-S2	Gastrocnemius

recommendations include the use of EMG in conjunction with radiography and palpation for optimized pedicle screw placement.

Regarding anesthetic agents, EMG is resistant to their effects and, as such, there are few limitations to maintain adequate monitoring conditions besides limiting or avoiding neuromuscular blocking agents.

ANESTHETIC EFFECTS ON NEUROPHYSIOLOGIC MONITORING

Neurophysiology and its use in scoliosis repair provide multiple challenges for anesthesiologists attempting to ensure patient comfort and safety while providing an anesthetic that minimally affects monitoring techniques. The impact of anesthetics on neurophysiologic recordings cannot be overstated. All anesthetics depress synaptic activity and axonal conduction in a dose-dependent manner with prominent alterations seen in cortically generated responses.[48] The difference in the severity of the decreased amplitude and increased latency seen from anesthetics relate to an individual agent's lipid solubility, which has traditionally been considered a gauge of an anesthetic's potency. Generally speaking, increasing lipid solubility resulted in increased cortical depression.[28]

The neurophysiologic effects of the commonly used volatile anesthetics are summarized as follows. Isoflurane, sevoflurane, and desflurane all produce an initial excitation with increased alpha wave activity. With increased exposure, slowing occurs with eventual burst suppression noted. All halogenated inhalational agents produce dose-dependent decrease in amplitude and increase in latency for SSEPs with cortical responses affected to a larger degree than subcortical and peripheral nerve responses.[41] Although isoflurane is most potent given its lipophilicity, studies with sevoflurane and desflurane suggest similar effects on EEG and potential recordings. Doses up to 0.5 minimum alveolar concentration (MAC) can be used if subcortical responses are adequate, whereas the use of cortical SSEP recordings restricts use of these anesthetics.[41] With increasing concentrations of halogenated agents, a prominent effect on the anterior horn is noted with cMAP responses being eliminated.[49] Concentrations as low as 0.2 MAC largely abolish TcMEPs, relegating these agents suboptimal for use in cases where IONM is used.[40,49,50]

Nitrous oxide (N_2O) causes profound reduction in amplitude with increased latency in all neurophysiologic monitoring with suppression of cortical responses that mimic halogenated agents. Given its synergistic effects on SSEPs when combined with volatile anesthetics, use of this insoluble agent should be limited, although techniques with N_2O and opioids have been described.[35,51]

Intravenous opioids produce minimal depression of cortical SSEPs and TcMEP recordings. Studies have shown mild amplitude decreases and latency increases with opioids thought secondary to the action at the μ receptor via G protein–mediated activity, resulting in depressed electrical excitability.[41,52] Considering their minimal neurophysiologic effects and superior analgesic properties, an opioid-based anesthetic for scoliosis cases requiring monitoring seems beneficial.

Ketamine, via its N-methyl-D-aspartate receptor inhibition, and etomidate, via its γ-aminobutyric acid A ($GABA_A$) receptor inhibition, differ from halogenated agents in that they cause increases in cortical amplitudes of SSEP and MEP, making them agents of choice when monitoring responses to stimulation are difficult.[53,54] Ketamine provides superb analgesia and hypnosis, but its use must be weighed against potential dissociative effects and its effects on patients with intracranial pathology. Etomidate can be used as a constant infusion to enhance SSEP cortical recordings, but lack of analgesia, potential for enhanced seizure activity, and adrenal suppression are factors to consider with its use.[55]

Benzodiazepines and midazolam, in particular, can be used for cortical SSEP monitoring because only mild effects are seen when used at induction doses.[56] These agents also seem to have minimal effect on subcortical and peripheral responses. Use of benzodiazepines in TcMEP monitoring results in significant depression of motor potentials, necessitating caution if midazolam is used for induction.[56,57]

Propofol does not result in amplitude enhancement. This agent produces amplitude depression on induction with isoelectric EEGs seen in those given large doses. This is transient given propofol's rapid metabolism. This rapid metabolism makes propofol an excellent agent for total intravenous anesthesia (TIVA) and for rapid titration of anesthetic depth, thereby minimally effecting evoked potentials.[50]

Dexmedetomidine is a specific α_2-receptor agonist that provides anxiolysis and analgesia without depression of respiration. At clinically relevant doses, there is little effect on neurophysiologic monitoring.[58–60] This ability to minimally affect IONM in combination with its MAC-sparing ability for volatile agents makes dexmedetomidine an appealing adjunct when cases require IONM.[61,62] There are 2 reported cases of significant impairment on neurophysiologic monitoring because of dexmedetomidine's effect on TcMEP, but further analysis of the study revealed dosing well above the clinical recommendations.[63–65]

NEUROPHYSIOLOGIC CONSIDERATIONS FOR SPECIAL POPULATIONS

In neuromuscular scoliosis and associated conditions, such as cerebral palsy and Down syndrome, IONM is still possible although there is debate about its utility and reliability in patients with these conditions. SSEP monitoring has been successfully accomplished in this patient population with rates approaching 85% to 95%, but failure rates with TcMEP monitoring in those with cerebral palsy ranged from 40% to 60% based on the severity of their cerebral palsy.[66–69] Congenital scoliosis occurs at a time when a still developing nervous system may be encountered, potentially rendering IONM less reliable. Recent prospective data, however, document reliable and successful IONM in infants and young children using a TIVA technique.[70,71] When encountering scoliosis patients who fall outside the common diagnosis of idiopathic scoliosis, addition of ketamine and/or etomidate to the anesthetic plan should be considered to assist neurophysiologic monitoring.

SUMMARY

The intraoperative management of patients presenting for scoliosis repair presents many challenges for anesthesiologists. Along with normal intraoperative and perioperative concerns for a procedure that involves hemodynamic fluctuations, potentially large intraoperative blood losses, and long operating times in the prone position, there is the added challenge of providing an anesthetic regimen that permits neurophysiologic monitoring to assess for intraoperative neurologic compromise. Commonly used anesthetic techniques for scoliosis repair include combinations of opioid with propofol infusions to allow for SSEP and TcMEP monitoring. If volatile agents are administered, they should be used in low concentrations with communication to the neurophysiologist. Patients in whom there may be difficulty obtaining reliable intraoperative signals because of preexisting neurologic deficits or because of immature neurologic development may require the use of etomidate or ketamine infusions to improve SSEP amplitudes. Anesthesiologists taking care of these patients must have a comprehensive understanding of the effects of anesthetic agents on monitoring techniques, including SSEPs, TcMEPs, EMG, and the intraoperative wake-up test. Appropriate anesthetic regimens should allow for rapid emergence in case of the need to wake a patient intraoperatively to assess neurologic function and should therefore use anesthetic agents that are known to have minimal effects on the monitoring technique used.

REFERENCES

1. Owen JH. The application of intraoperative monitoring during surgery for spinal deformity. Spine (Phila Pa 1976) 1999;24(24):2649–62.
2. Pajewski TN, Arlet V, Phillips LH. Current approach on spinal cord monitoring: the point of view of the neurologist, the anesthesiologist and the spine surgeon. Eur Spine J 2007;16(Suppl 2):S115–29.
3. Sloan T. Anesthesia and intraoperative neurophysiological monitoring in children. Childs Nerv Syst 2010;26(2):227–35.
4. Altaf F, et al. Adolescent idiopathic scoliosis. BMJ 2013;30(346):f2508.
5. Yamada K, Yamamoto H, Nakagawa Y, et al. Etiology of idiopathic scoliosis. Clin Orthop Relat Res 1984;(184):50–7.
6. Machida M. Cause of idiopathic scoliosis. Spine (Phila Pa 1976) 1999;24(24): 2576–83.
7. Giampietro PF, Blan RD, Raggio CL, et al. Congenital and idiopathic scoliosis: clinical and genetic aspects. Clin Med Res 2003;1(2):125–36.
8. Bosmia AN, Hogan E, Loukas M, et al. Blood supply to the human spinal cord. I. Anatomy and hemodynamics. Clin Anat 2013. [Epub ahead of print].
9. Motoyama EK, Davis P. Smith's anesthesia for infants and children. 7th edition. Philadelphia: Mosby; 2006. xxvii, 1256 p.
10. Gregory GA. Pediatric anesthesia. 3rd edition. New York: Churchill Livingstone; 1994. xvi, 942 p.
11. Dawson EG, Sherman JE, Kanim LE, et al. Spinal cord monitoring. Results of the scoliosis research society and the European Spinal Deformity Society survey. Spine (Phila Pa 1976) 1991;16(Suppl 8):S361–4.
12. MacEwen GD, Bunnell WP, Sriram K. Acute neurological complications in the treatment of scoliosis. A report of the Scoliosis Research Society. J Bone Joint Surg Am 1975;57(3):404–8.
13. Qiu Y, Wang S, Wang B, et al. Incidence and risk factors of neurological deficits of surgical correction for scoliosis: analysis of 1373 cases at one Chinese institution. Spine (Phila Pa 1976) 2008;33(5):519–26.
14. Coe JD, Arlet V, Donaldson W, et al. Complications in spinal fusion for adolescent idiopathic scoliosis in the new millennium. A report of the Scoliosis Research Society Morbidity and Mortality Committee. Spine (Phila Pa 1976) 2006;31(3):345–9.
15. Hamilton DK, Smith JS, Sansur CA, et al. Rates of new neurologicsal deficit associated with spine surgery based on 108,419 procedures: a report of the scoliosis research society morbidity and mortality committee. Spine (Phila Pa 1976) 2011;36(15):1218–28.
16. Labrom RD, Hoskins M, Reilly CW, et al. Clinical usefulness of somatosensory evoked potentials for detection of brachial plexopathy secondary to malpositioning in scoliosis surgery. Spine (Phila Pa 1976) 2005;30(18): 2089–93.
17. Uribe JS, Kolla J, Omar H, et al. Brachial plexus injury following spinal surgery. J Neurosurg Spine 2010;13(4):552–8.
18. Zuber WF, Gaspar MR, Rothschild PD. The anterior spinal artery syndrome–a complication of abdominal aortic surgery: report of five cases and review of the literature. Ann Surg 1970;172(5):909–15.

19. Harrington PR. Treatment of scoliosis. Correction and internal fixation by spine instrumentation. J Bone Joint Surg Am 1962;44-A:591–610.
20. Mendiratta A, Emerson RG. Neurophysiologic intraoperative monitoring of scoliosis surgery. J Clin Neurophysiol 2009;26(2):62–9.
21. Vauzelle C, Stagnara P, Jouvinroux P. Functional monitoring of spinal cord activity during spinal surgery. Clin Orthop Relat Res 1973;(93):173–8.
22. Diaz JH, Lockhart CH. Postoperative quadriplegia after spinal fusion for scoliosis with intraoperative awakening. Anesth Analg 1987;66(10):1039–42.
23. Schwartz DM, Auerbach JD, Dormans JP, et al. Neurophysiological detection of impending spinal cord injury during scoliosis surgery. J Bone Joint Surg Am 2007;89(11):2440–9.
24. Tamaki T, Yamane T. Proceedings: clinical utilization of the evoked spinal cord action potential in spine and spinal cord surgery. Electroencephalogr Clin Neurophysiol 1975;39(5):539.
25. Nash CL Jr, Lorig RA, Schatzinger LA, et al. Spinal cord monitoring during operative treatment of the spine. Clin Orthop Relat Res 1977;(126):100–5.
26. Gonzalez AA, Jeyanandarajan D, Hansen C, et al. Intraoperative neurophysiological monitoring during spine surgery: a review. Neurosurg Focus 2009;27(4):E6.
27. Browning JL, Heizer ML, Baskin DS. Variations in corticomotor and somatosensory evoked potentials: effects of temperature, halothane anesthesia, and arterial partial pressure of CO_2. Anesth Analg 1992;74(5):643–8.
28. Sloan TB. Anesthetic effects on electrophysiologic recordings. J Clin Neurophysiol 1998;15(3):217–26.
29. Nuwer MR, Dawson EG, Carlson LG, et al. Somatosensory evoked potential spinal cord monitoring reduces neurologic deficits after scoliosis surgery: results of a large multicenter survey. Electroencephalography and Clinical Neurophysiology/Evoked Potentials Section January 1995;96(1):6–11.
30. Chatrian GE, Berger MS, Wirch AL. Discrepancy between intraoperative SSEP's and postoperative function. Case report. J Neurosurg 1988;69(3):450–4.
31. Lesser RP, Raudzens P, Lüders H, et al. Postoperative neurological deficits may occur despite unchanged intraoperative somatosensory evoked potentials. Ann Neurol 1986;19(1):22–5.
32. Bejjani GK, Nora PC, Vera PL, et al. The predictive value of intraoperative somatosensory evoked potential monitoring: review of 244 procedures. Neurosurgery 1998;43(3):491–8 [discussion: 498–500].
33. Merton PA, Morton HB. Stimulation of the cerebral cortex in the intact human subject. Nature 1980;285(5762):227.
34. Hicks R, Burke D, Stephen J, et al. Corticospinal volleys evoked by electrical stimulation of human motor cortex after withdrawal of volatile anaesthetics. J Physiol 1992;456:393–404.
35. Taniguchi M, Nadstawek J, Pechstein U, et al. Total intravenous anesthesia for improvement of intraoperative monitoring of somatosensory evoked potentials during aneurysm surgery. Neurosurgery 1992;31(5):891–7 [discussion: 897].
36. Taniguchi M, Cedzich C, Schramm J. Modification of cortical stimulation for motor evoked potentials under general anesthesia: technical description. Neurosurgery 1993;32(2):219–26.
37. Burke D, Hicks R, Stephen J. Anodal and cathodal stimulation of the upper-limb area of the human motor cortex. Brain 1992;115(Pt 5):1497–508.
38. Taylor BA, Fennelly ME, Taylor A, et al. Temporal summation–the key to motor evoked potential spinal cord monitoring in humans. J Neurol Neurosurg Psychiatry 1993;56(1):104–6.

39. Woodforth IJ, Hicks RG, Crawford MR, et al. Variability of motor-evoked potentials recorded during nitrous oxide anesthesia from the tibialis anterior muscle after transcranial electrical stimulation. Anesth Analg 1996;82(4):744–9.
40. Sekimoto K, Nishikawa K, Ishizeki J, et al. The effects of volatile anesthetics on intraoperative monitoring of myogenic motor-evoked potentials to transcranial electrical stimulation and on partial neuromuscular blockade during propofol/fentanyl/nitrous oxide anesthesia in humans. J Neurosurg Anesthesiol 2006; 18(2):106–11.
41. Sloan TB, Heyer EJ. Anesthesia for intraoperative neurophysiologic monitoring of the spinal cord. J Clin Neurophysiol 2002;19(5):430–43.
42. MacDonald DB, Janusz M. An approach to intraoperative neurophysiologic monitoring of thoracoabdominal aneurysm surgery. J Clin Neurophysiol 2002; 19(1):43–54.
43. Devlin VJ, Schwartz DM. Intraoperative neurophysiologic monitoring during spinal surgery. J Am Acad Orthop Surg 2007;15(9):549–60.
44. Calancie B, Lebwohl N, Madsen P, et al. Intraoperative evoked EMG monitoring in an animal model. A new technique for evaluating pedicle screw placement. Spine (Phila Pa 1976) 1992;17(10):1229–35.
45. Raynor BL, Lenke LG, Kim Y, et al. Can triggered electromyograph thresholds predict safe thoracic pedicle screw placement? Spine (Phila Pa 1976) 2002; 27(18):2030–5.
46. Hicks JM, Singla A, Shen FH, et al. Complications of pedicle screw fixation in scoliosis surgery: a systematic review. Spine (Phila Pa 1976) 2010;35(11): E465–70.
47. Raynor BL, Lenke LG, Bridwell KH, et al. Correlation between low triggered electromyographic thresholds and lumbar pedicle screw malposition: analysis of 4857 screws. Spine (Phila Pa 1976) 2007;32(24):2673–8.
48. Toleikis JR, American Society of Neurophysiological Monitoring. Intraoperative monitoring using somatosensory evoked potentials. A position statement by the American Society of Neurophysiological Monitoring. J Clin Monit Comput 2005;19(3):241–58.
49. Zentner J, Albrecht T, Heuser D. Influence of halothane, enflurane, and isoflurane on motor evoked potentials. Neurosurgery 1992;31(2):298–305.
50. Pechstein U, Nadstawek J, Zentner J, et al. Isoflurane plus nitrous oxide versus propofol for recording of motor evoked potentials after high frequency repetitive electrical stimulation. Electroencephalogr Clin Neurophysiol 1998;108(2): 175–81.
51. Sloan T, Sloan H, Rogers J. Nitrous oxide and isoflurane are synergistic with respect to amplitude and latency effects on sensory evoked potentials. J Clin Monit Comput 2010;24(2):113–23.
52. Lee VC. Spinal and cortical evoked potential studies in the ketamine-anesthetized rabbit: fentanyl exerts component-specific, naloxone-reversible changes dependent on stimulus intensity. Anesth Analg 1994;78(2):280–6.
53. Kano T, Shimoji K. The effects of ketamine and neuroleptanalgesia on the evoked electrospinogram and electromyogram in man. Anesthesiology 1974; 40(3):241–6.
54. Glassman SD, Shields CB, Linden RD, et al. Anesthetic effects on motor evoked potentials in dogs. Spine (Phila Pa 1976) 1993;18(8):1083–9.
55. Hildreth AN, Mejia VA, Maxwell RA, et al. Adrenal suppression following a single dose of etomidate for rapid sequence induction: a prospective randomized study. J Trauma 2008;65(3):573–9.

56. Sloan TB, Fugina ML, Toleikis JR. Effects of midazolam on median nerve somatosensory evoked potentials. Br J Anaesth 1990;64(5):590–3.
57. Schonle PW, Isenberg C, Crozier TA, et al. Changes of transcranially evoked motor responses in man by midazolam, a short acting benzodiazepine. Neurosci Lett 1989;101(3):321–4.
58. Tobias JD, Goble TJ, Bates G, et al. Effects of dexmedetomidine on intraoperative motor and somatosensory evoked potential monitoring during spinal surgery in adolescents. Paediatr Anaesth 2008;18(11):1082–8.
59. Kajiyama S, Nakagawa I, Hidaka S, et al. Effect of dexmedetomidine on intraoperative somatosensory evoked potential monitoring. Masui 2009;58(8):966–70 [in Japanese].
60. Bala E, Sessler DI, Nair DR, et al. Motor and somatosensory evoked potentials are well maintained in patients given dexmedetomidine during spine surgery. Anesthesiology 2008;109(3):417–25.
61. Aho M, Erkola O, Kallio A, et al. Dexmedetomidine infusion for maintenance of anesthesia in patients undergoing abdominal hysterectomy. Anesth Analg 1992;75(6):940–6.
62. Ngwenyama NE, Anderson J, Hoernschemeyer DG, et al. Effects of dexmedetomidine on propofol and remifentanil infusion rates during total intravenous anesthesia for spine surgery in adolescents. Paediatr Anaesth 2008;18(12): 1190–5.
63. Mahmoud M, Sadhasivam S, Sestokas AK, et al. Loss of transcranial electric motor evoked potentials during pediatric spine surgery with dexmedetomidine. Anesthesiology 2007;106(2):393–6.
64. Mahmoud M, Sadhasivam S, Salisbury S, et al. Susceptibility of transcranial electric motor-evoked potentials to varying targeted blood levels of dexmedetomidine during spine surgery. Anesthesiology 2010;112(6):1364–73.
65. Li BH, Lohmann JS, Schuler HG, et al. Preservation of the cortical somatosensory-evoked potential during dexmedetomidine infusion in rats. Anesth Analg 2003;96(4):1155–60 [table of contents].
66. Owen JH, Sponseller PD, Szymanski J, et al. Efficacy of multimodality spinal cord monitoring during surgery for neuromuscular scoliosis. Spine (Phila Pa 1976) 1995;20(13):1480–8.
67. Hammett TC, Boreham B, Quraishi NA, et al. Intraoperative spinal cord monitoring during the surgical correction of scoliosis due to cerebral palsy and other neuromuscular disorders. Eur Spine J 2013;22(Suppl 1):S38–41.
68. Patel AJ, Agadi S, Thomas JG, et al. Neurophysiologic intraoperative monitoring in children with Down syndrome. Childs Nerv Syst 2013;29(2):281–7.
69. DiCindio S, Theroux M, Shah S, et al. Multimodality monitoring of transcranial electric motor and somatosensory-evoked potentials during surgical correction of spinal deformity in patients with cerebral palsy and other neuromuscular disorders. Spine (Phila Pa 1976) 2003;28(16):1851–5 [discussion: 1855–6].
70. Yang J, Huang Z, Shu H, et al. Improving successful rate of transcranial electrical motor-evoked potentials monitoring during spinal surgery in young children. Eur Spine J 2012;21(5):980–4.
71. Skaggs DL, Choi PD, Rice C, et al. Efficacy of intraoperative neurologic monitoring in surgery involving a vertical expandable prosthetic titanium rib for early-onset spinal deformity. J Bone Joint Surg Am 2009;91(7):1657–63.

Brain Monitoring in Children

Michael Sury, MB, BS, FRCA, PhD

KEYWORDS

- Near infrared spectroscopy • Electroencephalography • Bispectral Index
- Amplitude-integrated electroencephalography • Oxygen • Cerebral function
- Cardiopulmonary bypass

KEY POINTS

- Electroencephalography (EEG) monitors are potential surrogate markers of conscious level and may detect effect of anesthesia on the cerebral cortex.
- Near infrared spectroscopy (NIRS) estimates cerebral oxygenation, which is affected by the balance between oxygen supply and demand.
- There is only weak evidence to support routine use of EEG or NIRS monitors to improve patient outcome.

INTRODUCTION

An anesthetist tries to keep a patient both alive and asleep during surgery. Monitoring is important to ensure that these objectives are met. Current practice is to prioritize the monitoring to ensure that anesthesia interventions maintain vital functions, such as arterial oxygen saturation, end-tidal carbon dioxide concentration, heart rate, and blood pressure. From these measurements, adequate oxygen delivery to the brain and other vital organs can be inferred. The adequacy of anesthesia can be judged by a combination of clinical observations of immobility and autonomic quiescence and also by the estimation of the concentration of anesthesia drug in the brain. These strategies are achievable and are standard, yet they may not be enough in some circumstances, and their accuracy is not certain.

Measuring unconsciousness is an ideal. Efficacy of anesthesia depends to a large extent on the concentration of anesthesia in the brain. Yet, this is not a simple concept. First, there is uncertainty about the concentration in blood. The assumption about an insoluble vapor achieving a steady state concentration in blood and therefore the brain is not supported by data, although few data are available to strengthen or weaken our assumptions. Data in adults measuring the washin and washout of 1% isoflurane show that there are delays between expired breath and blood concentrations, and, more importantly, there are wide limits of agreement within a patient group, which makes

Department of Anaesthesia, Great Ormond Street Hospital, Great Ormond Street, London WC1N 3JH, UK
E-mail address: mike.sury@gosh.nhs.uk

Anesthesiology Clin 32 (2014) 115–132
http://dx.doi.org/10.1016/j.anclin.2013.10.013
1932-2275/14/$ – see front matter © 2014 Elsevier Inc. All rights reserved. anesthesiology.theclinics.com

the prediction of blood concentration, from expired breath analysis, weaker than expected.[1] Similar variation exists between target and measured blood concentrations of propofol.[2]

The effective dose is guided by minimal alveolar concentration (MAC). Because MAC is a median value, it should be expected that some patients are not adequately anesthetized, and that the dose needs to be increased. Conversely, some patients are excessively anesthetized, perhaps with dangerous cardiovascular depression, and the dose needs to be decreased. The measurement of MAC itself has many problems.[3] Efficacy of a chosen dose can, to a degree, be assumed from immobility, yet, movement itself may be largely related to lack of suppression of the spinal cord rather than the brain.[4] It may be assumed, from our understanding of MAC studies, that the dose required to cause unconsciousness is lower than that required for immobility, which is reassuring, but the use of muscle relaxants removes the usefulness of immobility.

The sum of these considerations is that anesthesiologists should not be 100% confident about the effects of a specified anesthesia dose on the brain. This dose is too much for some patients and too little for others. This review examines monitoring devices that may help to reduce this uncertainty in children. Moreover, it focuses on direct brain monitoring rather than discussion of monitors of vital cardiorespiratory or autonomic functions, which are important but are indirect monitors of brain function.

The usefulness of direct monitoring may be best shown in the scenario of uncertainty about the adequacy of oxygen delivery to the brain. For example, hypotension is a common phenomenon in anesthesia,[5] and yet there is uncertainty about the lower limit of blood pressure that ensures safe brain oxygenation. If hypotension is assumed to be caused by cardiovascular depression by an excessive dose of anesthesia, what is the dose that is compatible with both safe brain oxygenation and unconsciousness? This problem may be one of the main causes for accidental awareness under anesthesia. Awareness in children[6] is uncommon, but the ability to monitor the brain, which helps to detect and prevent awareness, is a long-held aspiration for the specialty.

Brain monitoring for anesthesia needs to be simple, robust, and reliable. Monitors that use noninvasive skin sensors, placed on the scalp, should have these qualities. Monitors of the following are considered in this article:

- Cerebral electrical activity
- Cortical oxygenation

Monitors of blood flow are also important. Monitoring cardiac output and cerebral blood flow is valuable but these topics not considered in this article because they are not direct monitors of brain function. Moreover, they are not sufficiently developed, as yet, to be practicable in small infants in a wide range of settings.

ELECTRICAL ACTIVITY
Electroencephalography

Before discussing processed electroencephalography (EEG), an understanding of the raw EEG is essential. The EEG is believed to represent a composite of the postsynaptic potentials of the cerebral cortex. The origin of this activity, whether it is from central or peripheral parts of the brain, remains unclear, but there is evidence that thalamic signals play a key role in the arousal of the cortex. The EEG is a complex random-looking waveform and has many constituent oscillations of varying amplitude and frequency.

Signals are detected from skin electrodes placed on the scalp. The signal amplitude is smaller than the electrocardiogram (ECG) (microvolts compared with millivolts), and therefore, the electrodes must have a secure contact on the skin so that the imped-ance does not vary. The electromyogram (EMG) has oscillations of higher amplitude than the EEG, and, because the EMG has wide frequency band, it can easily obscure the EEG. Muscle activity is a problem and makes interpretation of the underlying EEG uncertain, and electrical equipment (eg, diathermy) can cause large interference.

Frontal electrodes are favored for practical reasons, but the amplitude of oscillations from centroparietal electrodes is larger. Three simple features of the EEG can be visualized:

- Steady oscillations
  - A complex waveform that seems to be continuous
- Accidentals
  - Sudden short-lived oscillations often of higher amplitude (eg, epileptiform activity)
- Silence
  - Periods of inactivity may be continuous or intermittent. Intermittent silence alternating with high-amplitude oscillations is called burst suppression (perhaps more easily understood as bursts and suppressions)

Visualizing the EEG requires expertise, but it allows immediate recognition of small and irregular changes. For example, δ (<4 Hz), θ (4–7 Hz), α (8–13 Hz), and β (15–30 Hz) waves, can be identified on short samples. Some degree of processing, using Fourier analysis principles, enables long samples (a few seconds) to be assessed, and the amplitude of constituent frequencies can be estimated. Using both the visual expert eye and Fourier analysis, changes in the EEG during anesthesia have been described. In children older than 6 months, the awake EEG is low amplitude and irregular with α waves on a background of fast oscillations (**Table 1**).

With anesthesia induction (eg, sevoflurane), the EEG becomes more regular. As depth increases, the oscillations increase in amplitude. Lower-frequency, large-ampli-tude oscillations become prominent. Deeper anesthesia causes burst suppression; periods of silence become longer until there is no EEG activity. EEG changes during sevoflurane washout and emergence are usually the same but in reverse. Propofol and other vapor anesthetics are believed to have similar effects on the EEG. Ketamine and nitrous oxide cause low-amplitude, high-frequency oscillations. Opioids, in clin-ical doses, have an effect on the EEG that is probably indirect, in that they counter the arousal activity related to pain.

The EEG of awake and naturally sleeping infants less than 6 months old is different mainly in terms of lower amplitude and the presence of irregular periods of low activity frequently seen before the age of 3 months, known as trace alternant (**Table 2**).[7,8] Few researchers have investigated the effects of anesthesia on the EEG in young infants.[9] There are 4 studies published on the effects of sevoflurane or isoflurane in infants and small children. Constant and colleagues[10] induced sevoflurane anesthesia in children aged 2 to 12 years old. As the dose increased, the total spectral power increased, especially in low-frequency bands, and 14-Hz to 30-Hz oscillations were common. Emergence was studied by Davidson and colleagues[8] (in infants, toddlers, and chil-dren) and Lo and colleagues[11] (in children aged 22 days to 3.6 years). Both studies found that infants younger than 6 months have low EEG power during anesthesia, but in older infants, there is appreciable power between 2 and 30 Hz. However, 1 study reported that the power within the 2-Hz to 20-Hz range decreased,[8] and in the other study,[11] power within the 8-Hz to 30-Hz range increased. A recent observation study of sevoflurane washout in infants found that anesthesia was associated with appre-ciable power between frequencies 5 and 20 Hz and that this decreased as sevoflurane

Table 1 EEG characteristics during wakefulness, natural sleep, and anesthesia after 6 months of age		
State	Dominant EEG Oscillations	EMG
Alert wakefulness	30–50 Hz (low amplitude)	High
Relaxed wakefulness	8–13 Hz	Reduced
Non-REM sleep		
Stage 1	2–3 s of 4–8 Hz and sharp waves over vertex	Reduced
Stage 2	Sleep spindles appear 1–3/min Up to 20% of epoch high-amplitude δ waves K complexes appear	Minimal
Stage 3	20%–50% of epoch δ waves	Minimal
Stage 4	>50% of epoch δ waves	Minimal
REM sleep	Irregular 30–50 Hz (low amplitude) Sharp waves replaced by saw tooth waves at 2–5 Hz	Sporadic bursts
Sedation through to light anesthesia	Continuous oscillations of low amplitude and mixed frequency Progressing to higher amplitude (1–4 Hz) and middle amplitude (8–16 Hz) (approximately) oscillations	Minimal
Anesthesia through to excessively deep anesthesia	Burst suppression (alternating periods of high-amplitude mainly low-frequency oscillations with suppression), increasing length of suppression until electrical silence	Minimal

Abbreviation: REM, rapid eye movement.

washed out (**Fig. 1**).[12] Moreover, the band power during anesthesia was age related, and only infants older than 3 months had appreciable band power (**Figs. 2** and **3**). Whether or not band power is useful enough to assess level of consciousness is not known; nevertheless, it is possible that EEG power changes indicate that an anesthetic drug is having a pharmacologic effect on the brain, and this may be useful in some circumstances. For example, in the development of target controlled infusion pharmacokinetic models, the effect site concentration is assumed to peak based on EEG changes.

Processed EEG

Given that the raw EEG may be difficult for nonneurophysiologists to interpret, there has been, and continues to be, a demand for a simple EEG variable that is useful in the assessment of conscious level. In addition, both the practical constraints of scalp electrodes and the technical complexities of signal interference, filtration, and amplification have prevented widespread use of EEG monitors during anesthesia. Clinicians need a robust monitor, easy to set up and reliable under the conditions of an operating theater rather than an EEG laboratory.

Amplitude-integrated EEG

In the 1960s, the cerebral function monitor (CFM) was developed.[13] It amplified and filtered a single EEG channel to create a fast (within seconds) visual printout of the trend of median and the range of the amplitude of a wide frequency band. The band amplitude was represented on a logarithmic scale. The observer could see simple characteristics of the EEG, for example, the minimum amplitude, reflected the

Table 2
EEG characteristics of natural sleep in infants younger than 6 months

Gestation	EEG
Maternal transabdominal recordings of fetal EEG (from 12 wk)	Continuous low-amplitude irregular activity unrelated to body movement
24–27 wk	*Tracé discontinu* Bursts of high-amplitude slow waves lasting 2–6 s mainly over the occipital cortex followed by depressed activity lasting 4–8 s
28 wk	REM-like Bursts of low-amplitude high-frequency oscillations
32–36 wk	*Tracé discontinu* becomes associated with quiet sleep
36 wk	*Tracé discontinu* is replaced by *tracé alternant* 3-s to 8-s bursts of high-amplitude slow-frequency activity interspersed with low-amplitude mixed-frequency oscillations Disappears by 48 wk
37 wk	REM-like becomes more continuous and associated with eye movements
Term–3 mo	Active sleep (eyes closed) Mixed irregular activity and EMG prominent Quiet sleep Single pattern of high-amplitude low-frequency Awake (eyes open) Low-amplitude, irregular activity
3–6 mo	Non-REM and REM sleep develop gradually from 3 mo from quiet sleep and active sleep, respectively Sleep spindles Appear by 4 wk of age Become characteristic of non-REM sleep by 3 mo K complexes appear by 6 mo

Abbreviation: REM, rapid eye movement.

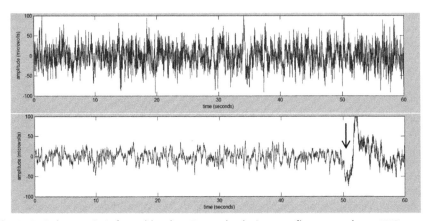

Fig. 1. EEG changes in infant older than 3 months during sevoflurane washout. EEG recordings from centroparietal channel. Top trace is during sevoflurane anesthesia after surgery (end-tidal sevoflurane 2.5%). Bottom trace is 5 minutes later: note that the amplitude has decreased. The arrow marks movement artifact at the point of awakening.

A

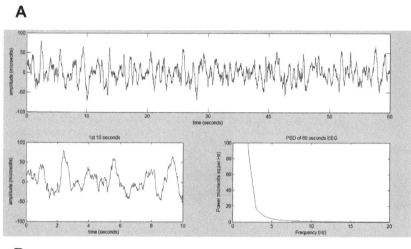

B

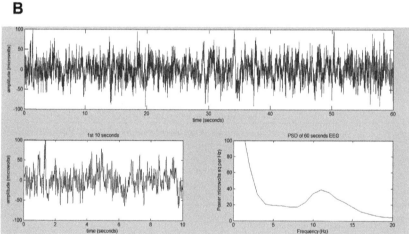

Fig. 2. Power spectrum of EEG during anesthesia in infants. EEG recordings and power spectrum density (PSD) taken during sevoflurane anesthesia after surgery from a centroparietal channel in 2 infants: (A) aged 45 weeks and (B) aged 66 weeks (postmenstrual age). Note that the older infant has appreciable power in frequency band 5 to 20 Hz, unlike the younger infant.

presence of EEG suppression, and zero minimum amplitude coincident with a high maximum amplitude indicated burst suppression. Epileptiform activity could also be easily distinguished. The CFM algorithm used was restricted for commercial reasons, and a monitor with a similar algorithm, known as the amplitude-integrated EEG (aEEG), is now frequently used in neonatal intensive care[14] and has been used in trials as an important outcome variable to test the usefulness of hypothermic protection after hypoxic ischemic encephalopathy[15] and to detect cortical suppression and convulsion activity.[16] Some neonatologists urge caution in its interpretation.[17] aEEG detection of cerebral ischemia during or after cardiopulmonary bypass (CPB) is poor.[18] Few studies have been undertaken to test its use in discerning depth of anesthesia in children, and results have not been promising.[19]

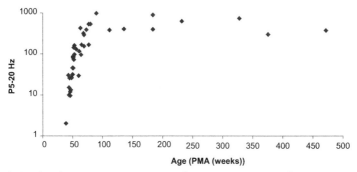

Fig. 3. Relationship between EEG power and age. Age is in weeks postmenstrual age. P5-20 Hz is the EEG band power (μV^2) between the frequencies 5 to 20 Hz recorded from a centroparietal channel.

Spectral edge frequency

Spectral edge frequency (SEF) is the frequency at lower than which 90% (SEF90) of the EEG power exists (or other specified % cutoff); it is a commonly studied variable calculated from the frequency spectrum. Hayashi and colleagues[20] studied SEF90 in neonates and infants during sevoflurane concentrations between 0.5% and 2%. In children aged 6 months to 2 years, SEF90 was inversely related to sevoflurane concentration, but this was less so in younger infants. In children younger than 3 months, SEF90 was always low.

A common problem with processing EEG is that any simple variable may miss the appearance of burst suppression. Consequently, as the concentration of anesthesia increases, the EEG power (and SEF) first increases and then decreases as periods of electrical silence dominate (**Fig. 4**).

Bispectral Index and other processed EEG

The Bispectral Index (BIS) (Covidien, Mansfield, MA), Entropy (E-Entropy, GE Healthcare, Milwaukee, WI), and Narcotrend (Narcotrend-Compact M, MonitorTechnik, GmbH & Co, Bad Bramstedt, Germany) monitors are 3 examples of sophisticated processed EEG monitors that rely on forehead electrodes. Each monitor has its algorithm to process the EEG and create a score from 0 to 100, representing the extremes of coma

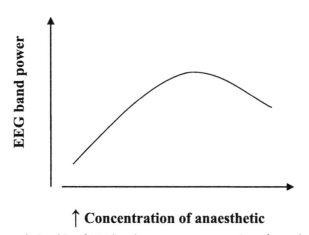

Fig. 4. Common relationship of EEG band power to concentration of anesthetic.

and full wakefulness; the scores correlate with depth of sedation and anesthesia. The BIS uses a combination of power in various frequency bands, phase synchronization between common frequencies, EMG, and burst suppression.[21–24] Entropy measures the predictability (or the sinusoidal nature) of 2 wide EEG frequency bands: 0.8 to 30 Hz for state entropy and 0.8 to 47 Hz for response entropy[25]; the latter incorporates the frontalis EMG.[26] The Narcotrend algorithm has not been published.[27] All have been developed to produce scores that decrease with both decreasing conscious level (as defined by a validated scale of behavior)[28,29] and also with increasing doses of propofol and concentrations of common inhalational agents.[30–32] All monitors of EEG are poor predictors of movement during surgery. This situation is not only because the monitor takes at least 15 seconds to calculate a score but also because pain activates spinal reflexes that remain present even in major brain damage.[33] Also, a major consideration is that an anesthesia drug can have an immobilizing effect at the spinal cord in addition to cortical effects.[4] For example, in a study, comparing the effects of equi-MAC doses of halothane and sevoflurane, the BIS scores were higher during halothane,[34] and this may be because halothane has a greater immobilizing action at the spinal cord than sevoflurane rather than because halothane has a different effect on the EEG and BIS.[35–37]

Evidence of usefulness in maintaining adequate depth of sedation or anesthesia A BIS score of 40 to 60 is said to be compatible with absence of explicit recall. Large trials have been conducted in adults. Myles and colleagues[38] showed that adults who could not receive high-dose anesthesia (eg, patients with cardiac disease, known difficult intubation, obstetric emergencies) had a reduced chance of accidental awareness if their anesthesia was directed by BIS. Avidan and colleagues[39] showed that, in protecting against awareness, BIS was equivalent to monitoring end-tidal anesthesia vapor concentration (maintaining a level >0.7 MAC). More recent studies showed no benefit of BIS in reducing awareness.[40,41] Nevertheless a UK National Institute for Health and Care Excellence technology evaluation[42] recommended that BIS and similar monitors may be helpful "for avoiding excessively light or deep anesthesia in patients at high risk of adverse outcomes from general anesthesia" and should be considered especially in total intravenous anesthesia (TIVA) techniques.

The distinction between explicit recall and awareness is important, and Russell has shown that when the BIS (or the Narcotrend) monitor is tested with the isolated forearm technique, neither monitor is able to distinguish between patients who can communicate and those who cannot.[43–45] Further studies may show that the cutoff BIS score (and equivalent) may be important. BIS may (or may not) help to reduce explicit recall, but it does not detect intraoperative awareness in patients who are pain free. There are no studies showing the effect on the EEG of awareness during painful surgery.

BIS can mislead. Changes may not be caused by anesthetic drugs. BIS can change with ischemia,[46] epileptiform activity,[47] muscle relaxants,[48] and hypoglycemia.[49] Ketamine[50] and nitrous oxide[51] tend to increase the BIS score and increase depth of anesthesia.

BIS scores correlate with isoflurane concentration in children older than 1 year similarly to adults.[52] However, several studies have reported that BIS scores are less reliable in infants and small children.[53–60] Given equi-MAC concentrations of sevoflurane, BIS scores are slightly higher in infants than in children.[56] In another study of sevoflurane,[61] the highest BIS scores tended to be in the youngest infants, and BIS increased paradoxically when sevoflurane increased from 3% to 4%. Comparing 3-month-old with 6-month-old infants with 7-month-old to 12-month-old infants, given equal doses of sevoflurane, BIS scores were lower in the youngest infants.[62] This situation may be because there is a special feature of young infants or perhaps because the BIS algorithm is not appropriate for their EEG. The unprocessed EEG needs to be seen to help to explain these changes.

At the end of anesthesia, BIS correlates with conscious level poorly in infants[59] and in children.[57] Infants who are not in pain (eg, who have an effective caudal local anesthetic block) need only very small concentrations of sevoflurane to keep BIS low.[55] Davidson and colleagues[58] measured BIS and Entropy in children having cardiac angiography and found that the youngest patients had the widest variation of scores and awakening occurred at lowest scores. In a study of children recovering after circumcision, infants often awoke spontaneously at low BIS scores.[53]

In a study of 60 children receiving anesthesia with propofol and remifentanil,[63] EEG variables were similarly predictive of awakening in children older than 1 year but were least reliable in infants. The prediction of conscious level in a sedation technique using propofol was poor, and this shows that BIS is not useful in directing the dose of propofol to achieve a certain level of sedation.[64] Probably, the presence of pain is influential in the steadiness of the BIS score.

The Narcotrend was used successfully to predict recovery in children older than 1 year.[65] Three other studies showed that Entropy and BIS are similar in monitoring conscious level in children older than 1 year.[26,58,59]

Evidence of usefulness in avoiding excessive depth of anesthesia There are 2 studies that support the concept that low BIS scores (perhaps related to excessive doses of anesthesia), in adults, are associated with poor long-term outcomes.[66,67] Whether these findings are related directly to low BIS scores or perhaps the finding relates to a vulnerable population has yet to be determined, but BIS and other monitors may protect vulnerable adults from long-term harm. In infants, studies of excessive depth may be important in avoiding potential harm of neuroapoptosis, but this problem has been shown only in young animals after heavy and prolonged anesthesia exposure, and the EEG effects of deep anesthesia have not been studied.

Evoked Potentials

Auditory evoked potentials (AEP) are EEG signals provoked by a noise (a click) and detected from EEG scalp electrodes. Noise causes a neural transmission through the brainstem, the midbrain, and the cortex. Averaging the EEG over many clicks removes background EEG; a typical accurate recording (used for assessment of hearing deficit) may use 1024 clicks at 6 Hz and take 2 to 3 minutes to achieve. The AEP waveform has characteristic peaks and troughs, which are time related to brainstem, early cortical, and late cortical transmission.[68,69] The brainstem component is resistant to anesthesia, and the late cortical component disappears easily at low doses of anesthetic. However, the early cortical waveform is suppressed by anesthesia (peaks are delayed) in a dose-dependent manner and is therefore useful as a depth monitor.[68–70] The Alaris AEP monitor can estimate the shape of the AEP within 2 to 6 seconds by autoregressive modeling.[71] From the AEP waveform, an algorithm calculates an index from 0 to 100 (representing deep coma and fully awake states, respectively).

This method is vulnerable to non-EEG interference; EMG, in particular, caused by contraction of the posterior auricular muscle, is triggered by noise, and therefore, the AEP is least reliable when muscle relaxants are not used.[68] A study of children older than 2 years found that AEP was as reliable as in adults,[72] but ECG interference is a problem in infants.[73]

EEG-evoked activity from pain may be detected in preterm infants whose background EEG is low amplitude.[74]

Learning points on EEG monitors

- EEG monitors are potential surrogate markers of conscious level and may be rational indicators of effect of anesthesia on the cerebral cortex
- They can be misleading; ischemia and hypoglycemia cause EEG suppression
- In respect of processed EEG and monitoring conscious level during anesthesia, monitoring inhaled anesthetic vapor concentration is equally effective (or perhaps more so); EEG monitors do not detect awareness shown by the isolated forearm technique
- Processed EEG monitors may be useful in some situations, perhaps with TIVA, in which monitoring blood level is not possible
- BIS monitoring in children (not infants) is similar to adults (BIS monitoring is less reliable in infants)
- The EEG in young infants is irregular and low amplitude
- aEEG is potentially useful as a simple monitor of seizure activity in intensive care

---

OXYGENATION MEASURED BY NEAR INFRARED SPECTROSCOPY
Validation

Near infrared spectroscopy (NIRS) measures and monitors nonpulsatile regional tissue oxygenation ($rSatHbo_2$) continuously. ($rSatHbo_2$ is used throughout this article to represent the % of saturated hemoglobin [Hb] relative to the total Hb assumed to be present in the cerebral cortex and surrounding tissue.) Light is beamed from a forehead scalp sensor into underlying tissue, and the wavelength spectrum of light reflected back is measured and processed to estimate the amount of oxygenated Hb in the cerebral cortex. Some monitors estimate the % of Hb saturated relative to the total Hb, and others monitor the absolute amount of saturated Hb.[75] Comparison of these 2 types of monitors in adult patients showed that there were large differences in $rSatHbo_2$.[76]

NIRS also detects the redox state of cytochrome, which in theory is useful, except that the contribution of this to the signal may be too small to be useful.[77] All the tissue components underlying the sensor make a contribution to the $rSatHbo_2$ and have different oxygen saturations. The venous and arterial blood, for example, make different contributions to $rSatHbo_2$, and the tissue itself, which consumes oxygen, has an $rSatHbo_2$ less than 100%. Various NIRS machines are calibrated to assume that tissue has a fixed volume contribution of venous and arterial blood. Cerebral vasoconstriction and dilatation, of capillaries, arteries, and veins, may have a large influence on the $rSatHbo_2$. Normal $rSatHbo_2$ in noncyanotic infants breathing air is approximately 70%, and this is reduced in cyanotic children to 40% to 60%.[78] Inactive cerebral tissue (perhaps as a result of cooling or irreversible cortical damage) may have $rSatHbo_2$ close to 100%, and excessively active cortical tissue (such as in status epilepticus) may have low $rSatHbo_2$, despite adequate oxygen supply. Regional brain metabolic activity and blood flow are linked, and in neonates the ratio is higher than in older infants, which means that neonates may be more vulnerable to ischemia.[79]

The mixed venous saturation has been used to detect cerebral hypoxia and may therefore help to validate $rSatHbo_2$. In cyanotic children, some investigators have reported a good correlation with $rSatHbo_2$[80] and others have not.[81,82] The use of jugular venous saturation ($Sjvo_2$) should be more closely related to $rSatHbo_2$, yet the evidence does not support this idea. $Sjvo_2$ and $rSatHbo_2$ were poorly correlated in 1 study in children (except in infants),[83] but others found that correlation was high.[84–86] In a comparison of both mixed venous and jugular bulb saturations, $SjvO_2$ was found to correlate with $rSatHbo_2$ least.[87]

$rSatHbo_2$ During Cardiac Surgery

Typically, CPB increases $rSatHbo_2$ close to 100%, because cerebral oxygen demand has been reduced by anesthesia and hypothermia.[75,88,89] As brain circulation is interrupted, $rSatHbo_2$ falls to 70% of the baseline by approximately 20 to 40 minutes, and then reperfusion should restore $rSatHbo_2$ to normal (**Fig. 5**).[88] In some neonates and infants, long deep hypothermic cardiac arrest (DHCA) times delay the recovery of $rSatHbo_2$.[90,91] Reduced $rSatHbo_2$ may be caused by increased cerebral metabolism as result of a metabolic debt.[79]

Kurth and colleagues[92,93] studied the $rSatHbo_2$ in a piglet model. Baseline $rSatHbo_2$ was 68%, and $rSatHbo_2$ was highly correlated with sagittal sinus oxygen saturation. As oxygen levels were reduced, cerebral lactate levels began to increase at $rSatHbo_2$ of 44%, major EEG change occurred at 37%, and brain adenosine triphosphate decreased at 33%. Sakamoto and colleagues[94,95] exposed piglets to DHCA and showed that hypothermia slowed the reduction of $rSatHbo_2$ during circulatory arrest and that at 15°C animals could tolerate 25 minutes of cerebral circulatory arrest without obvious neurologic harm.

In a study of neonates and infants having repair of aortic coarctation, $rSatHbo_2$ decreased during aortic clamping and the decrease was greatest in neonates, although this may have been related to the possible presence of collateral circulation in older infants.[96,97]

Outcome After Cardiac Surgery

The incidence of severe brain damage after CPB surgery has decreased over the decades, largely because of improvements in the management of CPB.[98–100] The causes of global delay and epilepsy seen after CPB may be related to ischemia and inflammation from emboli[101] or from underlying congenital brain defects and genetic factors.[102] The institution of low-flow CPB (either continuous or intermittent) during what would otherwise be circulatory arrest has been shown, in randomized controlled trials, to reduce early postoperative seizures[103] and, at age 1 year, to improve neurologic assessment scores.[104]

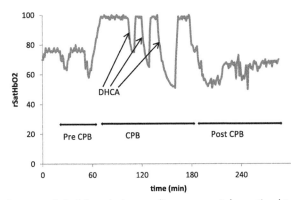

Fig. 5. Typical changes of $rSatHbo_2$ during cardiac surgery. Schematized typical changes in $rSatHbo_2$ with time in an infant undergoing cardiac surgery under CPB and deep hypothermic cardiac arrest (DHCA). (*Adapted from* Andropoulos DB, Stayer SA, Diaz LK, et al. Neurological monitoring for congenital heart surgery. Anesth Analg 2004;99(5):1369; with permission.)

With this background, the use of NIRS and transcranial Doppler assessment of cerebral blood flow was begun, in 1 center, without a control group, and may have improved outcome.[105] Nevertheless, the potential of NIRS[106] is uncertain and debated. Many hospitals have decided to use NIRS as a standard monitor, yet, others have not.[106] The evidence for improved outcome is limited to small studies. In a study of 26 children undergoing DHCA,[88] 3 patients, all with low rSatHbo$_2$, had seizures or prolonged coma. In a larger study of 250 patients, 41% had prolonged low rSatHbo$_2$ ($\geq$20% decrease from baseline) and 25% of these had prolonged coma, seizures, or hemiparesis.[105] Andropoulos and colleagues[75] reported that approximately 90% of all interventions to improve cerebral oxygenation during cardiac surgery are triggered by low rSatHbo$_2$ rather than EEG or other monitors. In another review, Hirsch and colleagues[107] concluded that NIRS may contribute to multimodal monitoring of cerebral perfusion and function, but evidence is lacking for its value as an isolated monitor. A recent review in respect of adult cardiac surgery concluded that current evidence for improved outcome using NIRS was low level.[108]

Notwithstanding all the debate, cerebral white matter changes, infarction, and hemorrhage are seen on magnetic resonance imaging scans in about a third of neonates after CBP.[109]

Usefulness in Neonatal Intensive Care

NIRS is being used as trend monitor of cerebral oxygenation in neonatal intensive care.[110] Only small studies so far have tested the usefulness of NIRS; in a study of 18 preterm infants, of whom 9 died of cerebral deterioration, rSatHbo$_2$ increased, as a result of reduced cerebral oxygen consumption, in those with a poor outcome.[111]

Overview of the usefulness of cerebral oxygenation monitors
- rSatHbo$_2$ estimates cortical oxygenation and is affected by the balance between oxygen supply and demand
- Isolated readings should be interpreted after consideration of the clinical circumstances
- It may be useful as a trend monitor and for goal-directed management
- It may be more useful in detection of cortical function when combined with other monitors of EEG and blood flow

SUMMARY

Applying scalp sensors in the operating theater, intensive care, or resuscitation scenarios to detect and monitor brain function is achievable, practical, and affordable. However, the clinician needs to understand that the modalities are complex and the output of the monitor needs careful interpretation. The monitor itself may have technical problems, and a single reading must be considered with caution. These monitors may have a use for monitoring trends in specific situations, but good evidence does not yet support their widespread use. Nevertheless, research should continue to investigate their role. Future techniques and treatments may show that these monitors can monitor brain function and prevent harm.

REFERENCES

1. Frei FJ, Zbinden AM, Thomson DA, et al. Is the end-tidal partial pressure of isoflurane a good predictor of its arterial partial pressure? Br J Anaesth 1991;66(3): 331–9.

2. Rigouzzo A, Servin F, Constant I. Pharmacokinetic-pharmacodynamic modeling of propofol in children. Anesthesiology 2010;113(2):343–52.
3. Aranake A, Mashour GA, Avidan MS. Minimum alveolar concentration: ongoing relevance and clinical utility. Anaesthesia 2013;68(5):512–22.
4. Antognini JF, Carstens E. In vivo characterization of clinical anaesthesia and its components. Br J Anaesth 2002;89(1):156–66.
5. Nafiu OO, Kheterpal S, Morris M, et al. Incidence and risk factors for preincision hypotension in a noncardiac pediatric surgical population. Paediatr Anaesth 2009;19(3):232–9.
6. Davidson AJ, Smith KR, Blusse Van Oud-Alblas HJ, et al. Awareness in children: a secondary analysis of five cohort studies. Anaesthesia 2011;66(6):446–54.
7. Constant I, Sabourdin N. The EEG signal: a window on the cortical brain activity. Paediatr Anaesth 2012;22(6):539–52.
8. Davidson AJ, Sale SM, Wong C, et al. The electroencephalograph during anesthesia and emergence in infants and children. Paediatr Anaesth 2008;18(1):60–70.
9. Davidson AJ. Measuring anesthesia in children using the EEG. Paediatr Anaesth 2006;16(4):374–87.
10. Constant I, Dubois MC, Piat V, et al. Changes in electroencephalogram and autonomic cardiovascular activity during induction of anesthesia with sevoflurane compared with halothane in children. Anesthesiology 1999;91(6):1604–15.
11. Lo SS, Sobol JB, Mallavaram N, et al. Anesthetic-specific electroencephalographic patterns during emergence from sevoflurane and isoflurane in infants and children. Paediatr Anaesth 2009;19(12):1157–65.
12. Sury MR, Worley A, Boyd S. EEG power spectra in infants during sevoflurane washout: changes related to maturation. Br J Anaesth, in press.
13. Schwartz MS, Colvin MP, Prior PF, et al. The cerebral function monitor. Its value in predicting the neurological outcome in patients undergoing cardiopulmonary by-pass. Anaesthesia 1973;28(6):611–8.
14. Toet MC, van der Meij W, de Vries LS, et al. Comparison between simultaneously recorded amplitude integrated electroencephalogram (cerebral function monitor) and standard electroencephalogram in neonates. Pediatrics 2002;109(5):772–9.
15. Gluckman PD, Wyatt JS, Azzopardi D, et al. Selective head cooling with mild systemic hypothermia after neonatal encephalopathy: multicentre randomised trial. Lancet 2005;365(9460):663–70.
16. van Rooij LG, Toet MC, Osredkar D, et al. Recovery of amplitude integrated electroencephalographic background patterns within 24 hours of perinatal asphyxia. Arch Dis Child Fetal Neonatal Ed 2005;90(3):F245–51.
17. Tao JD, Mathur AM. Using amplitude-integrated EEG in neonatal intensive care. J Perinatol 2010;30(Suppl):S73–81.
18. Andropoulos DB, Mizrahi EM, Hrachovy RA, et al. Electroencephalographic seizures after neonatal cardiac surgery with high-flow cardiopulmonary bypass. Anesth Analg 2010;110(6):1680–5.
19. McKeever S, Johnston L, Davidson AJ. An observational study exploring amplitude-integrated electroencephalogram and spectral edge frequency during paediatric anaesthesia. Anaesth Intensive Care 2012;40(2):275–84.
20. Hayashi K, Shigemi K, Sawa T. Neonatal electroencephalography shows low sensitivity to anesthesia. Neurosci Lett 2012;517(2):87–91.
21. Rampil IJ. A primer for EEG signal processing in anesthesia. Anesthesiology 1998;89:980–1002.

22. Todd MM. EEGs, EEG processing, and the bispectral index. Anesthesiology 1998;89(4):815–7.
23. Dumermuth G, Huber PJ, Kleiner B, et al. Analysis of the interrelations between frequency bands of the EEG by means of the bispectrum. A preliminary study. Electroencephalogr Clin Neurophysiol 1971;31(2):137–48.
24. Sigl JC, Chamoun NG. An introduction to bispectral analysis for the electroencephalogram. J Clin Monit 1994;10(6):392–404.
25. Jantti V, Alahuhta S, Barnard J, et al. Spectral entropy–what has it to do with anaesthesia, and the EEG? Br J Anaesth 2004;93(1):150–2.
26. Davidson AJ, Kim MJ, Sangolt GK. Entropy and bispectral index during anaesthesia in children. Anaesth Intensive Care 2004;32(4):485–93.
27. Schultz B, Grouven U, Schultz A. Automatic classification algorithms of the EEG monitor Narcotrend for routinely recorded EEG data from general anaesthesia: a validation study. Biomed Tech (Berl) 2002;47(1–2):9–13.
28. Katoh T, Suzuki A, Ikeda K. Electroencephalographic derivatives as a tool for predicting the depth of sedation and anesthesia induced by sevoflurane. Anesthesiology 1998;88(3):642–50.
29. Kreuer S, Biedler A, Larsen R, et al. The Narcotrend–a new EEG monitor designed to measure the depth of anaesthesia. A comparison with bispectral index monitoring during propofol-remifentanil-anaesthesia. Anaesthesist 2001;50(12):921–5.
30. Schwender D, Daunderer M, Klasing S, et al. Power spectral analysis of the electroencephalogram during increasing end-expiratory concentrations of isoflurane, desflurane and sevoflurane. Anaesthesia 1998;53(4):335–42.
31. Vanluchene AL, Vereecke H, Thas O, et al. Spectral entropy as an electroencephalographic measure of anesthetic drug effect: a comparison with bispectral index and processed midlatency auditory evoked response. Anesthesiology 2004;101(1):34–42.
32. Struys M, Versichelen L, Mortier E, et al. Comparison of spontaneous frontal EMG, EEG power spectrum and bispectral index to monitor propofol drug effect and emergence. Acta Anaesthesiol Scand 1998;42(6):628–36.
33. Rampil IJ, Mason P, Singh H. Anesthetic potency (MAC) is independent of forebrain structures in the rat. Anesthesiology 1993;78(4):707–12.
34. Schwab HS, Seeberger MD, Eger EI, et al. Sevoflurane decreases bispectral index values more than does halothane at equal MAC multiples. Anesth Analg 2004;99(6):1723–7 table.
35. Antognini JF, Carstens E. Increasing isoflurane from 0.9 to 1.1 minimum alveolar concentration minimally affects dorsal horn cell responses to noxious stimulation. Anesthesiology 1999;90(1):208–14.
36. Antognini JF, Carstens E, Atherley R. Does the immobilizing effect of thiopental in brain exceed that of halothane? Anesthesiology 2002;96(4):980–6.
37. Jinks SL, Martin JT, Carstens E, et al. Peri-MAC depression of a nociceptive withdrawal reflex is accompanied by reduced dorsal horn activity with halothane but not isoflurane. Anesthesiology 2003;98(5):1128–38.
38. Myles PS, Leslie K, McNeil J, et al. Bispectral index monitoring to prevent awareness during anaesthesia: the B-Aware randomised controlled trial. Lancet 2004;363(9423):1757–63.
39. Avidan MS, Zhang L, Burnside BA, et al. Anesthesia awareness and the bispectral index. N Engl J Med 2008;358(11):1097–108.
40. Avidan MS, Jacobsohn E, Glick D, et al. Prevention of intraoperative awareness in a high-risk surgical population. N Engl J Med 2011;365(7):591–600.

41. Mashour GA, Shanks A, Tremper KK, et al. Prevention of intraoperative aware-ness with explicit recall in an unselected surgical population: a randomized comparative effectiveness trial. Anesthesiology 2012;117(4):717–25.
42. Smith D, Andrzejowski J, Smith A. Certainty and uncertainty: NICE guidance on 'depth of anaesthesia' monitoring. Anaesthesia 2013;68(10):1000–5.
43. Russell IF. The Narcotrend 'depth of anaesthesia' monitor cannot reliably detect consciousness during general anaesthesia: an investigation using the isolated forearm technique. Br J Anaesth 2006;96(3):346–52.
44. Russell IF. BIS-guided isoflurane/relaxant anaesthesia monitored with the iso-lated forearm technique. Br J Anaesth 2008;100:875–6.
45. Russell IF. BIS-guided TCI propofol/remifentanil anaesthesia monitored with the isolated forearm technique. Br J Anaesth 2008;100:876.
46. Estruch-Perez MJ, Barbera-Alacreu M, Ausina-Aguilar A, et al. Bispectral index variations in patients with neurological deficits during awake carotid endarterec-tomy. Eur J Anaesthesiol 2010;27(4):359–63.
47. Sandin M, Thorn SE, Dahlqvist A, et al. Effects of pain stimulation on bispectral index, heart rate and blood pressure at different minimal alveolar concentration values of sevoflurane. Acta Anaesthesiol Scand 2008;52(3):420–6.
48. Messner M, Beese U, Romstock J, et al. The bispectral index declines during neuromuscular block in fully awake persons. Anesth Analg 2003;97(2):488–91 table.
49. Alkire MT. Quantitative EEG correlations with brain glucose metabolic rate dur-ing anesthesia in volunteers. Anesthesiology 1998;89(2):323–33.
50. Sakai T, Singh H, Mi WD, et al. The effect of ketamine on clinical endpoints of hypnosis and EEG variables during propofol infusion. Acta Anaesthesiol Scand 1999;43(2):212–6.
51. Barr G, Jakobsson JG, Owall A, et al. Nitrous oxide does not alter bispectral in-dex: study with nitrous oxide as sole agent and as an adjunct to i.v. anaesthesia. Br J Anaesth 1999;82(6):827–30.
52. Whyte S, Booker PD. Bispectral index during isoflurane anesthesia in pediatric patients. Anesth Analg 2004;98(6):1644–9.
53. Davidson AJ, McCann ME, Devavaram P, et al. The differences in the bispectral index between infants and children during emergence from anesthesia after circumcision surgery. Anesth Analg 2001;93(2):326–30.
54. Degoute CS, Macabeo C, Dubreuil C, et al. EEG bispectral index and hypnotic component of anaesthesia induced by sevoflurane: comparison between chil-dren and adults. Br J Anaesth 2001;86(2):209–12.
55. Bannister CF, Brosius KK, Sigl JC, et al. The effect of bispectral index monitoring on anesthetic use and recovery in children anesthetized with sevoflurane in nitrous oxide. Anesth Analg 2001;92(4):877–81.
56. Denman WT, Swanson EL, Rosow D, et al. Pediatric evaluation of the bispectral index (BIS) monitor and correlation of BIS with end-tidal sevoflurane concentra-tion in infants and children. Anesth Analg 2000;90(4):872–7.
57. Rodriguez RA, Hall LE, Duggan S, et al. The bispectral index does not correlate with clinical signs of inhalational anesthesia during sevoflurane induction and arousal in children. Can J Anaesth 2004;51(5):472–80.
58. Davidson AJ, Huang GH, Rebmann CS, et al. Performance of entropy and Bis-pectral Index as measures of anaesthesia effect in children of different ages. Br J Anaesth 2005;95(5):674–9.
59. Klockars JG, Hiller A, Ranta S, et al. Spectral entropy as a measure of hypnosis in children. Anesthesiology 2006;104(4):708–17.

60. Kern D, Fourcade O, Mazoit JX, et al. The relationship between bispectral index and endtidal concentration of sevoflurane during anesthesia and recovery in spontaneously ventilating children. Paediatr Anaesth 2007;17(3):249–54.
61. Kim HS, Oh AY, Kim CS, et al. Correlation of bispectral index with end-tidal sevoflurane concentration and age in infants and children. Br J Anaesth 2005;95(3): 362–6.
62. Kawaraguchi Y, Fukumitsu K, Kinouchi K, et al. Bispectral index (BIS) in infants anesthetized with sevoflurane in nitrous oxide and oxygen. Masui 2003;52(4): 389–93 [in Japanese].
63. Jeleazcov C, Schmidt J, Schmitz B, et al. EEG variables as measures of arousal during propofol anaesthesia for general surgery in children: rational selection and age dependence. Br J Anaesth 2007;99(6):845–54.
64. Powers KS, Nazarian EB, Tapyrik SA, et al. Bispectral index as a guide for titration of propofol during procedural sedation among children. Pediatrics 2005; 115(6):1666–74.
65. Weber F, Hollnberger H, Gruber M, et al. The correlation of the Narcotrend Index with endtidal sevoflurane concentrations and hemodynamic parameters in children. Paediatr Anaesth 2005;15(9):727–32.
66. Monk TG, Saini V, Weldon BC, et al. Anesthetic management and one-year mortality after noncardiac surgery. Anesth Analg 2005;100(1):4–10.
67. Lindholm ML, Traff S, Granath F, et al. Mortality within 2 years after surgery in relation to low intraoperative bispectral index values and preexisting malignant disease. Anesth Analg 2009;108(2):508–12.
68. Thornton C, Sharpe RM. Evoked responses in anaesthesia. Br J Anaesth 1998; 81(5):771–81.
69. Thornton C, Newton DE. The auditory evoked potential: a measure of depth of anaesthesia. Ballieres Clin Anaesthesiol 1989;3:559–85.
70. Gajraj RJ, Doi M, Mantzaridis H, et al. Comparison of bispectral EEG analysis and auditory evoked potentials for monitoring depth of anaesthesia during propofol anaesthesia. Br J Anaesth 1999;82(5):672–8.
71. Jensen EW, Lindholm P, Henneberg SW. Autoregressive modeling with exogenous input of middle-latency auditory-evoked potentials to measure rapid changes in depth of anesthesia. Methods Inf Med 1996;35(3):256–60.
72. Daunderer M, Feuerecker MS, Scheller B, et al. Midlatency auditory evoked potentials in children: effect of age and general anaesthesia. Br J Anaesth 2007; 99(6):837–44.
73. Bell SL, Smith DC, Allen R, et al. Recording the middle latency response of the auditory evoked potential as a measure of depth of anaesthesia. A technical note. Br J Anaesth 2004;92(3):442–5.
74. Slater R, Worley A, Fabrizi L, et al. Evoked potentials generated by noxious stimulation in the human infant brain. Eur J Pain 2010;14(3):321–6.
75. Andropoulos DB, Stayer SA, Diaz LK, et al. Neurological monitoring for congenital heart surgery. Anesth Analg 2004;99(5):1365–75.
76. Yoshitani K, Kawaguchi M, Tatsumi K, et al. A comparison of the INVOS 4100 and the NIRO 300 near-infrared spectrophotometers. Anesth Analg 2002;94(3):586–90.
77. Sakamoto T, Jonas RA, Stock UA, et al. Utility and limitations of near-infrared spectroscopy during cardiopulmonary bypass in a piglet model. Pediatr Res 2001;49(6):770–6.
78. Kurth CD, Steven JM, Nicholson SC, et al. Kinetics of cerebral deoxygenation during deep hypothermic circulatory arrest in neonates. Anesthesiology 1992; 77:656–61.

79. Greeley WJ, Kern FH. Cerebral blood flow and metabolism during infant cardiac surgery. Paediatr Anaesth 1994;4:285–99.
80. Ranucci M, Isgro G, De la TT, et al. Near-infrared spectroscopy correlates with continuous superior vena cava oxygen saturation in pediatric cardiac surgery patients. Paediatr Anaesth 2008;18(12):1163–9.
81. Ricci Z, Garisto C, Favia I, et al. Cerebral NIRS as a marker of superior vena cava oxygen saturation in neonates with congenital heart disease. Paediatr Anaesth 2010;20(11):1040–5.
82. Knirsch W, Stutz K, Kretschmar O, et al. Regional cerebral oxygenation by NIRS does not correlate with central or jugular venous oxygen saturation during interventional catheterisation in children. Acta Anaesthesiol Scand 2008;52(10):1370–4.
83. Daubeney PE, Pilkington SN, Janke E, et al. Cerebral oxygenation measured by near-infrared spectroscopy: comparison with jugular bulb oximetry. Ann Thorac Surg 1996;61(3):930–4.
84. Abdul-Khaliq H, Troitzsch D, Berger F, et al. Regional transcranial oximetry with near infrared spectroscopy (NIRS) in comparison with measuring oxygen saturation in the jugular bulb in infants and children for monitoring cerebral oxygenation. Biomed Tech (Berl) 2000;45(11):328–32.
85. Abdul-Khaliq H, Troitzsch D, Schubert S, et al. Cerebral oxygen monitoring during neonatal cardiopulmonary bypass and deep hypothermic circulatory arrest. Thorac Cardiovasc Surg 2002;50(2):77–81.
86. Yoxall CW, Weindling AM, Dawani NH, et al. Measurement of cerebral venous oxyhemoglobin saturation in children by near-infrared spectroscopy and partial jugular venous occlusion. Pediatr Res 1995;38(3):319–23.
87. Nagdyman N, Fleck T, Schubert S, et al. Comparison between cerebral tissue oxygenation index measured by near-infrared spectroscopy and venous jugular bulb saturation in children. Intensive Care Med 2005;31(6):846–50.
88. Kurth CD, Steven JM, Nicolson SC. Cerebral oxygenation during pediatric cardiac surgery using deep hypothermic circulatory arrest. Anesthesiology 1995; 82:74–82.
89. Daubeney PE, Smith DC, Pilkington SN, et al. Cerebral oxygenation during paediatric cardiac surgery: identification of vulnerable periods using near infrared spectroscopy. Eur J Cardiothorac Surg 1998;13(4):370–7.
90. Toet MC, Flinterman A, Laar I, et al. Cerebral oxygen saturation and electrical brain activity before, during, and up to 36 hours after arterial switch procedure in neonates without pre-existing brain damage: its relationship to neurodevelopmental outcome. Exp Brain Res 2005;165(3):343–50.
91. Greeley WJ, Bracey VA, Ungerleider RM, et al. Recovery of cerebral metabolism and mitochondrial oxidation state is delayed after hypothermic circulatory arrest. Circulation 1991;84(Suppl 5):III400–6.
92. Kurth CD, Levy WJ, McCann J. Near-infrared spectroscopy cerebral oxygen saturation thresholds for hypoxia-ischemia in piglets. J Cereb Blood Flow Metab 2002;22(3):335–41.
93. Kurth CD, McCann JC, Wu J, et al. Cerebral oxygen saturation-time threshold for hypoxic-ischemic injury in piglets. Anesth Analg 2009;108(4):1268–77.
94. Sakamoto T, Zurakowski D, Duebener LF, et al. Combination of alpha-stat strategy and hemodilution exacerbates neurologic injury in a survival piglet model with deep hypothermic circulatory arrest. Ann Thorac Surg 2002;73(1):180–9.
95. Sakamoto T, Hatsuoka S, Stock UA, et al. Prediction of safe duration of hypothermic circulatory arrest by near-infrared spectroscopy. J Thorac Cardiovasc Surg 2001;122(2):339–50.

96. Polito A, Ricci Z, Di CL, et al. Bilateral cerebral near infrared spectroscopy monitoring during surgery for neonatal coarctation of the aorta. Paediatr Anaesth 2007;17(9):906–7.

97. Berens RJ, Stuth EA, Robertson FA, et al. Near infrared spectroscopy monitoring during pediatric aortic coarctation repair. Paediatr Anaesth 2006;16(7):777–81.

98. Fallon P, Aparicio JM, Elliott MJ, et al. Incidence of neurological complications of surgery for congenital heart disease. Arch Dis Child 1995;72(5):418–22.

99. Ferry PC. Neurologic sequelae of cardiac surgery in children. Am J Dis Child 1987;141(3):309–12.

100. Menache CC, du Plessis AJ, Wessel DL. Current incidence of acute neurologic complications after open-heart operations in children. Ann Thorac Surg 2002; 73(6):1752–8.

101. du Plessis AJ. Mechanisms of brain injury during infant cardiac surgery. Semin Pediatr Neurol 1999;6(1):32–47.

102. Wernovsky G, Newburger J. Neurologic and developmental morbidity in children with complex congenital heart disease. J Pediatr 2003;142(1):6–8.

103. Newburger JW, Jonas RA, Wernovsky G, et al. A comparison of the perioperative neurologic effects of hypothermic circulatory arrest versus low-flow cardiopulmonary bypass in infant heart surgery. N Engl J Med 1993;329(15):1057–64.

104. Bellinger DC, Jonas RA, Rappaport LA, et al. Developmental and neurologic status of children after heart surgery with hypothermic circulatory arrest or low-flow cardiopulmonary bypass. N Engl J Med 1995;332(9):549–55.

105. Austin EH III, Edmonds HL Jr, Auden SM, et al. Benefit of neurophysiologic monitoring for pediatric cardiac surgery. J Thorac Cardiovasc Surg 1997; 114(5):707–15, 717.

106. Kasman N, Brady K. Cerebral oximetry for pediatric anesthesia: why do intelligent clinicians disagree? Paediatr Anaesth 2011;21(5):473–8.

107. Hirsch JC, Charpie JR, Ohye RG, et al. Near-infrared spectroscopy: what we know and what we need to know–a systematic review of the congenital heart disease literature. J Thorac Cardiovasc Surg 2009;137(1):154–9.

108. Zheng F, Sheinberg R, Yee MS, et al. Cerebral near-infrared spectroscopy monitoring and neurologic outcomes in adult cardiac surgery patients: a systematic review. Anesth Analg 2013;116(3):663–76.

109. Andropoulos DB, Hunter JV, Nelson DP, et al. Brain immaturity is associated with brain injury before and after neonatal cardiac surgery with high-flow bypass and cerebral oxygenation monitoring. J Thorac Cardiovasc Surg 2010;139(3): 543–56.

110. Toet MC, Lemmers PM. Brain monitoring in neonates. Early Hum Dev 2009; 85(2):77–84.

111. Toet MC, Lemmers PM, van Schelven LJ, et al. Cerebral oxygenation and electrical activity after birth asphyxia: their relation to outcome. Pediatrics 2006; 117(2):333–9.

Anesthetic Neurotoxicity

Erica P. Lin, MD[a],*, Sulpicio G. Soriano, MD[b],
Andreas W. Loepke, MD, PhD[a]

KEYWORDS

- Anesthetics • Anesthesia • Neurodegeneration • Neurotoxicity • Infant
- Learning impairment

KEY POINTS

- All routinely used sedatives and anesthetics have been found to be neurotoxic in a wide variety of animal species, including nonhuman primates.
- The neurotoxic effects observed in animals include apoptotic neuronal cell death, diminished neuronal density, decreased neurogenesis and gliogenesis, alterations in dendritic architecture, diminution of neurotrophic factors, mitochondrial degeneration, cytoskeletal destabilization, abnormal reentry into the cell cycle, as well as learning and memory impairment.
- Several epidemiologic human studies have observed an association between anesthesia exposure in patients younger than 3 to 4 years and subsequent learning disabilities and language abnormalities, whereas others have not found this link.
- It remains unresolved whether anesthetic exposure or other factors, such as the underlying medical condition, surgery, inflammatory response, pain, physiologic abnormalities during surgery, or other unknown factors, are causative for the observed abnormalities.
- Additional animal and clinical research is urgently needed to identify the phenomenon's underlying mechanisms, to assess human applicability, and to devise mitigating strategies.

ANESTHESIA: WITHOUT SENSATION

Since its inception more than a century ago, anesthesia has become a mainstay of modern medicine for its ability to render patients insensate to the trauma and stress associated with surgery. Because millions of children across the world are anesthetized annually for surgeries, painful procedures, and imaging studies,[1] it has been widely thought that once the anesthetic effects dissipate, the brain returns to its

Funding Sources. None.
Conflicts of Interest. None to disclose.
[a] Department of Anesthesiology, Cincinnati Children's Hospital Medical Center, University of Cincinnati College of Medicine, 3333 Burnet Ave, MLC 2001, Cincinnati, OH 45229, USA;
[b] Department of Anesthesiology, Perioperative, and Pain Medicine, Harvard Medical School, Boston Children's Hospital, 300 Longwood Ave, Boston, MA 02115, USA
* Corresponding author.
E-mail address: erica.lin@cchmc.org

baseline preanesthetic state. More recently, however, a growing body of work, largely arising from laboratory research, has suggested that sedatives and anesthetics may have long-lasting effects on the brain. Numerous animal studies have observed histologic evidence for widespread apoptotic brain cell death (an inborn cell suicide program) immediately following anesthetic exposure early in life. Several laboratory studies have also demonstrated subsequent neurocognitive impairment. Although it remains unknown whether the phenomenon's mechanism parallels that of the anesthetic state, these findings have raised substantial disquiet within the anesthesia community, as well as among parents and government regulators, about the safety of clinical pediatric anesthesia practice. Accordingly, this article provides an overview of the currently available data from both animal experiments and human clinical studies regarding the effects of sedatives and anesthetics on the developing brain.

HISTORICAL PEDIATRIC ANESTHESIA: NOCICEPTIVE RESPONSE OF THE IMMATURE BRAIN TO SURGERY

Before the 1980s, general anesthetics were routinely withheld from critically ill neonates to avoid hemodynamic deterioration and myocardial depression. Instead, perioperative drug regimens were oftentimes limited to muscle relaxants and nitrous oxide,[2] termed the *Liverpool technique*, because neonates were widely thought to be incapable of perceiving or localizing pain. However, with the recognition that painful stimulation can also lead to dramatic metabolic and endocrine responses in premature infants,[3] an analgesic component was introduced into neonatal anesthesia practice to blunt the nociceptive response to surgery.[4]

Robinson and Gregory[5] showed that fentanyl analgesia can be safely administered in neonates and is effective in blunting response to surgical stimulation. A randomized study in newborn patients undergoing ligation of a patent ductus arteriosus further demonstrated that the addition of fentanyl to the minimalist, conventional approach of nitrous oxide and paralytic blunted the hormonal response to surgery and improved the postoperative outcome by decreasing circulatory and metabolic complications.[4] Since then, the advent of modern analgesics and anesthetics, including the development of volatile anesthetics with less myocardial depressant effects, combined with better monitoring techniques has afforded critically ill infants the benefits of amnesia and analgesia, while enabling surgeons to undertake more extensive and effective interventions in one of the most vulnerable of patient populations. General anesthesia for stressful procedures may even lead to immediate improvement in outcomes because a small retrospective study noted that patients undergoing ward reduction of gastroschisis without general anesthesia had a higher incidence of serious adverse events, such as bowel ischemia, need for total parenteral nutrition, and unplanned reoperation, compared with neonates receiving anesthesia for the same procedure.[6] Moreover, untreated painful stimulation early in life has been demonstrated to be associated with subsequent diminished cognition and motor function.[7,8]

Importantly, widespread neuronal cell death has been found following repetitive painful stimulation in neonatal animals[9] and resulted in adverse neurologic outcomes, including altered pain processing, changes in behavioral and cognitive function that increase vulnerability to stress- and anxiety-mediated disorders, and chronic pain syndromes.[10] Concomitant administration of a small dose of ketamine significantly reduced pain-induced neuronal degeneration.[9] Furthermore, preemptive morphine analgesia administered in neonatal rats before an inflammatory injury facilitated recovery from the insult and attenuated subsequent injury-induced hypoalgesia in adolescence and adulthood.[11]

Taken together, both animal and human data suggest that pain-related stress early in life is deleterious to nervous system development and that blunting this stress pharmacologically may interrupt some of these degenerative effects.

DELETERIOUS EFFECTS OF ANESTHETIC EXPOSURE ON THE DEVELOPING BRAIN

Concerns regarding the potentially debilitating effects of general anesthesia on neurologic function initially arose in the 1950s based on personality changes, such as increased temper tantrums, night terrors, fear behaviors, and bed wetting, that were observed especially in younger children following exposure to vinyl ether, cyclopropane, or ethyl chloride for otolaryngologic surgery.[12] Because these abnormalities were partially alleviated by the timely administration of preoperative sedative medication before induction, it was thought that these behavioral abnormalities were more psychological in nature than a representation of underlying structural defects. Several decades later, animal studies investigating the potential occupational health hazards for pregnant health care workers chronically exposed to low levels of anesthetic waste gases observed delayed synaptogenesis and behavioral abnormalities in offspring born to rats exposed to subclinical doses of halothane during their intrauterine life.[13,14]

Approximately 10 years ago, potentially deleterious effects of anesthetics on young children garnered interest, first, in a ground-breaking study observing widespread neuronal degeneration following repeated N-methyl-D-aspartate (NMDA) antagonist exposure in neonatal rat pups[15] and later in a sentinel article by Jevtovic-Todorovic and colleagues[16] focusing on the deleterious effects of a combination of the gamma-aminobutyric acid (GABA)-agonist midazolam, the combined GABA-agonist and NMDA-antagonist isoflurane, and the NMDA-antagonist nitrous oxide. Neonatal rats exposed to doses sufficient to maintain a surgical depth of anesthesia experienced both immediate brain cell loss and impaired long-term neurocognitive function. Subsequent studies by a variety of research groups have documented acute neuronal cell loss, altered dendritic architecture, reduced synaptic density, decreased levels of neurotrophic factors, mitochondrial degeneration, destabilization of the cytoskeleton, and cell cycle abnormalities following exposure to all routinely used anesthetics and sedatives in several immature animal species, including chicks, mice, rats, guinea pigs, swine, sheep, and rhesus monkeys (reviewed in[17]). Of these deleterious effects during anesthetic exposure, the most obvious manifestation is widespread neuronal cell death.

APOPTOTIC NEURONAL CELL DEATH: PHYSIOLOGIC AND PATHOLOGIC

Brain architecture is not static, and both expanding and regressing processes are integral to proper brain development. In utero and postnatally during infancy, the human brain undergoes rapid growth. The resulting overabundance of neurons and neuronal connections is followed by neuronal cell death and synaptic regression, resulting in less than half the neurons generated during development actually surviving into adulthood.[18] This naturally occurring, cellular suicide process of programed cell death, termed *apoptosis*, is required for normal central nervous system structure and function; disruptions to this process can result in brain malformation and intrauterine demise.[19] Across species, apoptotic cell death is characteristic of normal tissue turnover, embryonic cell death, and metamorphosis. Cells that are either functionally redundant or potentially detrimental are eliminated. For example, apoptosis is responsible for the embryonal cell death of interdigital mesenchymal tissue separating the digits of hands and feet as well as the ablation of tail tissue as part of tadpole metamorphosis in amphibians. In contrast to the other main cell death process, necrosis, apoptosis represents an active, energy-consuming process. This built-in cell death program involves cascades of caspases, which are specialized enzymes that break down cells by chromatin aggregation, nuclear and cytoplasmic condensation, deconstruction of cellular debris into apoptotic bodies, and removal of this material without the need for an extensive inflammatory response.[20]

Physiologic apoptotic cell death also occurs in the developing brain, but its distribution is not uniform across all regions because it is regulated by the age and maturational stage of the neurons. Specifically, 2 main waves of natural apoptosis take place: one involving progenitor cells occurs during early embryonic development and another, later apoptotic surge affects early postmitotic neurons.[21] The former wave of neuronal elimination is thought to regulate the neuronal precursor pool size, whereas the latter adjusts the size of neuronal populations to their functional target fields.[22] Furthermore, it also fine tunes the neuronal wiring of developing networks by eliminating neurons with erroneous or inadequate projections and selectively removing long axon collaterals.[23] Throughout this process, the development of neighboring cells is largely unaffected.

Given the central role of physiologic apoptosis in the immature brain, cell death triggered by pathologic insults during development, such as hypoxia and ischemia, may also heavily depend on this process and manifest with mixed characteristics of both apoptosis and necrosis.[22] As an example, although early hypoxic-ischemic injury in the striatum and cortex of neonatal rats seems necrotic, later injury in the thalamus, white matter tracts, and synaptic terminal fields remote from the primary injury is more consistent with apoptosis, suggesting that neuronal death outside of the immediate infarct area may heavily depend on apoptotic pathways.[24]

APOPTOSIS: TRIGGERED BY ANESTHETICS

A widespread and dramatic increase in neuronal cell death has been observed immediately following anesthetic exposure in a wide variety of animal species when compared with unanesthetized littermates. The cell death pathway has been delineated as using both intrinsic and extrinsic apoptotic pathways.[25] The final step of this process involves activated caspase 3, which has been repeatedly used as a marker in laboratory studies to assess and quantify anesthesia-induced neuroapoptosis. Caspase 3 expression is dose- and exposure-time dependent and has been observed as early as 1 hour into an isoflurane anesthetic exposure.[26] All commonly clinically used anesthetics and sedatives, such as ketamine, desflurane, enflurane, halothane, isoflurane, sevoflurane, xenon, diazepam, midazolam, chloral hydrate, pentobarbital, and propofol, have been found in either in vivo or in vitro experiments to dramatically increase neuroapoptosis. These observations have been made in such diverse species as nematodes, chicks, mice, rats, guinea pigs, piglets, and rhesus monkeys. Neurotoxic effects are amplified when several sedatives and anesthetics acting by different mechanism are combined in that midazolam and nitrous oxide by themselves do not seem to trigger neuroapoptosis but dramatically increase neuroapoptosis when administered in combination with isoflurane.[16] Even though of great concern, given the inability to directly assess human brain histology immediately following exposure, it remains unclear whether similar neurodegeneration occurs in infants and children undergoing anesthesia.

LONG-TERM BRAIN CELL VIABILITY AND NEUROLOGIC FUNCTION FOLLOWING ANESTHESIA IN ANIMALS

Even in animals, whereby brain injury can be assessed histologically, it remains unclear whether neuronal elimination early in life leads to permanent cell loss and dysfunction or can be compensated for by the developing brain's capacity for repair. Only a few studies have examined neonatal neuroapoptosis and adult neuronal density and function. In a neonatal rat model, a 6-hour exposure to midazolam, isoflurane, and nitrous oxide early in life dramatically increased neuroapoptosis immediately following the exposure and led to impaired learning in the Morris water maze in young adulthood and older age[16] as well as decreased adult neuronal density in brain regions affected by neonatal neuroapoptosis.[27] In the same animals, however, other tests of behavior and learning, such as acoustic startle response, sensorimotor tests, spontaneous locomotor behavior, and learning and memory in the radial arms maze, were unaffected, making it unclear which specific neurocognitive domains are affected long-term by neonatal anesthetic exposure. Although another study in neonatal mice also demonstrated dramatically increased apoptotic cellular degeneration in several brain regions immediately following a 6-hour isoflurane exposure, subsequent neuronal density in the corresponding brain regions was unaltered, and Morris water maze learning and memory function remained intact into adulthood.[28] Thus, it remains unresolved whether differences in species or anesthetic regimen can lead to differential effects on the neurocognitive outcome. In a different study involving isoflurane exposure in neonatal rats, neuronal apoptosis was observed after 2 hours of exposure. However, long-term neurologic abnormalities only appeared after 4 hours of anesthesia exposure.[29] Furthermore, in this same study, 4 hours of carbon dioxide–induced hypercarbia induced substantial apoptotic cell death but did not result in long-term deficits and actually improved spatial reference and working memory.[29] Accordingly, this study calls into question the relationship between early neuronal cell death and subsequent neurologic sequelae; it remains to be determined whether there exists a threshold exposure time after which neurologic abnormalities occur. Similar uncertainty exists regarding a possible threshold dose of intravenous anesthetic necessary to induce permanent neurologic damage. Exposure to 20 to 50 mg/kg/h of ketamine for 24 hours in newborn rhesus monkeys has been demonstrated to lead to long-term impairment of memory tasks and motivation,[30] but this dosing far exceeds routine clinical regimens.

THE CLINICAL RELEVANCE OF EXPERIMENTAL CONDITIONS: CAN ANIMAL STUDIES BE DIRECTLY TRANSLATED TO HUMANS?

The mounting evidence of neurotoxic effects following anesthetic exposure in animal models is undeniable. However, it remains highly questionable whether these findings can be directly translated from bench to bedside (or operating room). Anesthetic management in rodent models is vastly different when compared with clinical practice, in particular the lack of continuous monitoring and airway management. The neonatal animals' diminutive size precludes continuous hemodynamic monitoring as well as repeated blood measurements of acid-base status and glucose levels, both standard practices in clinical anesthesia for human neonates. In small rodents, anesthetic exposure can result in extensive hypercarbia, metabolic acidosis, and hypoglycemia,[28,29,31] derangements that would not be tolerated without acute intervention in clinical practice and can lead to neurologic deficits.[32]

Most laboratory studies also do not include continuous stimulation of the central nervous system by surgical stress and pain, which is frequently encountered during human perioperative care. The effects of surgical anesthesia in children, in the face of these noxious stimuli, may be different than prolonged unstimulated anesthetic exposure in the animal laboratory. Animal studies attempting to address this question, however, by introducing caustic injections or tail clamping as nociceptive stimuli have provided conflicting results. One study showed increased neuroapoptosis following isoflurane anesthesia exposure with painful stimulation.[33] Another study noted that a small anesthetic dose of ketamine alleviated the deleterious effects of painful stimulation,[9] whereas a separate report showed that concurrent noxious stimulus mitigated the expected neuroapoptosis associated with a large dose of ketamine.[34] Finally, a study using isoflurane did not demonstrate any differences between stimulated and unstimulated animals.[35] Importantly, when factoring in long-term outcomes, neonatal stress in animals has been found to obviate adult behavioral impairment because of neonatally administered morphine.[36]

The anesthetic dose required to cause injury is also a point of controversy that limits the immediate application of animal data to human practice. Unlike in pediatric anesthesia, clinical doses of volatile anesthetics for only a few hours can be lethal in a significant percentage of small rodents.[28,29] Furthermore, the doses of intravenous agents necessary to generate neuronal injury far exceed those used in clinical practice, by a factor of 10 for ketamine and a factor of 20 to 30 for propofol, using weight-based comparisons. Even when accounting for differential body size and metabolic rates among species, doses in animal studies still remain higher than those routinely clinically used.[17] Accordingly, plasma concentrations of ketamine leading to increased neuronal cell death in a nonhuman primate model were 5 to 10 times higher than those measured in humans.[37]

It remains controversial whether the duration of anesthetic exposure should be expressed as a fraction of the animal's life expectancy or as an absolute number. If applying the former strategy, exposure times in rodent models clearly represent a much larger fraction of the animal's life than that of a human's. Although it is probably an oversimplification to compare exposure times like dog years, it is undeniable that a multi-hour anesthetic in rodents covers a much larger portion of the functionally important brain growth spurt during the first 2 weeks of rodent life, compared with the equivalent fraction of brain development that occurs over several years in humans. It would, therefore, also be conceivable that brain damage caused in rodents cannot be repaired in the relatively short remaining time of rapid brain development, thereby becoming functionally relevant, whereas human brain function following a similar injury may fully recover because of the substantially longer brain developmental period during which repair mechanisms can occur. Alternatively, the much greater complexity of human brain development and the higher level of brain function may render humans more vulnerable to potential injury compared with lower animals, following similar neurotoxic insults.

EFFECTS OF ANESTHETIC EXPOSURE ON SUBSEQUENT LEARNING AND BEHAVIOR IN YOUNG CHILDREN

In light of the emerging experimental evidence that anesthetic exposure causes neurodegeneration across a wide variety of animal species and that anesthesia-induced neuronal cell loss may be associated with subsequent neurologic abnormalities, the possibility of this phenomenon also occurring in humans cannot be ignored. Because it is impossible to examine brain tissue in healthy children, human studies have relied on assessing neurologic function. However, these studies have thus far not been able to produce any prospective data and are obviously hampered by the inability to randomize young children to undergo painful procedures without anesthesia and analgesia. Furthermore, exposure to anesthetic agents cannot be justified without a surgical or diagnostic indication, rendering it difficult to distinguish the respective contributions of the underlying condition, the surgical procedure, and anesthesia on the neurologic outcome. Therefore, currently available human data rely heavily on postoperative behavioral studies, epidemiologic analyses, and studies into long-term neurologic outcomes in children suffering from illnesses requiring the administration of anesthetics and sedatives during surgery and intensive care.

It is widely known that surgery and anesthesia in young children can lead to prolonged behavioral changes (eg, attention seeking, crying, temper tantrums, sleep disturbances, anxiety). These maladaptive behaviors usually occur early in the postoperative course and decrease significantly during the first month.[38] Predictors for these behaviors have included younger age, severity of postoperative pain, previous negative experience with health care, and patient and parental anxiety.[38–40] Although the precise mechanism underlying these behavioral changes is unknown, it presumably involves psychological factors and not structural brain abnormalities because the administration of preoperative benzodiazepines did not worsen postoperative maladaptive behaviors as would be expected for a cytotoxic cause, but instead significantly ameliorated behavioral symptoms.[41] However, these behavioral studies heavily relied on parental reporting and did not include professional assessment or long-term neurocognitive outcome evaluations, adding uncertainty to the permanent sequelae of these abnormal behaviors.

Conversely, a patient population whose neurocognitive development has been followed closely long-term with neurologic testing tools are neonates and infants who have undergone palliative or corrective congenital heart surgery early in life, such as children with hypoplastic left heart syndrome or transposition of the great arteries. Neurocognitive impairment is well documented in these populations, and its underlying cause is likely multifactorial.[42] Many newborns with complex heart defects may already present with abnormal brain structure and function preoperatively.[43] Perioperative diminution of oxygenation and cardiac output, compounded by intraoperative techniques interfering with physiologic homeostasis, including nonpulsatile flow during cardiopulmonary bypass, deep hypothermia, circulatory arrest, and regional cerebral perfusion, may all contribute to poor neurologic outcomes. In cohorts of patients who underwent neonatal arterial switch operation, follow-up standardized testing at 12 months,[44] preschool and school age,[45–48] and adolescence[49] have demonstrated abnormalities in motor and cognitive development. These persistent neurologic abnormalities, despite improved surgical and supportive techniques, raise the possibility that the repeated obligatory anesthetic exposures in many of these children may contribute to poor outcomes. None of the aforementioned referenced studies, however, specified the anesthetic techniques used. A smaller study in 95 survivors of neonatal cardiac surgery aiming to address these concerns found no effects of cumulative anesthetic doses and exposure times on neurologic performance, adaptive behavior, or vocabulary at 18 to 24 months.[50] However, because of a switch in the neurocognitive measuring tool during the study, the investigators were unable to use their testing tool as a continuous variable, thereby significantly limiting the study's assessment of subtle neurologic abnormalities.

Other cohort studies involving critically ill neonates with necrotizing enterocolitis[51,52] and patent ductus arteriosus[53] have demonstrated that subsets of patients requiring surgical intervention with anesthesia experienced significant growth delay and adverse neurodevelopmental outcomes compared with their counterparts who were managed with medical therapies alone. However, some of these results could be skewed by selection bias because some of the extremely low-birth-weight study participants requiring surgery seemed sicker and required higher inotropic support.[51]

In order to examine the long-term neurodevelopmental implications of pediatric anesthetic exposure in comparably healthy children, several research groups have conducted retrospective analyses of large-scale epidemiologic data. DiMaggio and coworkers[54] used the *International Classification of Diseases, Ninth Revision* (*ICD-9*) procedural code for inguinal hernia repair to query the New York State Medicaid database for patients who underwent general anesthesia for this procedure during the first 3 years of life (n = 383), comparing them with an age-matched cohort of 5050 children who had no history of hernia repair.[54] After controlling for gender and birth-related complications, children who underwent inguinal hernia repair who were younger than 3 years were more than twice as likely to subsequently be diagnosed with a developmental or behavioral disorder. To control for environmental confounders (eg, home environment, parenting style, education system), a subsequent study by the same group focused on a sibling birth cohort of 10,450 of whom 304 had surgery/anesthesia before 3 years of age.[55] Using both proportional hazards modeling and pair-matched analysis, they found evidence linking surgery with anesthesia to a poor neurodevelopmental outcome. A single exposure did not increase the risk of behavioral/developmental abnormalities (hazard ratio [HR] 1.1 [95% confidence interval (CI): 0.8, 1.4]). Two exposures increased the risk (HR 2.9 [95% CI: 2.5, 3.1]), and 3 or more anesthetics increased it even further (HR 4.0 [95% CI: 3.5, 4.5]).

To further correct for environmental and genetic confounders, Bartels and colleagues[56] conducted a retrospective study in 1142 monozygotic twin pairs, demonstrating that twin pairs in which one or both siblings were exposed to anesthesia before 3 years of age had significantly lower educational achievement scores and more cognitive problems than twins not exposed to anesthesia. Strikingly, however, in discordant twins whereby one twin was exposed to anesthesia but not the other, school performance was identical among siblings, suggesting no direct causal relationship between anesthesia exposure and later learning-related difficulties but perhaps indicating a genetic component that increases both the need for surgery and the risk for poor school performance.

In another set of studies, the Mayo Clinic anesthesia group used an existing birth cohort in Olmstead County, Minnesota to perform several anesthesia-related epidemiologic analyses. In a study of 5357 children, of whom 593 received general anesthesia before 4 years of age, Wilder and colleagues[57] used the subsequent development of learning disabilities as the primary end point, defined as low performance on standardized aptitude tests administered by the school district. Compared with those not exposed to anesthesia, which consisted predominantly of halothane and nitrous oxide, a singular exposure was not a significant risk factor for developing a learning disability. Conversely, multiple anesthetic exposures incrementally increased this risk, concomitant with an increased cumulative duration of anesthesia. However, the principal use of the now-obsolete anesthetic halothane and the lack of pulse oximetry monitoring in many of the children temper the direct applicability of these findings to contemporary pediatric anesthesia.

Using the same cohort, the research group also examined anesthetic exposures before the second birthday.[58] Similar to the patients exposed up to their fourth birthday, the risk for developing a learning disability did not increase following a single anesthetic exposure in the younger children. However, after adjustment for health status, multiple anesthetic exposures before the age of 2 years represented a significant independent risk factor (HR 2.12 [95% CI: 1.26–3.54]).

In another study, the same group assessed the neurocognitive implications of a brief anesthetic exposure even earlier in life, just before delivery by cesarean section. School and health data from almost 5000 children delivered via vaginal delivery were compared with data from approximately 200 neonates born via cesarean section with general anesthesia (consisting primarily of sodium thiopental, halothane, and nitrous oxide) and 300 neonates born via cesarean section with regional anesthesia.[59] Children exposed to general or regional anesthesia for cesarean delivery were not at a higher risk for developing learning disabilities when compared with their counterparts who were vaginally delivered, suggesting that a brief peripartum anesthetic exposure had no lasting impact on neurodevelopment. This finding was not entirely expected, given that infants in the general-anesthesia group experienced lower birth weights, lower gestational ages, lower Apgar scores, and their deliveries were more commonly complicated by hemorrhage, eclampsia/preeclampsia, and emergent circumstances than their peers delivered without anesthesia.

In a study involving Danish birth cohorts from 1986 to 1990, Hansen and co-workers[60] assessed the academic performance of 2689 children with a history of inguinal hernia repair in infancy with that of a randomly selected, age-matched 5% population sample.[60] After an adjustment for known confounders, no difference in test scores on a standardized, nationwide ninth grade general examination of academic achievement was observed between the previously exposed children and the population sample. However, previously exposed children were more likely to not sit for the examination, which could mean that they were either academically or otherwise unable to do so.

Finally, using the Western Australian Pregnancy Cohort in Perth, Australia, Ing and colleagues[61] found an association between a single previous exposure to surgery with anesthesia in infants and toddlers and deficits in abstract reasoning and language development when measured at 10 years of age. Raven's Colored Progressive Matrices and Clinical Evaluation of Language (CELF) tests were used as measures for abstract reasoning and language (receptive, expressive, and total language) development, respectively. After an adjustment for confounders, any anesthetic exposure to children younger than 3 years increased the risk ratio for disability to between 1.7 and 2.1. However, several other domains, such as tests of vocabulary, behavior, and motor functions, were not affected by exposure.

In summary, the clinical evidence of anesthetic neurotoxicity in humans is not entirely clear. Several retrospective studies have found an association between anesthetic exposure early in life and abnormal subsequent neurocognitive function, whereas others have not (**Table 1**). Rigorous prospective, randomized, placebo-controlled clinical trials are unfeasible; retrospective studies are limited by multiple confounders, both known and unknown. The currently available retrospective data in humans have relied heavily on group-administered tests assessing school performance or the need for remediating services. Moreover, several of the retrospective epidemiologic studies collected data in an era before the anesthetic standard of care included continuous pulse oximetry and when inhalational anesthetics with profound cardiovascular effects, such as halothane, were commonly used.[57] Knowing that the at-risk population of neonates and infants has higher incidences of oxygen desaturations, hypercarbia, or hypocarbia[62] introduces physiologic instabilities related to surgery/anesthesia as potential contributing factors for adverse neurologic outcomes.[32,63] On the other hand, most studies using validated neurocognitive testing tools have examined severely ill patients with multiple confounders and have not described the used anesthetic or sedative regimens. Study design and medical ethics preclude the separation of the respective effects of the surgical procedure from those related only to the anesthetic exposure. Surgery is commonly associated with neurohumoral and inflammatory responses, which have been found to influence neurocognitive outcomes. Moreover, any congenital malformations or morbidities associated with the underlying disease process requiring surgical intervention may also increase the risk of poor neurodevelopmental performance regardless of surgery/anesthesia exposure.

Table 1
Clinical and epidemiologic studies into the effect of surgery with anesthesia early in life on subsequent neurologic function

Study Design	Study Group	Control Group	Number of Patients	Age During Exposure	Age During Neurologic Assessment	Neurologic Assessment Tools	Neurologic Sequelae in Study Group	Reference
Survey study	General anesthesia for general surgery, ENT, gastroenter-ology, plastics surgery, orthopedics	None, some sibling controls	1027	3–12 y	3 and 30 d postanes-thesia	PHBQ	Behavioral changes in 24% on day 3 after surgery, 16% on day 30, including anxiety and regression, apathy or withdrawal, and separation anxiety	Stargatt et al,[40] 2006
Case series	ASO	None, comparison with normative values	30	Neonatal	12 mo	BSID3, structural assessment with MRI	Diminished language composite was within population norm, lower scores correlated with higher cumulative midazolam dose	Andropoulos et al,[44] 2012
Case series	ASO	None, comparison with normative values	60	Neonatal	3–14 y	Kiphard and Schilling Body Coordination Test, Kaufman Assessment Battery for Children, Oral and Speech Motor Control Test, Mayo Test of Speech and Oral Apraxia	Assessor not blinded: increased prevalence of neurologic impairment (27%), speech impairment (40%), motor dysfunction, language impairment; no difference in intelligence	Hövels-Gürich[45,46]

Study design	Group	Control	N	Population	Age at testing	Tests	Outcomes	Reference
Prospective, randomized trial	ASO with DHCA	ASO with LF-CPB or general population	155	Neonatal	1.0, 2.5, 4.0, 8.0 y	WISC 3, WIAT, TRF, CBCL, WCST, TOVA, Mayo Test for Apraxia of Speech, Goldman-Fristoe Test of Articulation	Lower Full-Scale IQ, Perceptual Organization, and Freedom from Distractibility scores, WIAT Reading and Mathematics Composites, Memory Screening Index, WCST, TOVA scores; most differences were <1 SD	Bellinger et al,[47,49]
Case series	Congenital heart surgery	None, examined effect of cumulative doses of anesthetics/sedatives	95	Infant ≤6 wk	18–24 mo	BSID2 & 3	No evidence for association between dose and duration of sedation/analgesia adverse neurodevelopmental outcomes	Guerrra et al,[50]
Case-control study	NEC requiring laparotomy	No NEC or NEC managed medically	115	26–27 wk PCA, VLBW	12 mo, 3 y, and 5 y	GMDS, SBIS	No blinded assessor: higher incidence of neurodevelopmental impairment; use of inotropes and TPN dependence more prevalent after laparotomy	Tobiansky et al,[51] 1995
Cohort study, case-control study	Laparotomy	Peritoneal drain placement	3725	Neonatal, ELBW	18–22 mo	Neurologic examination, BSID2	Blinded assessor: higher frequency of CP and lower BSID 2; no difference between medically treated patients with or without NEC	Hintz et al,[52] 2005

(continued on next page)

Table 1
(continued)

Study Design	Study Group	Control Group	Number of Patients	Age During Exposure	Age During Neurologic Assessment	Neurologic Assessment Tools	Neurologic Sequelae in Study Group	Reference
Cohort study, case-control study	PDA ligation	Indomethacin treatment	340	84% neonatal (25–29 wk PCA), ELBW	18 mo	Neurologic examination, BSID2	Increase in cerebral palsy, cognitive delay, hearing loss, bilateral blindness	Kabra et al,[53] 2007
Matched cohort study	ICD-9 procedural code for inguinal hernia without preexisting developmental/ behavioral diagnosis	Children in birth cohort without procedural code for inguinal hernia	5433	Younger than 3 y	n/a	Diagnostic code for unspecified delay or behavioral disorder, mental retardation, autism, and language or speech problems	Not individually specified, increased hazard ratio for diagnosis following multiple exposures	DiMaggio et al,[54]
Cohort study	ICD-9 procedural codes for anesthesia/ surgery without preexisting developmental/ behavioral diagnosis	Siblings in birth cohort without anesthesia/ surgery	10,450	Younger than 3 y	n/a	Diagnostic code for autism, unsocial and social conduct, developmental delay, reading and language disorders, attention deficit and hyperkinetic disorders	Not individually specified, increased HR for diagnosis following multiple exposures but not in sibling pairs discordant for exposure	DiMaggio et al,[55]

Study type	Exposure to anesthesia	Other unexposed	Number	Age at exposure	Age at outcome	Outcome measures	Findings	Reference
Cohort study	Exposure to anesthesia according to parent	Other unexposed monozygotic twin pairs or unexposed co-twin	1142 twin pairs	Younger than 3 y	12 y	CITO test assessing language, mathematics, information processing, and world orientation	Lower educational achievement scores and cognitive problems compared with unexposed twin pairs but no difference within co-twins discordant for exposure	Bartels et al,[56] 2009
Cohort study	Any surgical procedure as identified by hospital and county records	Unanesthetized members of the birth cohort	5357	Younger than 4 y	Any learning disability before 19 y of age	Included standardized school aptitude tests, WISC, and/or Woodcock Johnson	Educational achievement >1.75 SD deviations less than predicted score more frequently observed following multiple anesthetic exposures but not single exposure	Wilder et al,[57] 2009
Matched cohort study	Any surgical procedure as identified by hospital and county records	Unanesthetized, matched members of the birth cohort	1050	Younger than 2 y	Any learning disability before 19 y of age	Included standardized school aptitude tests, WISC, and/or Woodcock Johnson	More frequent learning disabilities and need for individualized education program for speech/language impairment in children with multiple, but not single exposures	Flick et al,[58] 2011

(continued on next page)

Table 1
(continued)

Study Design	Study Group	Control Group	Number of Patients	Age During Exposure	Age During Neurologic Assessment	Neurologic Assessment Tools	Neurologic Sequelae in Study Group	Reference
Cohort study	Birth by cesarean section with general anesthesia	Birth by cesarean section with regional anesthesia or by spontaneous vaginal delivery without any anesthesia	5320	Neonatal	Any learning disability before 19 y of age	Included standardized school aptitude tests, WISC, and/or Woodcock Johnson	Equal risk of developing learning disability in children born via vaginal delivery or by cesarean section with general anesthesia	Sprung et al,[59] 2009
Cohort study	Inguinal hernia repair	Unanesthetized, age-matched members of the birth cohort	17,264	Infancy	15–16 y	Ninth grade school exit examination	No difference in scores, but exposed children less likely to sit for examination	Hansen et al,[60] 2011
Cohort study	Any anesthetic exposure	Unanesthetized members of the birth cohort	2868	Younger than 3 y	10 y	Individually administered tests of language development (CELF) and cognition (CPM)	Even single anesthetic exposure associated with increased risk of language and abstract reasoning deficits	Ing et al,[61] 2012

Abbreviations: ASO, arterial switch operation; BSID, Bayley Scales of Infant Development; CBCL, Achenbach Child Behavior Checklist Parental Assessment; CITO, Centraal Instituut voor Toetsontwikkeling; CP, cerebral palsy; CPM, Colored Progressive Matrices; CTRS-R, Connor's Teacher Rating Scale-Revised; DHCA, deep hypothermic circulatory arrest; ELBW, extremely low birth weight (<1000 g); ENT, ears, nose, and throat; GMDS, Griffiths Mental Development Scales; LF-CPB, low flow-cardiopulmonary bypass; MRI, magnetic resonance imaging; NEC, necrotizing enterocolitis; PCA, post-conceptual age; PDA, patent ductus arteriosus; PHBQ, Vernon Post Hospitalization Behavior Questionnaire; SBIS, Stanford-Binet Intelligence Scales; TOVA, Test of Variables of Attention; TPN, total parenteral nutrition; TRF, Teacher's Report Form; VLBW, very low birth weight (≤1500 g); WCST, Wisconsin Card Sorting Test of problem solving; WIAT, Wechsler Individual Achievement Test; WISC 3, Wechsler Intelligence Scale for Children, Third Edition.

Data from Refs.[40,44–61]

CHALLENGING STANDARD THERAPIES: THE UTILITY OF PROSPECTIVE RANDOMIZED CONTROLLED TRIALS

Prospective randomized controlled trials remain the gold standard for determining the efficacy and identifying complications associated with a specific intervention. Certainly, prospective studies neutralize the confounding factors that are inherent to retrospective analyses by precise stratification of the treatment groups. Furthermore, this type of study not only determines the utility and consequences of a routine treatment modality but can also uncover unexpected sequelae of the therapy.

The well-publicized line of investigation into the effect of routine dexamethasone therapy for bronchopulmonary dysplasia in premature neonates highlights the usefulness of prospective randomized controlled trials. Much like the routine use of general anesthetic for neonatal surgery, dexamethasone had been the standard treatment regimen for the prevention of bronchopulmonary dysplasia in premature neonates and led to decreased pulmonary-related morbidity and mortality. However, this practice was associated with increased incidences of gastrointestinal bleeding, hyperglycemia, hypertension, cardiomyopathy, and cerebral palsy. These observations fueled a rigorous double-blind placebo-controlled trial in premature neonates requiring mechanical ventilation. The initial analysis of these patients at 2 years of age revealed adverse effects on neuromotor function and somatic growth.[64] A follow-up evaluation of these children at school age demonstrated significant decrements in height, head circumference, motor skills and coordination, visual-motor integration, and IQ scores for the dexamethasone-treated group.[65] These unexpected findings resulted in published guidelines against the routine use of prophylactic dexamethasone in this setting by the American Academy of Pediatrics (AAP).[66] Subsequently, a 15-year follow-up neurodevelopmental evaluation of a similar cohort resulted in no observed differences between the treatment groups.[67] Given these conflicting findings, the AAP reissued a consensus statement confirming the link between high-dose dexamethasone treatment and neurodevelopmental deficits and advocating studies of low-dose dexamethasone.[68]

At present, there are several investigations into the effects of anesthetic exposure early in life. The GAS study, which is an ongoing National Institute of Health–funded prospective clinical study that compares regional and general anesthesia for effects on neurodevelopmental outcome and apnea in infants, has recruited more than 700 infants randomized to either a general or spinal anesthetic for inguinal hernia surgery in 7 countries.[69] In a neonatal rat model comparing general and spinal anesthesia, prolonged exposure to isoflurane clearly increased neuroapoptosis, whereas a short exposure to isoflurane or a bupivacaine spinal anesthetic did not.[70] Given these findings in the laboratory, the GAS study intends to examine the effect of a general anesthetic (sevoflurane) versus a spinal anesthetic (bupivacaine) on neurocognitive performance at 2 and 5 years using a battery of individually administered neurocognitive tests. Further analysis of the data collected from this international study will likely demonstrate the effects of these different anesthetic techniques on other clinical and technical variables. The GAS study has completed enrollment; but given the substantial duration between exposure and testing, the initial results are not expected before 2017.

Another approach has been taken by the Pediatric Anesthesia and Neurodevelopmental Assessment study, a multicenter ambidirectional trial comparing the performance of existing sibling cohorts discordant for anesthetic exposure for inguinal hernia repair in children younger than 3 years in prospectively administered neurocognitive function tests, including the developmental neuropsychological assessment tool

NEPSY-II, which assesses attention, executive function, language, learning, memory, sensorimotor development, social perception, and visuospatial processing.[71] This trial is still enrolling children, and the initial results are anticipated in 2014.

A third study currently being performed, the Mayo Safety in Kids study, compares the performance of children previously exposed to one or multiple anesthetics before 3 years of age to those never anesthetized using an extensive battery of neurocognitive tests, including the operant test battery previously used by researchers at the National Center for Toxicologic Research in nonhuman primates. This particular study has just started enrolling and testing children, and preliminary results are not expected before 2015.

IMMEDIATE LESSONS FROM ANIMAL STUDIES: ARE THERE ANY SAFE DRUGS OR NONTOXIC EXPOSURE TIMES OR DOSES?

The expanding evidence for the neurotoxic effects of many commonly used anesthetic agents in animals, the emerging epidemiologic evidence for a potential association between exposures early in life and learning abnormalities, and the current dearth of prospective studies addressing these concerns led to 2 clinically very important questions: do there exist any anesthetic drugs that the developing brain can be safely exposed to and, if not, are there any differences in toxic potency among different anesthetics? The latter question has been recently addressed for several inhaled anesthetics, whereby equal anesthetic potency can be assessed as the minimum alveolar concentration (MAC). Unfortunately, the findings have not been uniform. Liang and coworkers[72] observed that the relatively small dose of 0.75% isoflurane when administered for 6 hours in 7-day-old mice caused greater neurodegeneration than an exposure to 1.1% sevoflurane, although neither of these exposures altered subsequent memory and learning abilities in adult animals.[72] Using higher doses of 7.4%, 1.5%, or 2.9% for desflurane, isoflurane, or sevoflurane, respectively, (all representing 0.6 MAC equivalents) for 6 hours in 7- to 8-day-old mice, Istaphanous and colleagues[73] did not observe any differences among the 3 volatile agents. Conflicting results were reported by Kodama and colleagues[74] who observed similar degrees of neuroapoptosis in 6-day-old mice following 6 hours of 3% sevoflurane and 2% isoflurane, compared with the higher neurotoxic effects of 8% desflurane, which led to subsequent short-term memory impairment in addition to the long-term memory abnormalities that were observed in all exposed animals. Accordingly, these discrepant findings are unable to guide clinical recommendations regarding the selection of one particular inhaled anesthetic over another. However, the combined findings suggest that the toxic potency may be more closely linked to anesthetic properties or related functions, rather than the absolute concentration, because desflurane did not cause 4 times the degree of neuroapoptosis of isoflurane while being administered in 4 times the dose. Moreover, although the sevoflurane concentration was generally higher than the isoflurane concentration, none of the studies observed a higher degree of neurotoxicity when comparing the two agents. It remains to be determined whether differences between the studies may be explained by the methodological complexities of quantifying the 3-dimensional cell death pattern and differential counting methodologies.

Comparing the neuroapoptotic properties of injectable anesthetics with each other or with inhaled anesthetics is even more difficult because in small animal studies injectable anesthetics are frequently administered as intermittent boluses, and maintenance of the anesthetic state cannot be guaranteed. Moreover, even when administered by infusion, the equipotency of injectable drugs with inhaled anesthetics may be difficult to prove. When the injectable anesthetic ketamine was administered for 5 hours in newborn rhesus monkeys, it elicited a 3.8-fold increase in neuroapoptosis compared with control animals,[75] whereas a 5-hour exposure to isoflurane raised the neuronal degeneration to 12-fold that observed in controls.[76] However, although both animal groups were reported to be in a surgical stage of anesthesia, an exactly equipotent depth of anesthesia could not be verified.

Toxic effects have been demonstrated in newborn mice as early as 1 hour after initiation of 2% isoflurane,[26] suggesting that any potential nontoxic exposure time in rodents may be brief. Longer exposures of 2 to 6 hours at 0.6 to 1.0 MAC of all commonly used inhaled anesthetics have been found to cause neurodegeneration.[29,73] Several studies using injectable anesthetics have tried to determine a toxic threshold for single-dose administration in developing animals. However, translation of these data is complicated by the fact that the doses of these drugs needed to anesthetize small animals, such as mice and rats, are much larger than similar doses for humans. When adjusting the drug doses administered to animals according to allometric scaling techniques,[77] single doses equivalent to greater than 6 or 7 mg/kg of propofol were found to lead to neuronal degeneration in newborn rats[78] and mice,[79] respectively. Only a single dose equivalent of less than a 2 mg/kg was found devoid of immediate toxic effects in mice. Ketamine has been found neurotoxic in mice at a dose equivalent of 3 mg/kg.[79] By comparison, a single dose that would be akin to up to 18 mg/kg in humans did not cause any acute neurodegeneration in rats.[80] Similarly, mice were more sensitive to a single dose of midazolam (1.1 mg/kg equivalent),[81] whereas up to 2.1 mg/kg did not cause neuroapoptosis in neonatal rats.[16] However, most of these studies did not assess subsequent neurologic function; even in studies that did, neurodegeneration has not consistently led to neurocognitive abnormalities. In contrast to this growing body of evidence demonstrating toxic effects of all routinely used general anesthetics and sedatives, the relatively mild sedative dexmedetomidine, in limited studies, has been found to not cause neuroapoptosis and to potentially protect from isoflurane-induced neurotoxicity.[82]

PERIOD OF VULNERABILITY: IS THERE A SAFE AGE FOR GENERAL ANESTHESIA?

Anesthetic neurotoxicity was initially described in very young animals, occurring between 4 to 10 days of age in small rodents,[25,73] around midgestation in guinea pigs,[83] and before 35 days of age in rhesus macaques.[37] Using now-dated brain developmental data, the corresponding maturational state of the human brain during this peak of vulnerability was estimated to range from the third trimester to the first 3 to 4 years of life.[84] However, more contemporary models using computational brain developmental data have equated brain maturation in these animal models to premature humans during mid to late gestation.[85,86]

Although these previous findings would place the potentially vulnerable period to anesthetic exposures for humans in utero, more recent animal studies have demonstrated anesthesia-induced neuronal cell death to also occur in adult mice following exposures to isoflurane or propofol.[87,88] These novel findings may be explained by recent observations that the age of the animal during exposure may be less relevant to the phenomenon's underlying mechanism than previously thought and that the age of the neuron during exposure may be a better predictor for neurodegeneration. In agreement with this hypothesis, dentate granule cells were recently found to be particularly vulnerable to isoflurane-induced degeneration when exposed before 18 days of neuronal age.[87] Complementary to these results, differential windows of vulnerability have been observed for different brain regions, in line with the specific region's peak in neurogenesis.[89] In brain regions with ongoing neurogenesis throughout life, such as the dentate gyrus and olfactory bulb, vulnerability to the phenomenon occurs throughout life, albeit to a reduced degree at an older age. This point suggests that no safe period for anesthetic exposure may exist, but rather the brain regions most susceptible to the toxic effects change depending on the age of most of the neurons within each region and that the heightened vulnerability of neonatal animals can be explained by their greater number of immature neurons. By extension, these findings further suggest that anesthetic neurotoxicity may not only be relevant for young children but also for adults undergoing anesthesia.

In summary, all currently routinely used anesthetics and sedatives acting as $GABA_A$-receptor agonists and/or NMDA-receptor antagonists have demonstrated deleterious effects on neuronal survival, brain structure, and neurocognitive function. Several epidemiologic studies have associated anesthetic exposures for surgery early in life with subsequent learning abnormalities and language impairment. However, the relative contributions of surgery, pain, underlying medical conditions, and anesthetics to this phenomenon are unknown. Although anesthetic toxicity peaks at a very early age in animals, emerging research has found this process to extend into adulthood in brain regions with ongoing neurogenesis, suggesting that the phenomenon targets neurons of an immature state. Accordingly, no particular age can be designated as entirely safe for anesthetic exposures. Because pediatric surgery frequently has to be performed at an early age to save patients' lives or to improve their quality of life, additional research is urgently needed to clarify the phenomenon's human applicability, to elucidate its mechanism, and to devise mitigating strategies.

REFERENCES

1. DeFrances CJ, Cullen KA, Kozak LJ. National Hospital Discharge Survey: 2005 annual summary with detailed diagnosis and procedure data. Vital Health Stat 13 2007;(165):1–209.
2. Anand KJ, Aynsley-Green A. Metabolic and endocrine effects of surgical ligation of patent ductus arteriosus in the human preterm neonate: are there implications for further improvement of postoperative outcome? Mod Probl Paediatr 1985;23:143–57.
3. Anand KJ, Brown MJ, Causon RC, et al. Can the human neonate mount an endocrine and metabolic response to surgery? J Pediatr Surg 1985;20:41–8.
4. Anand KG, Sippell WG, Aynsley-Green A. Randomised trial of fentanyl anaesthesia in preterm babies undergoing surgery: effects on the stress response. Lancet 1987;1:243–8.
5. Robinson S, Gregory GA. Fentanyl-air-oxygen anesthesia for ligation of patent ductus arteriosus in preterm infants. Anesth Analg 1981;60:331–4.
6. Rao SC, Pirie S, Minutillo C, et al. Ward reduction of gastroschisis in a single stage without general anaesthesia may increase the risk of short-term morbidities: results of a retrospective audit. J Paediatr Child Health 2009;45:384–8.
7. Grunau R. Early pain in preterm infants. A model of long-term effects. Clin Perinatol 2002;29:373–94.
8. Grunau RE, Whitfield MF, Petrie-Thomas J, et al. Neonatal pain, parenting stress and interaction, in relation to cognitive and motor development at 8 and 18 months in preterm infants. Pain 2009;143:138–46.
9. Anand KJ, Garg S, Rovnaghi CR, et al. Ketamine reduces the cell death following inflammatory pain in newborn rat brain. Pediatr Res 2007;62: 283–90.

10. Anand KJ, Coskun V, Thrivikraman KV, et al. Long-term behavioral effects of repetitive pain in neonatal rat pups. Physiol Behav 1999;66:627–37.
11. Laprairie JL, Johns ME, Murphy AZ. Preemptive morphine analgesia attenuates the long-term consequences of neonatal inflammation in male and female rats. Pediatr Res 2008;64:625–30.
12. Eckenhoff JE. Relationship of anesthesia to postoperative personality changes in children. AMA Am J Dis Child 1953;86:587–91.
13. Quimby KL, Katz J, Bowman RE. Behavioral consequences in rats from chronic exposure to 10 ppm halothane during early development. Anesth Analg 1975; 54:628–33.
14. Uemura E, Levin ED, Bowman RE. Effects of halothane on synaptogenesis and learning behavior in rats. Exp Neurol 1985;89:520–9.
15. Ikonomidou C, Bosch F, Miksa M, et al. Blockade of NMDA receptors and apoptotic neurodegeneration in the developing brain. Science 1999;283:70–4.
16. Jevtovic-Todorovic V, Hartman RE, Izumi Y, et al. Early exposure to common anesthetic agents causes widespread neurodegeneration in the developing rat brain and persistent learning deficits. J Neurosci 2003;23:876–82.
17. Loepke AW, Soriano SG. Impact of pediatric surgery and anesthesia on brain development. In: Gregory GA, Andropoulos DA, editors. Gregory's pediatric anesthesia. 5th edition. Hoboken (NJ): Blackwell Publishing Ltd; 2012. p. 1183–218.
18. Oppenheim RW. Cell death during development of the nervous system. Annu Rev Neurosci 1991;14:453–501.
19. Kuida K, Zheng TS, Na S, et al. Decreased apoptosis in the brain and premature lethality in CPP32-deficient mice. Nature 1996;384:368–72.
20. Zimmermann KC, Green DR. How cells die: apoptosis pathways. J Allergy Clin Immunol 2001;108:S99–103.
21. Kuan CY, Roth KA, Flavell RA, et al. Mechanisms of programmed cell death in the developing brain. Trends Neurosci 2000;23:291–7.
22. Blomgren K, Leist M, Groc L. Pathological apoptosis in the developing brain. Apoptosis 2007;12:993–1010.
23. Cowan WM, Fawcett JW, O'Leary DD, et al. Regressive events in neurogenesis. Science 1984;225:1258–65.
24. Northington FJ, Ferriero DM, Graham EM, et al. Early neurodegeneration after hypoxia-ischemia in neonatal rat is necrosis while delayed neuronal death is apoptosis. Neurobiol Dis 2001;8:207–19.
25. Yon JH, Daniel-Johnson J, Carter LB, et al. Anesthesia induces neuronal cell death in the developing rat brain via the intrinsic and extrinsic apoptotic pathways. Neuroscience 2005;135:815–27.
26. Johnson SA, Young C, Olney JW. Isoflurane-induced neuroapoptosis in the developing brain of non-hypoglycemic mice. J Neurosurg Anesthesiol 2008; 20:21–8.
27. Nikizad H, Yon JH, Carter LB, et al. Early exposure to general anesthesia causes significant neuronal deletion in the developing rat brain. Ann N Y Acad Sci 2007; 1122:69–82.
28. Loepke AW, Istaphanous GK, McAuliffe JJ, et al. The effects of neonatal isoflurane exposure in mice on brain cell viability, adult behavior, learning and memory. Anesth Analg 2009;108:90–104.
29. Stratmann G, May LD, Sall JW, et al. Effect of hypercarbia and isoflurane on brain cell death and neurocognitive dysfunction in 7-day-old rats. Anesthesiology 2009;110:849–61.

30. Paule MG, Li M, Allen RR, et al. Ketamine anesthesia during the first week of life can cause long-lasting cognitive deficits in rhesus monkeys. Neurotoxicol Teratol 2011;33:220–30.

31. Loepke AW, McCann JC, Kurth CD, et al. The physiologic effects of isoflurane anesthesia in neonatal mice. Anesth Analg 2006;102:75–80.

32. McCann ME, Soriano SG. Perioperative central nervous system injury in neonates. Br J Anaesth 2012;109:i60–7.

33. Shu Y, Zhou Z, Wan Y, et al. Nociceptive stimuli enhance anesthetic-induced neuroapoptosis in the rat developing brain. Neurobiol Dis 2012;45:743–50.

34. Liu JR, Liu Q, Li J, et al. Noxious stimulation attenuates ketamine-induced neuroapoptosis in the developing rat brain. Anesthesiology 2012;117:64–71.

35. Shih J, May LD, Gonzalez HE, et al. Delayed environmental enrichment reverses sevoflurane-induced memory impairment in rats. Anesthesiology 2012;116:586–602.

36. Boasen JF, McPherson RJ, Hays SL, et al. Neonatal stress or morphine treatment alters adult mouse conditioned place preference. Neonatology 2009;95:230–9.

37. Slikker W Jr, Zou X, Hotchkiss CE, et al. Ketamine-induced neuronal cell death in the perinatal rhesus monkey. Toxicol Sci 2007;98:145–58.

38. Kotiniemi LH, Ryhänen PT, Moilanen IK. Behavioural changes in children following day-case surgery: a 4-week follow-up of 551 children. Anaesthesia 1997;52:970–6.

39. Kain ZN, Caldwell-Andrews AA, Maranets I, et al. Preoperative anxiety and emergence delirium and postoperative maladaptive behaviors. Anesth Analg 2004;99:1648–54.

40. Stargatt R, Davidson AJ, Huang GH, et al. A cohort study of the incidence and risk factors for negative behavior changes in children after general anesthesia. Paediatr Anaesth 2006;16:846–59.

41. Kain ZN, Mayes LC, Wang SM, et al. Postoperative behavioral outcomes in children: effects of sedative premedication. Anesthesiology 1999;90:758–65.

42. Tabbutt S, Gaynor JW, Newburger JW. Neurodevelopmental outcomes after congenital heart surgery and strategies for improvement. Curr Opin Cardiol 2012;27:82–91.

43. Owen M, Shevell M, Majnemer A, et al. Abnormal brain structure and function in newborns with complex congenital heart defects before open heart surgery: a review of the evidence. J Child Neurol 2011;26:743–55.

44. Andropoulos DB, Easley RB, Brady K, et al. Changing expectations for neurological outcomes after the neonatal arterial switch operation. Ann Thorac Surg 2012;94:1250–5.

45. Hövels-Gürich HH, Seghaye MC, Däbritz S, et al. Cognitive and motor development in preschool and school-aged children after neonatal arterial switch operation. J Thorac Cardiovasc Surg 1997;114:578–85.

46. Hövels-Gürich HH, Seghaye MC, Schnitker R, et al. Long-term neurodevelopmental outcomes in school-aged children after neonatal arterial switch operation. J Thorac Cardiovasc Surg 2002;124:448–58.

47. Bellinger DC, Wypij D, Kuban KC, et al. Developmental and neurologic status of children at 4 years of age after heart surgery with hypothermic circulatory arrest or low-flow cardiopulmonary bypass. Circulation 1999;100:526–32.

48. Bellinger DC, Wypij D, duPlessis AJ, et al. Neurodevelopmental status at eight years in children with dextro-transposition of the great arteries: the Boston Circulatory Arrest Trial. J Thorac Cardiovasc Surg 2003;126:1385–96.

49. Bellinger DC, Wypij D, Rivkin MJ, et al. Adolescents with d-transposition of the great arteries corrected with the arterial switch procedure: neuropsychological assessment and structural brain imaging. Circulation 2011;124:1361–9.
50. Guerra GG, Robertson CM, Alton GY, et al. Neurodevelopmental outcome following exposure to sedative and analgesic drugs for complex cardiac surgery in infancy. Paediatr Anaesth 2011;21:932–41.
51. Tobiansky R, Lui K, Roberts S, et al. Neurodevelopmental outcome in very low birthweight infants with necrotizing enterocolitis requiring surgery. J Paediatr Child Health 1995;31:233–6.
52. Hintz SR, Kendrick DE, Stoll BJ, et al. Neurodevelopmental and growth outcomes of extremely low birth weight infants after necrotizing enterocolitis. Pediatrics 2005;115:696–703.
53. Kabra NS, Schmidt B, Roberts RS, et al. Neurosensory impairment after surgical closure of patent ductus arteriosus in extremely low birth weight infants: results from the Trial of Indomethacin Prophylaxis in Preterms. J Pediatr 2007;150: 229–34.
54. DiMaggio C, Sun LS, Kakavouli A, et al. A retrospective cohort study of the association of anesthesia and hernia repair surgery with behavioral and developmental disorders in young children. J Neurosurg Anesthesiol 2009;21:286–91.
55. DiMaggio C, Sun LS, Li G. Early childhood exposure to anesthesia and risk of developmental and behavioral disorders in sibling birth cohort. Anesth Analg 2011;113:1143–51.
56. Bartels M, Althoff RR, Boomsma DI. Anesthesia and cognitive performance in children: no evidence for causal relationship. Twin Res Hum Genet 2009;12: 246–53.
57. Wilder RT, Flick RP, Sprung J, et al. Early exposure to anesthesia and learning disabilities in a population-based birth cohort. Anesthesiology 2009;110: 796–804.
58. Flick RP, Katusik SK, Colligan RC, et al. Cognitive and behavioral outcomes after early exposure to anesthesia and surgery. Pediatrics 2011;128:e1053–61.
59. Sprung J, Flick RP, Wilder RT, et al. Anesthesia for cesarean delivery and learning disabilities in a population-based birth cohort. Anesthesiology 2009; 111:302–10.
60. Hansen TG, Pedersen JK, Henneberg SW, et al. Academic performance in adolescence after inguinal hernia repair in infancy: a nationwide cohort study. Anesthesiology 2011;114:1076–85.
61. Ing C, DiMaggio C, Whitehouse A, et al. Long-term differences in language and cognitive function after childhood exposure to anesthesia. Pediatrics 2012;130: e476–85.
62. Coté CJ, Rolf N, Liu LM, et al. A single-blind study of combined pulse oximetry and capnography in children. Anesthesiology 1991;74:980–7.
63. McCann ME, Schouten ANJ, Dobija N, et al. Infantile postoperative encephalopathy after general anesthesia. Pediatrics 2013 [forthcoming].
64. Yeh TF, Lin YJ, Huang CC, et al. Early dexamethasone therapy in preterm infants: a follow-up study. Pediatrics 1998;101:E7.
65. Yeh TF, Lin YJ, Lin HC, et al. Outcomes at school age after postnatal dexamethasone therapy for lung disease of prematurity. N Engl J Med 2004;350: 1304–13.
66. American Academy of Pediatrics, Committee on Fetus and Newborn. Postnatal corticosteroids to treat or prevent chronic lung disease in preterm infants. Pediatrics 2002;109:330–8.

67. Gross SJ, Anbar RD, Mettelman BB. Follow-up at 15 years of preterm infants from a controlled trial of moderately early dexamethasone for the prevention of chronic lung disease. Pediatrics 2005;115:681–7.
68. Watterberg KL, American Academy of Pediatrics, Committee on Fetus and Newborn. Policy statement—postnatal corticosteroids to prevent or treat bronchopulmonary dysplasia. Pediatrics 2010;126:800–8.
69. Davidson AJ, McCann ME, Morton NS, et al. Anesthesia and outcome after neonatal surgery: the role for randomized trials. Anesthesiology 2008;109: 941–4.
70. Yahalom B, Athiraman U, Soriano SG, et al. Spinal anesthesia in infant rats: development of a model and assessment of neurologic outcomes. Anesthesiology 2011;114:1325–35.
71. Sun L. Early childhood general anaesthesia exposure and neurocognitive development. Br J Anaesth 2010;105:i61–8.
72. Liang G, Ward C, Peng J, et al. Isoflurane causes greater neurodegeneration than an equivalent exposure of sevoflurane in the developing brain of neonatal mice. Anesthesiology 2010;112:1325–34.
73. Istaphanous GK, Howard J, Nan X, et al. Comparison of the neuroapoptotic properties of equipotent anesthetic concentrations of desflurane, isoflurane, or sevoflurane in neonatal mice. Anesthesiology 2011;114:578–87.
74. Kodama M, Satoh Y, Otsubo Y, et al. Neonatal desflurane exposure induces more robust neuroapoptosis than do isoflurane and sevoflurane and impairs working memory. Anesthesiology 2011;115:979–91.
75. Brambrink AM, Evers AS, Avidan MS, et al. Ketamine-induced neuroapoptosis in the fetal and neonatal rhesus macaque brain. Anesthesiology 2012;116:372–84.
76. Brambrink AM, Evers AS, Avidan MS, et al. Isoflurane-induced neuroapoptosis in the neonatal rhesus macaque brain. Anesthesiology 2010;112:834–41.
77. Reagan-Shaw S, Nihal M, Ahmad N. Dose translation from animal to human studies revisited. FASEB J 2008;22:659–61.
78. Pesić V, Milanović D, Tanić N, et al. Potential mechanism of cell death in the developing rat brain induced by propofol anesthesia. Int J Dev Neurosci 2009;27:279–87.
79. Fredriksson A, Pontén E, Gordh T, et al. Neonatal exposure to a combination of N-methyl-D-aspartate and gamma-aminobutyric acid type A receptor anesthetic agents potentiates apoptotic neurodegeneration and persistent behavioral deficits. Anesthesiology 2007;107:427–36.
80. Hayashi H, Dikkes P, Soriano SG. Repeated administration of ketamine may lead to neuronal degeneration in the developing rat brain. Paediatr Anaesth 2002;12: 770–4.
81. Young C, Jevtovic-Todorovic V, Qin YQ, et al. Potential of ketamine and midazolam, individually or in combination, to induce apoptotic neurodegeneration in the infant mouse brain. Br J Pharmacol 2005;146:189–97.
82. Sanders RD, Xu J, Shu Y, et al. Dexmedetomidine attenuates isoflurane-induced neurocognitive impairment in neonatal rats. Anesthesiology 2009;110:1077–85.
83. Rizzi S, Ori C, Jevtovic-Todorovic V. Timing versus duration: determinants of anesthesia-induced developmental apoptosis in the young mammalian brain. Ann N Y Acad Sci 2010;1199:43–51.
84. Dobbing J, Sands J. Comparative aspects of the brain growth spurt. Early Hum Dev 1979;3:79–83.
85. Clancy B, Finlay BL, Darlington RB, et al. Extrapolating brain development from experimental species to humans. Neurotoxicology 2007;28:931–7.

86. Workman AD, Charvet CJ, Clancy B, et al. Modeling transformations of neurodevelopmental sequences across mammalian species. J Neurosci 2013;33: 7368–83.
87. Hofacer RD, Deng M, Ward CG, et al. Cell age-specific vulnerability of neurons to anesthetic toxicity. Ann Neurol 2013;73:695–704.
88. Krzisch M, Sultan S, Sandell J, et al. Propofol anesthesia impairs the maturation and survival of adult-born hippocampal neurons. Anesthesiology 2013;118: 602–10.
89. Deng M, Hofacer R, Jiang C, et al. Brain regional vulnerability to anaesthesia-induced neuroapoptosis shifts with age at exposure and extends into adulthood for some regions. Br J Anaesth. In press.

The Anesthetic Management of Children with Pulmonary Hypertension in the Cardiac Catheterization Laboratory

Mark D. Twite, MB BChir*, Robert H. Friesen, MD

KEYWORDS

- Pulmonary hypertension • Cardiac catheterization laboratory • Anesthesia
- Children

KEY POINTS

- A new classification of pediatric pulmonary arterial hypertension (PAH) has been developed that incorporates abnormalities of lung growth and development as well as syndromes frequently contributing to PAH.
- Children with PAH will require cardiac catheterization to establish the diagnosis and monitor the response to therapy.
- Children receiving general anesthesia for cardiac catheterization are at significantly increased risk of perioperative complications such as a pulmonary hypertensive crisis.
- There is no one ideal anesthetic agent for children with PAH, and it is essential to understand the different hemodynamic effects of anesthetic agents and adopt a balanced anesthetic technique for children with PAH.

INTRODUCTION

Pulmonary hypertension has many different causes, which all share the final common pathway of elevated pulmonary arterial pressure (PAP). Pulmonary arterial hypertension (PAH) is due to abnormalities in the pulmonary arterial vasculature. Pulmonary venous hypertension is a result of left-sided heart disease, for example, pulmonary vein stenosis or left-side valvar heart disease. The treatments of PAH and pulmonary venous hypertension are different, so the distinction of one from the other is of obvious clinical importance.[1] This article focuses on PAH in children. PAH is a life-threatening disease which, if undiagnosed, will eventually culminate in irreversible elevation of

Neither author has any financial disclosures to make.
Department of Anesthesiology, University of Colorado School of Medicine, CO, USA
* Corresponding author. Department of Anesthesiology B090, Children's Hospital Colorado, University of Colorado Anschutz Medical Campus, 13123 East 16th Avenue, Aurora, CO 80045.
E-mail address: Mark.Twite@childrenscolorado.org

Anesthesiology Clin 32 (2014) 157–173
http://dx.doi.org/10.1016/j.anclin.2013.10.005   anesthesiology.theclinics.com

pulmonary vascular resistance (PVR), leading to right ventricular failure and death.[2] Unfortunately, delays in diagnosis and treatment are not uncommon because of nonspecific presenting symptoms, especially in young children, and the low incidence of the disease.[3] The estimated prevalence in adults is 15 to 50 cases per 1 million, whereas in children it is less than 10 cases per 1 million.[4,5]

Children with suspected PAH require invasive hemodynamic assessment in the cardiac catheterization laboratory to confirm the diagnosis of PAH and determine future therapy. To tolerate the procedure, most of these children will need general anesthesia provided by an anesthesiologist. It is essential, therefore, that the providing anesthesiologist understands the pathophysiology of PAH, which measurements are made in the catheterization laboratory, how anesthetic medications may affect these measurements, and how to manage a pulmonary hypertensive crisis.[6–9] Children with PAH, especially those with a new diagnosis who are not yet on any treatment, are at increased risk of complications under anesthesia in the cardiac catheterization laboratory. The cardiologist performing the procedure, the pediatric anesthesiologist, and the catheterization laboratory support staff must effectively communicate to provide safe perioperative care.

DEFINITION AND CLASSIFICATION

In normal, healthy individuals the mean pulmonary artery pressure (mPAP) at rest is around 15 mm Hg, and is independent of age, ethnicity, and gender. During exercise, mPAP increases and is dependent on the level of exertion and age. During mild exercise, mPAP is 20 ± 5 mm Hg in subjects younger than 50 years compared with 30 ± 5 mm Hg in subjects older 50, which makes it difficult to define normal mPAP during exercise; hence, the definition of PAH uses mPAP at rest.[10] PAH is defined as mPAP greater than 25 mm Hg at rest, with a normal pulmonary capillary wedge pressure (≤ 15 mm Hg) and increased pulmonary vascular resistance index (PVRI) greater than 3 Wood units per m[2].[11] The normal pulmonary capillary wedge pressure excludes patients with pulmonary venous hypertension from left-sided heart disease. In patients with suspected PAH, the initial investigation is usually a transthoracic echocardiogram that can estimate the mPAP and diagnose any congenital cardiac lesions that may be contributing to the PAH. Echocardiography may support the diagnosis of PAH with qualitative images of elevated right ventricular pressure, such as right ventricular hypertrophy and septal-wall flattening. Quantitative information may be obtained on echocardiography if there is tricuspid regurgitation during systole. In this case, the modified Bernoulli equation may be applied to estimate mPAP, with a tricuspid regurgitant velocity of greater than 2.8 m/s being highly indicative of PAH (**Box 1**).[10,12]

Transthoracic echocardiography is an attractive method to monitor children with PAH, and possibly enable the cardiologist to lengthen the interval between cardiac catheterizations that the child will require to monitor ongoing therapy. There are many echocardiographic techniques in the research and validation phase. One technique is to monitor the right ventricular systolic to diastolic duration ratio, whereby an increase has been shown to be associated with worse right ventricular function, exercise capability, and survival.[13] Another is to measure the degree of tricuspid annular plane systolic excursion (TAPSE), which has been shown to reflect right ventricular function and prognosis in PAH.[14,15]

In the absence of shunts, the pulmonary and systemic circulations receive the same amount of blood flow per minute. PVR beyond the newborn period is more than 10-fold lower than resistance in the systemic circulation, and the pressure in the venous bed draining the pulmonary arteries (pulmonary veins, left atrium) accounts

---

Box 1
Estimating mPAP from systolic tricuspid regurgitant jet velocity on echocardiography

Modified Bernouilli equation:

  sPAP = $4v^2$ + RAP

  eg, sPAP = 4 (2.8^2) + 10 = 41 mm Hg

Converting sPAP to mPAP

  mPAP = (0.61 × sPAP) + 2 mm Hg

  eg, mPAP = (0.61 × 41) + 2 = 27 mm Hg

Abbreviations: mPAP, mean pulmonary artery pressure; RAP, right atrial pressure; sPAP, systolic pulmonary artery pressure; v, tricuspid regurgitation velocity using Doppler on echocardiography.

---

for a much greater percentage of PAP (40%–60%) than the corresponding downstream venous pressure in the systemic circuit. Hence, pulmonary hypertension attributable to pulmonary venous hypertension from left-sided heart disease is the most common form of pulmonary hypertension in adults but not in children.[16]

Three factors can lead to an increase in mPAP: increases in left atrial pressure (LAP), cardiac output, or PVR. From these 3 parameters it is possible to consider 3 broad categories that cause elevated mPAP and pulmonary hypertension (**Box 2**).[2] The original classification of pulmonary hypertension was conceived at the 1998 World Health Organization (WHO) Symposium in Evian, and underwent subsequent revisions at symposia in Venice and Dana Point. However, using this WHO classification system for children has been problematic, as it often does not reflect the complex heterogeneity of factors that contribute to pediatric PAH. For example, children who are commonly evaluated for PAH may have been born prematurely and have chromosomal or genetic anomalies. In addition, such children may have congenital heart defects and acquired problems such as sleep-disordered breathing, chronic aspiration, and secondary lung disease. As a result, the Pulmonary Vascular Research Institute Pediatric Taskforce proposed a new classification of pediatric PAH at its meeting in Panama in 2011. The classification comprises 10 categories based on clinical pediatric practice (**Box 3**). The Panama classification includes an additional definition of pulmonary

---

Box 2
Deriving the potential causes of increased mPAP

Derived from Ohm's Law:

  PVR = ΔP/Flow

  ΔP (TPG)= mPAP − LAP

  PVR = (mPAP − LAP)/CO

  mPAP = LAP + (CO × PVR)

eg, ↑ LAP: left-side heart dysfunction; ↑ CO: congenital heart disease with a large left-to-right shunt; ↑ PVR: pulmonary parenchymal disease or thromboembolic disease

Abbreviations: ΔP, difference in pressure; CO, cardiac output; LAP, left atrial pressure; mPAP, mean pulmonary artery pressure; PVR, pulmonary vascular resistance; TPG, transpulmonary gradient.

Box 3
The 10 categories of pediatric pulmonary hypertensive vascular disease

Category	Description
1	Prenatal or developmental pulmonary hypertensive vascular disease
2	Perinatal pulmonary vascular maladaptation
3	Pediatric cardiovascular disease
4	Bronchopulmonary dysplasia
5	Isolated pediatric pulmonary hypertensive vascular disease
6	Multifactorial pulmonary hypertensive vascular disease in congenital malformation syndromes
7	Pediatric lung disease
8	Pediatric thromboembolic disease
9	Pediatric hypobaric hypoxic exposure
10	Pediatric pulmonary vascular disease associated with other system disorders

Adapted from Cerro MJ, Abman S, Diaz G, et al. A consensus approach to the classification of pediatric pulmonary hypertensive vascular disease: report from the PVRI Pediatric Taskforce, Panama 2011. Pulm Circ 2011;1:288; with permission.

---

hypertension for children with univentricular circulations: following a cavopulmonary anastomosis PAH is defined as a PVRI greater than 3 Wood units/m^2 or a transpulmonary gradient (mPAP − LAP) greater than 6 mm Hg even if the mPAP is less than 25 mm Hg (**Box 4**).[17,18]

PATHOPHYSIOLOGY AND TREATMENT

The factors leading to an increase in mPAP may all eventually result in pulmonary vascular remodeling and increased PVR. As the pulmonary vasculature remodels in PAH, changes occur that may be reactive or fixed. Reactive changes will result in vasodilation of the pulmonary vasculature to an exogenously administered pulmonary vasodilator such as inhaled nitric oxide (iNO). Fixed changes are unreactive to such pulmonary vasodilators. As the disease processes leading to PAH progress, the cross-sectional area of the pulmonary vasculature exponentially decreases according to Poiseuille's Law, leading to increased PVR. Poiseuille's Law states that the

---

Box 4
The modern definition of pulmonary arterial hypertension in children with biventricular and palliated univentricular circulations

Biventricular Circulation

  mPAP >25 mm Hg and PVRI >3 Wood units/m^2

  Positive vasodilator response, defined as a decrease in mPAP and PVRI by 20% with no change in CO

Univentricular Circulation

  Following palliation with a cavopulmonary anastomosis

  PVRI >3 Wood units/m^2 or TPG >6 mm Hg even if mPAP <25 mm Hg

Abbreviations: CO, cardiac output; mPAP, mean pulmonary artery pressure; PVRI, pulmonary vascular resistance index; TPG, transpulmonary gradient.

resistance of a vessel is proportional to the fourth power of the radius. In other words, as the pulmonary arterioles develop thickening of their walls and a smaller intraluminal radius, the resistance will increase exponentially. A pulmonary hypertensive crisis is an acute on chronic increase in PVR during the perioperative period resulting from an acute increase in vascular tone of the reactive portion of the pulmonary vasculature. Early recognition and appropriate management of a pulmonary hypertensive crisis can be life-saving.

The current treatment strategies for PAH are aimed at the 3 pathologic processes. Vasodilators treat reactive vasoconstriction, antiproliferative drugs attenuate vascular remodeling, and anticoagulation may be used to treat and prevent thrombosis from forming in narrowed vessels. Based on the understanding of abnormalities of the vascular endothelium, 3 classes of drugs have been studied for the treatment of PAH.[19] The prostanoids epoprostenol (Flolan), treprostinil (Remodulin), and iloprost (Ventavis) act via cyclic adenosine monophosphate in the smooth muscle cell to produce vasodilation, and may also have some antiproliferative effects. The nitric oxide pathway acts via a cyclic guanosine monophosphate (cGMP) pathway in the smooth muscle cell to produce vasodilation. This pathway may be stimulated directly with iNO, or the breakdown of cGMP may be inhibited by phosphodiesterase type 5 inhibitors such as sildenafil (Revatio) and tadalafil (Adcirca). Recently the US Food and Drug Administration issued a warning against the use of sildenafil for pediatric PAH, because of an apparent increase in mortality during long-term therapy.[20] The endothelin pathway acts via endothelin receptors, which are present on both the endothelial and smooth muscle cells. The endothelin type 1 receptor has 2 further subtypes, A and B. Bosentan (Tracleer) is a nonselective antagonist of both subtypes, whereas ambrisentan (Letairis) is a selective type A antagonist. Both endothelin receptor antagonists require close monitoring of liver function tests. Whereas therapy for PAH in adults is evidence-based, most therapy for PAH in children is extrapolated from the adult data and is based on the experience of clinicians.[18]

CARDIAC CATHETERIZATION

Despite advances in noninvasive imaging techniques, cardiac catheterization with vasodilator testing is necessary for the diagnosis, treatment stratification, and prognosis of PAH in children.[21] There are 3 objectives during the catheterization procedure: to obtain hemodynamic data, to test vasoreactivity, and to rule out any associated disease states.

Accurate hemodynamic data are essential for the diagnosis and ongoing monitoring of patients with PAH. End-hole or flow-directed catheters are used to obtain hemodynamic data. Catheters with multiple side holes are used for angiography to prevent myocardial staining during injection. During catheterization, baseline measures include right atrial pressure, PAP, systemic arterial pressure, mixed venous and systemic arterial saturation, cardiac output, and pulmonary artery occlusion pressure. From these measures, important calculations can be made for pulmonary-to-systemic flow ratio (Qp:Qs) (**Box 5**) and PVR (**Box 6**).[22] It is important for the cardiologist performing the catheterization procedure to exclude intracardiac defects. It is essential that the anesthesiologist maintain stability during these periods of measurement and that the conditions under which they are made is clearly communicated. Most cardiac catheterization laboratories will obtain baseline measurements in room air followed by 70% to 100% oxygen, and then introduce an acute vasodilator such as iNO 20 to 40 ppm. In a recent review of cardiac catheterization laboratory protocols and hemodynamic data in pediatric patients with PAH, general anesthesia was found

---

Box 5
Calculating Qp and Qs

Based on the Fick principle:

Qp:Qs = (Sat Ao − Sat MV)/(Sat PV − Sat PA)

Abbreviations: Qp, pulmonary blood flow; Qs, systemic blood flow; Sat Ao, aortic saturation; Sat MV, mixed venous saturation; Sat PA, pulmonary artery saturation; Sat PV, pulmonary vein saturation.

---

to lower systemic arterial pressure, but there was no difference between general anesthesia and procedural sedation regarding mPAP or PVRI. It also demonstrated that pediatric patients with PAH demonstrate a higher incidence of PAH associated with congenital heart disease and neonatal specific disorders in comparison with adults. Pediatric PAH patients had baseline mPAP of less than 40 mm Hg but greater than 50% of their systemic blood pressure, illustrating the difficulty of applying adult criteria to children with PAH.[23]

The degree to which mPAP and PVR can be decreased acutely by the administration of fast-acting, short-duration vasodilators reflects the extent to which vascular smooth muscle constriction is contributing to the hypertensive state. The response to vasodilators has important therapeutic implications in PAH, and almost all patients will undergo a vasodilator trial during their initial cardiac catheterization. Intravenous epoprostenol, intravenous adenosine, and iNO are commonly used for acute vasodilator testing. The definition of a positive vasodilator response in adults is a reduction in mPAP by at least 10 mm Hg, and this number must be lower than 40 mm Hg. The pediatric definition of a positive response to vasodilators is a decrease in mPAP and PVRI by 20% with no significant change or increase in cardiac index. Such responders are likely to have a beneficial hemodynamic and clinical response to treatment with calcium-channel blocking drugs. It is estimated that 70% to 90% of children with severe PAH are nonresponders to acute vasodilator testing, and therefore require therapy other than calcium-channel antagonists.[18,24]

A pediatric anesthesiologist should be present during the cardiac catheterization, as anesthesia may pose a significant risk to the pediatric patient with PAH. Studies of children with PAH have demonstrated a high incidence of perioperative cardiac arrest and death. A benchmark estimate of the incidence of perioperative cardiac arrest in all pediatric patients is 0.014%.[25] By comparison, children with PAH experienced an

---

Box 6
Calculating PVR

Based on Ohm's Law:

$$PVR = (P_{in} − P_{out})/Qp$$
$$= (mean\ PAP − mean\ LAP)/Qp$$

PVR is measured in Wood units = mm Hg/L/min

or 80 × Woods units = dyne/s/cm^5 (metric units)

Abbreviations: LAP, left atrial pressure (equivalent to pulmonary artery occlusion pressure); P, pressure; PAP, pulmonary artery pressure; PVR, pulmonary vascular resistance; Qp, pulmonary blood flow.

---

incidence of perioperative cardiac arrest of 1.6% associated with all types of procedures and 10% associated with major surgical procedures, including cardiac surgery.[26] Preoperative PAH has been shown to be significantly associated with perioperative death following pediatric open cardiac surgery.[27] The presence of PAH also adds significantly to perioperative risk in children undergoing cardiac catheterization (**Fig. 1**). The incidence of cardiac arrest during pediatric cardiac catheterization is reported to be 0.45%.[28] This incidence increases dramatically when only children with PAH undergoing cardiac catheterization are considered, with reports of 0.8%,[26] 1.2%,[29] and 5.7%.[30] Such morbidity is directly associated with the severity of PAH, with patients with suprasystemic PAH having a much greater incidence of major complications than those with systemic or subsystemic PAH (**Fig. 2**).[29]

ANESTHETIC MANAGEMENT

Cardiac catheterization is rarely tolerated in the awake child. Pediatric anesthesiologists working in the cardiac catheterization laboratory needs to consider some of the unique issues of their surrounding environment. The cardiac catheterization laboratory may be in a remote location away from the main operating rooms, and as a result there may be a delay in help arriving when it is called for. It is therefore essential to work closely with the team in the laboratory, as they may offer the most immediate help during an acute crisis.[31] The position of the cameras in the catheterization laboratory may hinder access to the patient, especially the airway, during a procedure. Usually the anterior-posterior camera may be swung out of the way for a mask induction of the patient, but this may be more difficult to achieve rapidly during a case if there is an airway problem. It is essential to have all necessary equipment and monitoring available. Standard intraoperative American Society of Anesthesiologists (ASA) monitoring should be used, and consideration given for additional monitoring such as a radial arterial line if the cardiologist performing the procedure does not plan to place a femoral arterial line. There may also be frequent interruptions in the invasive pressure wave form as catheters are changed in and out of the femoral arterial sheath, which may again influence placement of a dedicated radial arterial line. Children should be placed on a forced air-warming blanket, as the catheterization laboratory is usually kept cool because everyone is wearing a lead apron to protect against the radiation being used for taking images. Patient monitors such as pulse oximetry and

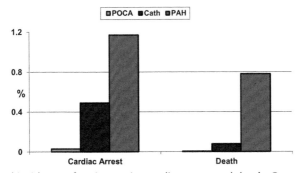

Fig. 1. Estimated incidence of perioperative cardiac arrest and death. Green bars, Perioperative Cardiac Arrest Registry (POCA), all children; blue bars, children undergoing cardiac catheterization (Cath); red bars, children with pulmonary arterial hypertension (PAH) undergoing cardiac catheterization. (*Data from* Refs.[25,28,29])

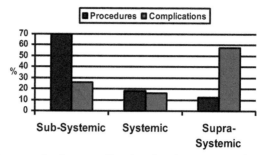

Fig. 2. Perioperative complications are directly related to severity of pulmonary hypertension. (*Adapted from* Carmosino MJ, Friesen RH, Doran A, et al. Perioperative complications in children with pulmonary hypertension undergoing noncardiac surgery or cardiac catheterization. Anesth Analg 2007;104:521–7; with permission.)

noninvasive blood-pressure cuff, in addition to peripheral vascular access, are generally best placed on an upper extremity, because the cardiologist will be accessing the femoral vessels. Appropriate drugs to manage a pulmonary hypertensive crisis should be readily available for each patient.[32,33]

The specific anesthetic technique and drugs chosen are probably less important than the attention to careful titration and maintaining hemodynamic stability. The ideal anesthetic drug for children with pulmonary hypertension would have pulmonary vasodilating effects, would not depress cardiac contractility, would maintain systemic vascular resistance and cardiac output, and would be short lasting and easy to titrate. Such an anesthetic agent, unfortunately, does not exist. Most anesthetics are associated with undesirable hemodynamic effects, depending on dosage and speed of administration, by altering heart rate or rhythm, cardiac contractility, systemic vascular resistance, or PVR (**Table 1**). The cardiovascular effects of anesthetic drugs pertinent to a discussion of pulmonary hypertension are summarized here.

Volatile Anesthetics

Volatile anesthetics cause a dose-dependent depression of cardiac contractility and a decrease in systemic vascular resistance (SVR),[34,35] and attenuate hypoxic pulmonary vasoconstriction during one-lung ventilation.[36] The ratio of pulmonary blood flow (Qp)

Table 1 Hemodynamic effects of anesthetic drugs					
	Contractility	MAP	SVR	PAP	PVR
Volatile	⇓	⇓	⇓⇓	⇓	⇓
Propofol	⇓	⇓	⇓⇓	⇓	⇓
Ketamine	⇒	⇒	⇑	⇑ ⇒	⇑ ⇒
Etomidate	⇒	⇒	⇒	⇑	⇑
Dexmedetomidine	⇒	⇑	⇑	⇒	⇒
Opioids	⇒	⇒	⇒	⇒	⇒
Benzodiazepines	⇒	⇒	⇒	⇒	⇒

Abbreviations: ⇓, decrease; ⇑, increase; ⇒, no significant change; MAP, mean arterial pressure; PAP, pulmonary artery pressure; PVR, pulmonary vascular resistance; SVR, systemic vascular resistance.

to systemic blood flow (Qs) remains unchanged in children with cardiac septal defects in response to halothane, sevoflurane, and isoflurane, so it is assumed that PVR has a similar response to that of SVR.[37]

Nitrous Oxide

Nitrous oxide may increase PVR during prolonged use in adults, but probably has no or little effect in children when it is used for a brief time to perform a mask induction of anesthesia.[38]

Propofol

Propofol causes dose-dependent depression of cardiac contractility.[39] In both adults and children with cardiac disease, propofol is associated with a marked decrease in SVR and mean arterial pressure (MAP), and a slight decrease in PVR and PAP.[40,41] In adults with artificial hearts, propofol causes vasodilation of systemic resistance and capacitance vessels, and a decrease in PAP.[42]

Ketamine

Whereas ketamine is supportive of hemodynamic stability and is frequently recommended as an anesthetic of choice in patients with cardiovascular impairment or instability, its use in patients with PAH is debated because of conflicting results from various studies conducted under a variety of conditions.[43] Study conditions have been varied (spontaneous vs controlled ventilation, natural airway vs endotracheal tube, room air vs added oxygen). A marked increase in PAP and PVR has been observed in children with PAH breathing room air through the natural airway.[44–46] On the other hand, no change in PAP or PVR has been observed in children with PAH during controlled ventilation or while receiving a pulmonary vasodilator, such as oxygen or sevoflurane.[47,48]

Etomidate

Etomidate is known to support systemic hemodynamics, but is associated with significant increases in both SVR and PVR. Despite the observed increase in PVR, etomidate is used as an anesthetic induction drug in patients with PAH because of its support of cardiac contractility and SVR. Only one pediatric study has been performed, which demonstrated a 28% increase in PVR.[49]

Dexmedetomidine

Dexmedetomidine is associated with acutely decreased heart rate and increased MAP and SVR, followed over time by a decrease in MAP.[50,51] These changes appear to be dose dependent. Despite the early significant increase in SVR, a similar pulmonary vasoconstrictor response was not observed in children with pulmonary hypertension.[52]

Opioids

Opioids have minimal hemodynamic effects. PVR remains unchanged in response to fentanyl.[53] Pulmonary vascular responses to remifentanil are clinically insignificant in adults with artificial hearts.[54]

Midazolam

Midazolam exerts clinically insignificant effects on the pulmonary vasculature of adults with cardiac disease.[55]

To minimize the undesired hemodynamic effects of a full anesthetic dose of a single anesthetic drug, it is preferable to use a balanced anesthetic technique; that is, administration of subanesthetic doses of several anesthetics. Thus an adequate depth of anesthesia can be achieved without marked hemodynamic changes. For most procedures the authors use midazolam, fentanyl, or remifentanil, and low-concentration sevoflurane or isoflurane. Dexmedetomidine can be added, especially when postoperative sedation is desirable, and high doses of fentanyl can be used if postoperative tracheal extubation is not anticipated. Judicious use of propofol at low infusion rates can be considered, and balancing propofol with ketamine may avoid the undesired effects on SVR of each drug alone. Sometimes hypotension can be observed despite a balanced technique, especially in children who are hypovolemic.

AIRWAY MANAGEMENT

Airway management techniques by the anesthesiologist are chosen as appropriate for the surgical or catheterization procedure. Although case reports have described pulmonary hypertensive crises in association with emergent tracheal intubation, the reports are unclear as to whether intubation caused the pulmonary vascular response or the patients were intubated because of impending cardiac arrest following pulmonary hypertensive crisis. Tracheal suctioning is associated with a significant increase in both PAP and PVR in children with pulmonary hypertension,[56] but with adequate topical and general anesthesia, the authors do not hesitate to intubate when indicated for the type of procedure or condition of the patient. The authors are more inclined to use tracheal intubation for long procedures, interventional cardiac catheterization procedures, or unstable patients.

Alternatively, airway management with a face mask, laryngeal mask airway, or the natural airway (with end-tidal CO_2 monitoring via nasal cannulas) can be chosen when indicated, and the authors often use these for shorter diagnostic catheterization procedures in stable children. It should be remembered that hypoxia and hypercarbia can be associated with a pulmonary hypertensive event, and that airway obstruction or hypoventilation during cardiac catheterization are more likely to occur during sedative techniques with a natural airway than during anesthesia with controlled ventilation.[57] Therefore, the anesthesiologist should consider all options for airway access and ventilatory support.

PULMONARY HYPERTENSIVE CRISIS

Cardiac arrest in children with PAH is often immediately preceded by an acute pulmonary hypertensive crisis, whereby an acute increase in PVR leads to right ventricular failure and a decrease in cardiac output. The self-perpetuating cycle of biventricular failure associated with a pulmonary hypertensive crisis is illustrated in **Fig. 3**. A pulmonary hypertensive crisis can be triggered by several stimuli that directly affect PVR, such as hypoxia,[58,59] acidosis,[60] noxious tracheal stimulation,[56] or events that cause ventricular dysfunction, such as inadequate coronary perfusion associated with systemic hypotension (**Box 7**). Early studies by Rudolph and Yuan[59] suggest that keeping an arterial pH higher than 7.40 and an arterial oxygen pressure (PaO_2) GREATER than 60 mmHg can avoid a severe increase in PVR (**Fig. 4**).

Treatment of a pulmonary hypertensive crisis is directed toward ameliorating the stimulating event and stabilizing hemodynamics (**Table 2**). Early use of a systemic vasoconstrictor, such as epinephrine, norepinephrine, or phenylephrine, or an inotrope, such as epinephrine or dopamine, can improve coronary perfusion and cardiac function, and may avert cardiac arrest. A pulmonary vasodilator should be administered.

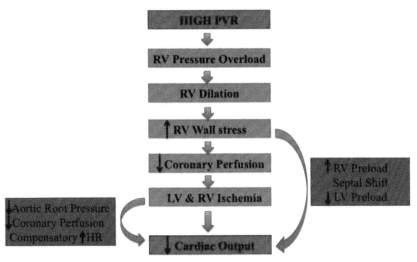

Fig. 3. Pathophysiologic changes during a pulmonary hypertensive crisis. HR, heart rate; LV, left ventricular; PVR, pulmonary vascular resistance; RV, right ventricular.

Because hypotension can be associated with acute administration of an intravenous vasodilator, it is preferable in an urgent setting to give pulmonary vasodilators by inhalation. This approach reduces the risk of systemic hypotension and coronary hypoperfusion by delivering the drug to the target pulmonary vasculature. iNO is the standard for inhaled pulmonary vasodilators, but inhaled prostacyclin analogues may be as effective. Once the cycle of increased PVR and decreased ventricular function begins, however, cardiac arrest may be difficult to prevent. If cardiac arrest occurs, Pediatric Advanced Life Support guidelines for cardiopulmonary resuscitation should be followed.[61] Cardiac arrest associated with pulmonary hypertensive crisis can be difficult to treat, and emergent use of extracorporeal membrane oxygenation (ECMO) may be necessary.[62] If emergent ECMO is required, improved outcomes are associated with shorter duration of cardiopulmonary resuscitation before ECMO, so an institutional protocol that anticipates the need for emergent ECMO in these situations is desirable.[63]

In addition to the avoidance of triggering stimuli, the risk of intraoperative cardiac arrest can be reduced by preoperative treatment with pulmonary vasodilator therapy. The odds ratio for children with PAH to develop a major perioperative complication was only 0.31 if they were chronically treated with a pulmonary vasodilator preoperatively.[26] Although the authors often use prophylactic administration of iNO during the

---

Box 7
Triggering stimuli for perioperative pulmonary hypertensive crisis

- Hypoxia
- Acidosis
- Hypercarbia
- Agitation and pain
- Tracheal suctioning
- Hypotension

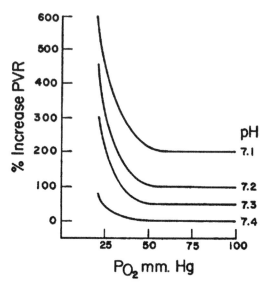

Fig. 4. Pattern of pulmonary vascular responses to changes of pH and Pao$_2$. The increases of pulmonary vascular resistance (PVR) are expressed as a percentage of the level at pH 7.4 and Pao$_2$ 100 mm Hg. The changes in PVR with changes in Pao$_2$ have been related at different levels of pH. (*From* Rudolph AM, Yuan S. Response of the pulmonary vasculature to hypoxia and H$^+$ ion concentration changes. J Clin Invest 1966;45:407; with permission.)

perioperative period for noncardiac surgical procedures, this is not usually done for diagnostic cardiac catheterization procedures in children with PAH, in which hemodynamic measurements under baseline conditions are measured.

When administration of a pulmonary vasodilator is indicated, the authors favor perioperative iNO over other pulmonary vasodilators for this purpose because it delivers drug directly to the pulmonary vascular bed, thus avoiding the systemic hypotension that can occur with acute intravenous administration of vasodilators. The authors administer iNO from beginning of induction of anesthesia into the recovery period,

Table 2 Treatment of pulmonary hypertensive crisis	
Treatment	**Rationale/Therapy**
Administer 100% O$_2$	↑ PAo$_2$ and Pao$_2$ will ↓ PVR
Hyperventilate	PVR is directly related to Paco$_2$
Exclude pneumothorax	Optimize ventilation
↓ Mean airway pressure	Avoid P$_{alv}$>P$_{art}$
Correct metabolic acidosis	PVR is directly related to H$^+$ level
Administer pulmonary vasodilators	iNO, magnesium
Analgesia	Decrease sympathetic mediated ↑ PVR
Support cardiac output	Phenylephrine, cautious volume, epinephrine
ECMO	Support cardiac output and oxygenation

Abbreviations: ECMO, extracorporeal membrane oxygenation; iNO, inhaled nitric oxide; P$_{alv}$, alveolar pressure; PAo$_2$, alveolar oxygen pressure; Pao$_2$, arterial oxygen pressure; P$_{art}$, arterial pressure; PVR, pulmonary vascular resistance.

when it can be administered by face mask or nasal cannulas.[64] Other pulmonary vasodilators that can be effectively administered by inhalation may emerge as satisfactory prophylactic perioperative drug therapy for children with pulmonary hypertension. These agents include the prostacyclin analogues epoprostenol,[65] iloprost,[66] and treprostinil,[67] the phosphodiesterase inhibitor milrinone, and nitroglycerin.[68]

POSTANESTHESIA RECOVERY

Children with PAH are at increased risk of adverse events following anesthesia.[69] Possible causes include increased pulmonary vascular tone, pulmonary hypertensive crisis, pulmonary thromboembolism, cardiac arrhythmia, and fluid shifts. All precautions should be taken to avoid hypoxemia, hypotension, and hypovolemia. Postoperative control of pain should be effective. Any therapy to decrease PVR, such as iNO, should be weaned with caution so as to avoid rebound increases in PVR.[70] It may be necessary to admit the child overnight to a unit where monitoring is available and immediate medical response is possible.

SUMMARY

Children with PAH undergoing cardiac catheterization are at increased risk of perioperative complications. This risk is greatest for those with suprasystemic pulmonary artery pressures and those with PAH who are not yet on any therapy. Although there are many factors that may contribute to the development of PAH, the final common pathway is elevated PAP. All currently available anesthetic agents will have an effect on the cardiovascular system. It is essential for the anesthesiologist to be aware of these effects and how they may change the data being acquired by the cardiologist. It is important to avoid factors that may trigger a pulmonary hypertensive crisis and, if one does occur, it is essential to respond appropriately. The most immediate available help in this situation may be the staff in the cardiac catheterization laboratory, making good communication important.

REFERENCES

1. Borlaug BA. Discerning pulmonary venous from pulmonary arterial hypertension without the help of a catheter. Circ Heart Fail 2011;4:235–7.
2. Strumpher J, Jacobsohn E. Pulmonary hypertension and right ventricular dysfunction: physiology and perioperative management. J Cardiothorac Vasc Anesth 2011;25:687–704.
3. Barst RJ, McGoon MD, Elliott CG, et al. Survival in childhood pulmonary arterial hypertension: insights from the registry to evaluate early and long-term pulmonary arterial hypertension disease management. Circulation 2012;125: 113–22.
4. Fraisse A, Jais X, Schleich JM, et al. Characteristics and prospective 2-year follow-up of children with pulmonary arterial hypertension in France. Arch Cardiovasc Dis 2010;103:66–74.
5. Humbert M, Sitbon O, Chaouat A, et al. Pulmonary arterial hypertension in France: results from a national registry. Am J Respir Crit Care Med 2006;173: 1023–30.
6. Fischer LG, Van Aken H, Burkle H. Management of pulmonary hypertension: physiological and pharmacological considerations for anesthesiologists. Anesth Analg 2003;96:1603–16.

7. Friesen RH, Williams GD. Anesthetic management of children with pulmonary arterial hypertension. Paediatr Anaesth 2008;18:208–16.

8. MacKnight B, Martinez EA, Simon BA. Anesthetic management of patients with pulmonary hypertension. Semin Cardiothorac Vasc Anesth 2008;12:91–6.

9. Shukla AC, Almodovar MC. Anesthesia considerations for children with pulmonary hypertension. Pediatr Crit Care Med 2010;11:S70–3.

10. Nef HM, Mollmann H, Hamm C, et al. Pulmonary hypertension: updated classification and management of pulmonary hypertension. Heart 2010;96:552–9.

11. Simonneau G, Galie N, Rubin LJ, et al. Clinical classification of pulmonary hypertension. J Am Coll Cardiol 2004;43:5S–12S.

12. Chemla D, Castelain V, Provencher S, et al. Evaluation of various empirical formulas for estimating mean pulmonary artery pressure by using systolic pulmonary artery pressure in adults. Chest 2009;135:760–8.

13. Alkon J, Humpl T, Manlhiot C, et al. Usefulness of the right ventricular systolic to diastolic duration ratio to predict functional capacity and survival in children with pulmonary arterial hypertension. Am J Cardiol 2010;106:430–6.

14. Forfia PR, Fisher MR, Mathai SC, et al. Tricuspid annular displacement predicts survival in pulmonary hypertension. Am J Respir Crit Care Med 2006;174:1034–41.

15. Koestenberger M, Nagel B, Avian A, et al. Systolic right ventricular function in children and young adults with pulmonary artery hypertension secondary to congenital heart disease and tetralogy of Fallot: tricuspid annular plane systolic excursion (TAPSE) and magnetic resonance imaging data. Congenit Heart Dis 2012;7:250–8.

16. Hoeper MM, Barbera JA, Channick RN, et al. Diagnosis, assessment, and treatment of non-pulmonary arterial hypertension pulmonary hypertension. J Am Coll Cardiol 2009;54:S85–96.

17. Cerro MJ, Abman S, Diaz G, et al. A consensus approach to the classification of pediatric pulmonary hypertensive vascular disease: report from the PVRI Pediatric Taskforce, Panama 2011. Pulm Circ 2011;1:286–98.

18. Ivy D. Advances in pediatric pulmonary arterial hypertension. Curr Opin Cardiol 2012;27:70–81.

19. Rashid A, Ivy D. Severe paediatric pulmonary hypertension: new management strategies. Arch Dis Child 2005;90:92–8.

20. Abman SH, Kinsella JP, Rosenzweig EB, et al. Implications of the U.S. Food and Drug Administration warning against the use of sildenafil for the treatment of pediatric pulmonary hypertension. Am J Respir Crit Care Med 2013;187:572–5.

21. Rosenzweig EB, Feinstein JA, Humpl T, et al. Pulmonary arterial hypertension in children: diagnostic work-up and challenges. Prog Pediatr Cardiol 2009;27:4–11.

22. Wilkinson JL. Haemodynamic calculations in the catheter laboratory. Heart 2001;85:113–20.

23. Hill KD, Lim DS, Everett AD, et al. Assessment of pulmonary hypertension in the pediatric catheterization laboratory: current insights from the magic registry. Catheter Cardiovasc Interv 2010;76:865–73.

24. McLaughlin VV, McGoon MD. Pulmonary arterial hypertension. Circulation 2006;114:1417–31.

25. Morray JP, Geiduschek JM, Ramamoorthy C, et al. Anesthesia-related cardiac arrest in children: initial findings of the Pediatric Perioperative Cardiac Arrest (POCA) Registry. Anesthesiology 2000;93:6–14.

26. Williams GD, Maan H, Ramamoorthy C, et al. Perioperative complications in children with pulmonary hypertension undergoing general anesthesia with ketamine. Paediatr Anaesth 2010;20:28–37.
27. Bando K, Turrentine MW, Sharp TG, et al. Pulmonary hypertension after operations for congenital heart disease: analysis of risk factors and management. J Thorac Cardiovasc Surg 1996;112:1600–7 [discussion: 1607–9].
28. Bennett D, Marcus R, Stokes M. Incidents and complications during pediatric cardiac catheterization. Paediatr Anaesth 2005;15:1083–8.
29. Carmosino MJ, Friesen RH, Doran A, et al. Perioperative complications in children with pulmonary hypertension undergoing noncardiac surgery or cardiac catheterization. Anesth Analg 2007;104:521–7.
30. Taylor CJ, Derrick G, McEwan A, et al. Risk of cardiac catheterization under anaesthesia in children with pulmonary hypertension. Br J Anaesth 2007;98: 657–61.
31. Mori Y, Nakazawa M, Yagihara T. Complications of pediatric cardiac catheterization and system of catheterization laboratories minimizing complications—a Japanese multicenter survey. J Cardiol 2010;56:183–8.
32. Hollinger I, Mittnacht A. Cardiac catheterization laboratory: catheterization, interventional cardiology, and ablation techniques for children. Int Anesthesiol Clin 2009;47:63–99.
33. Joe RR, Chen LQ. Anesthesia in the cardiac catheterization lab. Anesthesiol Clin North America 2003;21:639–51.
34. Hanouz JL, Massetti M, Guesne G, et al. In vitro effects of desflurane, sevoflurane, isoflurane, and halothane in isolated human right atria. Anesthesiology 2000;92:116–24.
35. Rivenes SM, Lewin MB, Stayer SA, et al. Cardiovascular effects of sevoflurane, isoflurane, halothane, and fentanyl-midazolam in children with congenital heart disease: an echocardiographic study of myocardial contractility and hemodynamics. Anesthesiology 2001;94:223–9.
36. Pagel PS, Fu JL, Damask MC, et al. Desflurane and isoflurane produce similar alterations in systemic and pulmonary hemodynamics and arterial oxygenation in patients undergoing one-lung ventilation during thoracotomy. Anesth Analg 1998;87:800–7.
37. Laird TH, Stayer SA, Rivenes SM, et al. Pulmonary-to-systemic blood flow ratio effects of sevoflurane, isoflurane, halothane, and fentanyl/midazolam with 100% oxygen in children with congenital heart disease. Anesth Analg 2002;95:1200–6 [table of contents].
38. Hickey PR, Hansen DD, Strafford M, et al. Pulmonary and systemic hemodynamic effects of nitrous oxide in infants with normal and elevated pulmonary vascular resistance. Anesthesiology 1986;65:374–8.
39. Gelissen HP, Epema AH, Henning RH, et al. Inotropic effects of propofol, thiopental, midazolam, etomidate, and ketamine on isolated human atrial muscle. Anesthesiology 1996;84:397–403.
40. Hammaren E, Hynynen M. Haemodynamic effects of propofol infusion for sedation after coronary artery surgery. Br J Anaesth 1995;75:47–50.
41. Williams GD, Jones TK, Hanson KA, et al. The hemodynamic effects of propofol in children with congenital heart disease. Anesth Analg 1999;89:1411–6.
42. Rouby JJ, Andreev A, Leger P, et al. Peripheral vascular effects of thiopental and propofol in humans with artificial hearts. Anesthesiology 1991;75:32–42.
43. Williams GD, Friesen RH. Administration of ketamine to children with pulmonary hypertension is safe: pro-con debate. Paediatr Anaesth 2012;22:1042–52.

44. Berman W Jr, Fripp RR, Rubler M, et al. Hemodynamic effects of ketamine in children undergoing cardiac catheterization. Pediatr Cardiol 1990;11:72–6.
45. Morray JP, Lynn AM, Stamm SJ, et al. Hemodynamic effects of ketamine in children with congenital heart disease. Anesth Analg 1984;63:895–9.
46. Wolfe RR, Loehr JP, Schaffer MS, et al. Hemodynamic effects of ketamine, hypoxia and hyperoxia in children with surgically treated congenital heart disease residing greater than or equal to 1,200 meters above sea level. Am J Cardiol 1991;67:84–7.
47. Hickey PR, Hansen DD, Cramolini GM, et al. Pulmonary and systemic hemodynamic responses to ketamine in infants with normal and elevated pulmonary vascular resistance. Anesthesiology 1985;62:287–93.
48. Williams GD, Philip BM, Chu LF, et al. Ketamine does not increase pulmonary vascular resistance in children with pulmonary hypertension undergoing sevoflurane anesthesia and spontaneous ventilation. Anesth Analg 2007;105: 1578–84 [table of contents].
49. Sarkar M, Laussen PC, Zurakowski D, et al. Hemodynamic responses to etomidate on induction of anesthesia in pediatric patients. Anesth Analg 2005;101: 645–50 [table of contents].
50. Jooste EH, Muhly WT, Ibinson JW, et al. Acute hemodynamic changes after rapid intravenous bolus dosing of dexmedetomidine in pediatric heart transplant patients undergoing routine cardiac catheterization. Anesth Analg 2010; 111:1490–6.
51. Mason KP, Zurakowski D, Zgleszewski SE, et al. High dose dexmedetomidine as the sole sedative for pediatric MRI. Paediatr Anaesth 2008;18:403–11.
52. Friesen RH, Nichols CS, Twite MD, et al. Hemodynamic response to dexmedetomidine loading dose in children with and without pulmonary hypertension. Anesth Analg 2013;17:953–9.
53. Hickey PR, Hansen DD, Wessel DL, et al. Pulmonary and systemic hemodynamic responses to fentanyl in infants. Anesth Analg 1985;64:483–6.
54. Ouattara A, Boccara G, Kockler U, et al. Remifentanil induces systemic arterial vasodilation in humans with a total artificial heart. Anesthesiology 2004;100:602–7.
55. Raza SM, Masters RW, Zsigmond EK. Comparison of the hemodynamic effects of midazolam and diazepam in patients with coronary occlusion. Int J Clin Pharmacol Ther Toxicol 1989;27:1–6.
56. Hickey PR, Hansen DD, Wessel DL, et al. Blunting of stress responses in the pulmonary circulation of infants by fentanyl. Anesth Analg 1985;64:1137–42.
57. Friesen RH, Alswang M. Changes in carbon dioxide tension and oxygen saturation during deep sedation for paediatric cardiac catheterization. Paediatr Anaesth 1996;6:15–20.
58. Chang AC, Zucker HA, Hickey PR, et al. Pulmonary vascular resistance in infants after cardiac surgery: role of carbon dioxide and hydrogen ion. Crit Care Med 1995;23:568–74.
59. Rudolph AM, Yuan S. Response of the pulmonary vasculature to hypoxia and H^+ ion concentration changes. J Clin Invest 1966;45:399–411.
60. Morray JP, Lynn AM, Mansfield PB. Effect of pH and PCO_2 on pulmonary and systemic hemodynamics after surgery in children with congenital heart disease and pulmonary hypertension. J Pediatr 1988;113:474–9.
61. Kleinman ME, Chameides L, Schexnayder SM, et al. Part 14: pediatric advanced life support: 2010 American Heart Association Guidelines for Cardiopulmonary Resuscitation and Emergency Cardiovascular Care. Circulation 2010;122:S876–908.

62. Allan CK, Thiagarajan RR, Armsby LR, et al. Emergent use of extracorporeal membrane oxygenation during pediatric cardiac catheterization. Pediatr Crit Care Med 2006;7:212–9.
63. Sivarajan VB, Best D, Brizard CP, et al. Duration of resuscitation prior to rescue extracorporeal membrane oxygenation impacts outcome in children with heart disease. Intensive Care Med 2011;37:853–60.
64. Ivy DD, Griebel JL, Kinsella JP, et al. Acute hemodynamic effects of pulsed delivery of low flow nasal nitric oxide in children with pulmonary hypertension. J Pediatr 1998;133:453–6.
65. Kelly LK, Porta NF, Goodman DM, et al. Inhaled prostacyclin for term infants with persistent pulmonary hypertension refractory to inhaled nitric oxide. J Pediatr 2002;141:830–2.
66. Rimensberger PC, Spahr-Schopfer I, Berner M, et al. Inhaled nitric oxide versus aerosolized iloprost in secondary pulmonary hypertension in children with congenital heart disease: vasodilator capacity and cellular mechanisms. Circulation 2001;103:544–8.
67. Voswinckel R, Enke B, Reichenberger F, et al. Favorable effects of inhaled treprostinil in severe pulmonary hypertension: results from randomized controlled pilot studies. J Am Coll Cardiol 2006;48:1672–81.
68. Singh R, Choudhury M, Saxena A, et al. Inhaled nitroglycerin versus inhaled milrinone in children with congenital heart disease suffering from pulmonary artery hypertension. J Cardiothorac Vasc Anesth 2010;24:797–801.
69. Blaise G, Langleben D, Hubert B. Pulmonary arterial hypertension: pathophysiology and anesthetic approach. Anesthesiology 2003;99:1415–32.
70. Namachivayam P, Theilen U, Butt WW, et al. Sildenafil prevents rebound pulmonary hypertension after withdrawal of nitric oxide in children. Am J Respir Crit Care Med 2006;174:1042–7.

Anesthesia and Analgesia for Pectus Excavatum Surgery

Jagroop Mavi, MD, David L. Moore, MD*

KEYWORDS

- Pectus excavatum • Nuss procedure • Thoracic epidural • Haller index
- Chest wall deformities • Multimodal analgesics

KEY POINTS

- Special attention is needed during surgical dissection across the mediastinum due to arrhythmias and potential viscus/vessel perforation.
- Deep extubation is preferable for avoidance of coughing and straining on the endotracheal tube, which can cause subcutaneous emphysema.
- Pain tends to be worse with increased age, because patients with ossified ribcages tolerate the procedure less.
- Multimodal analgesic techniques work best including nonnarcotic analgesics, narcotics, regional anesthesia, muscle relaxants, and anxiolytics.
- Aggressive physical therapy, particularly ambulation, improves dynamic pain control and may decrease chronic postoperative pain.

INTRODUCTION

Pectus deformities, mainly pectus excavatum, are the most common chest wall deformity seen by pediatricians and family practitioners.[1] Originally described by Ravitch in 1949, pectus repair was undertaken in the more severe instances to correct the existing deformity and to prevent its progression. It was believed at the time of surgical correction that younger patients had a higher chance for attaining a normal appearance with subsequent growth of the thoracic cage.[2]

These deformities are caused by defective growth of the sternum and surrounding costal cartilages. Although criticized by some as a cosmetic repair, other evidence supports surgical repair because of the increased likelihood of progressive cardiopulmonary dysfunction over time.

Disclosures: There are no disclosures to declare. Neither author has any direct financial interests in the subject matter or materials discussed in the article, or with a company making a competing product. No financial support except departmental salary support for the authors.
Department of Anesthesia, Cincinnati Children's Hospital Medical Center, 3333 Burnet Avenue, Cincinnati, OH 45229, USA
* Corresponding author.
E-mail address: david.moore@cchmc.org

After need for surgical repair has been established, the technique of choice for the last couple of decades has been the Nuss procedure.[3] This is a minimally invasive technique in which rigid metal bars are placed transthoracically beneath the sternum and costal cartilages for a period of time until permanent remodeling of the chest wall has occurred. That length of time tends to be 2 years before bars are removed.

During anesthesia, the three areas of focus include (1) potential for considerable blood loss, (2) potential for lethal arrhythmias, and (3) potential consequences of pneumothoraces. Postoperative pain is considerable, making multimodal analgesia the hallmark of postoperative pain control. Controversy exists regarding the best method of controlling postoperative pain, whether the emphasis is placed on patient-controlled analgesia (PCA) or regional anesthesia. Part of the answer may be found by examining patient outcomes. However, measuring patient outcomes depends on the identity of the enquirer. Surgeons, anesthesiologists, pain services, and hospital administration may all have different end points. Surgeons may look at optimal correction of the deformity followed by a short length of stay. The anesthesia team may be invested in a safe passage through anesthesia without complications. The pain service may focus on optimal postoperative pain control, and the hospital administration may be most concerned with cost and patient satisfaction scores.

EPIDEMIOLOGY

Pectus excavatum occurred in approximately 0.12% of patients in one autopsy series.[4] Researchers investigated the prevalence of pectus excavatum in teenage public school students in Brazil, and found it to be 1.275%.[5] Of the congenital chest wall deformities, between 3% and 4% fall under the umbrella of rare deformities (eg, pentalogy of Cantrell, Jeune syndrome, and Poland syndrome).[6] Pectus excavatum and pectus carinatum represent the remainder, with 90% of those being pectus excavatum.[1,6]

Gender distribution favors males, noted in different studies from a 2:1 ratio up to 9:1.[5,6] Although no genetic defect has specifically been discovered, positive family histories, up to 65.5% in one study, make this predisposition likely.[5]

Depending on the surgeon, the type of operation, and the presence of connective tissue disorders, recurrence occurs with unsatisfactory results thus requiring reoperation in 2% to 37%,[7] although most series claim recurrence rates of 2% to 10%.[8]

PATHOPHYSIOLOGY

The cause of pectus deformity is largely unknown. There are multiple hypotheses regarding the origin. The current dominant theory to explain the development of these two most common chest wall deformities is overgrowth of the costal cartilages.[9] Collagen type II is one of the major structural components of rib cartilage, but results of histologic and biochemical studies of costal cartilages in patients with pectus excavatum remain inconclusive.[9]

CLINICAL PICTURE

Patients with pectus excavatum, or "funnel chest" as it is known, typically present for repair during adolescence. There has been some discussion in the literature as to the best timing for surgical repair. In the past, these defects were repaired at an earlier age (4–6 years of age) using a Ravitch procedure,[2] which removes three to four overgrown cartilages and repositions the sternum.[10] Even Nuss tended to repair these defects prepubertally. His patients had an age range of 1 to 15 years old, with most in the

3- to 5-year range.[3] This contrasts with more recent studies involving the Nuss procedure, which have a mean age of between 13 and 23 years of age.[8,11–13]

Pectus repair can be problematic in very young children. Patients may be more active following discharge and have a greater rate of sustaining unexpected trauma.[3] Rib growth after early pectus correction can also be impaired in younger patients, sometimes to the point of minimizing chest wall movement, also known as asphyxiating thoracic chondrodystrophy.[3]

Repairs in older patients can be more difficult, with prolonged operating time and more blood loss.[3] The trend in current practice is to wait for patients to reach their middle teenage years to perform a pectus excavatum repair. This allows for the patients to complete their teenage growth spurt and have a less likely chance of recurrence. Nonetheless, older school-age children and younger teenagers with significant cardiorespiratory compromise affecting their ability to participate in aerobic sports could also be candidates for repair.

Patients with connective tissue disorders, such as Marfan syndrome and Ehlers-Danlos syndrome, are noted to have a higher incidence of recurrence.[7] Therefore, one might consider waiting to correct these deformities. However, this subset of patients is at risk for aortic dilation and aortic valve insufficiency. Patients with normal cardiac anatomy may have repair of their pectus excavatum on an elective basis, but those in need of aortic arch repair may need to have their pectus repaired at the time of open heart surgery, or deferred to a later date after cardiac repair.[14] Thus, the timing of surgery for patients with these connective tissues disorders must also be carefully assessed.

Reasons for postpubertal repair include body image issues that become manifest during puberty, recurrence of the defect, and progressive cardiopulmonary dysfunction. Patients may have dyspnea on exertion, shortness of breath, breathlessness, a feeling of heaviness in the chest, air hunger, and exercise intolerance.[14] These symptoms can be progressive, and may not be eminent until the patient or family notices difficulties in "keeping up with their peers."

Indications for surgery to correct a pectus excavatum include symptomatic patients, which includes exercise intolerance, decreased endurance, and pain; body image issues; Haller index greater than 3; caliper measurement depth greater than 2.5 cm; exercise-induced asthma; abnormal pulmonary function tests (PFTs); and compression of the right atrium or right ventricle on echocardiogram.[14]

Currently, the work-up for pectus excavatum repair includes a history and physical examination and frequently includes a computed tomography (CT) scan of the chest. Since the early 1990s, CT scans have been used to evaluate patients with pectus deformities for surgery. CT scans more clearly document the severity of the deformity, along with the degree of cardiac compression and displacement, the degree of lung compression, and other unexpected problems.[3] In patients with known cardiac issues, a cardiac magnetic resonance imaging has been used. Additional work-up may include echocardiography, caliper measurement of the depth of pectus deformity (>2.5 cm),[14] and PFTs. In general, most patients with significant pectus excavatum have low normal or below normal PFTs. Both static and exercise PFTs are useful in eliciting a physiologic effect of the pectus excavatum defect on the patient.

The Haller index is a measure of pectus excavatum severity using a CT scan measurement. The CT is used to demonstrate the abnormal ratio between the patient's transverse diameter and their anterior-posterior diameter.[10] An index of more than three is considered a moderately severe or greater defect.[10,14] The width of the chest between the ribs at the lowest level of the pectus defect is measured in centimeters and divided by the height of the chest from the anterior aspect of the spine to the back of the lowest part of the sternal defect. The quotient from this division is the Haller index (**Figs. 1** and **2**).

An echocardiogram may be useful to perform because it may show the depressed sternum compressing the right atrium and right ventricle, which may interfere with diastolic filling of these structures. Significant compression of the right heart chambers by the depressed sternum is an indication for surgical correction.[14] Mitral valve prolapse is also commonly seen in patients with pectus excavatum.

Patients with pectus excavatum should also be assessed for connective tissue disorders. Less than 1% of patients with pectus excavatum may have an underlying connective tissue disorder, such as Marfan syndrome, Ehlers-Danlos syndrome, or Loeys-Dietz syndrome. If this class of disorders is suspected then further genetic, cardiac, and ophthalmologic evaluations should be performed.[14]

Most pectus excavatum defects involve the lower end of the sternum with the turning down of the sternum and inward turning of costal cartilages four through seven. In regards to the Nuss procedure and surgical technique, two bars are more effective than a single bar but may cause overcorrection in some patients. Those with Marfan syndrome and other connective tissue diseases have soft bones and therefore require two bars to distribute the pressures over a wider area.[3]

The advantages of the minimally invasive technique include no anterior chest wall incision, no need to raise pectoralis muscle flaps, and no need to resect rib cartilages or perform sternal osteotomy. Other advantages include short operating time, minimal blood loss, early return to full activity, and excellent long-term cosmetic results.[3] Disadvantages of the Nuss minimally invasive technique include greater postoperative pain; longer inpatient length of stay; higher cost compared with other techniques; and more involved methods of pain control, including regional anesthesia.[13]

ANESTHESIA MANAGEMENT

The anesthesia management of pectus excavatum repairs can be divided into three main categories: (1) preoperative evaluation and preparation, (2) intraoperative management, and (3) postoperative analgesia.

Preoperatively, the degree of cardiac and pulmonary dysfunction is important to assess. This information can be obtained from a thorough history and physical examination focusing on exercise tolerance and symptomatology. Further knowledge of the cardiopulmonary insult can be obtained from the CT scan and Haller index,

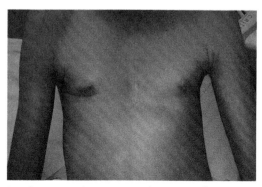

Fig. 1. Anterior photo of preoperative pectus patient. Note the incisional scar from original pectus repair at earlier age.

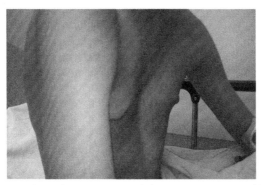

Fig. 2. Photo from more lateral aspect. Pectus deformity more noticeable from this aspect. Note the "rolling" forward of the shoulders and kyphosis, which are not unusual for these patients.

electrocardiogram, echocardiogram, and PFTs. Knowledge about cardiac compromise, arrhythmias, and pectus recurrence can only help to increase situational awareness.

Preparation before the case is essential, and the need to be prepared for potentially large blood loss is foremost. Type and screening of the patient's blood is necessary to receive emergency blood products in case of catastrophe. It is mandatory to receive confirmation of potential blood products in the operating room before proceeding with surgery.

Decisions concerning methods of postoperative pain control need to be made and addressed preoperatively. Typically, a postoperative pain service manages the patient's pain after the procedure. The pain service confers with surgery and anesthesia about the type of regional anesthesia and type of narcotic. Regional anesthesia includes anesthesia-driven blocks, such as thoracic epidural and paravertebral blocks; and surgeon-driven blocks, such as intercostal nerve blocks, wound catheter placement, and local infiltration. Anesthesia-driven blocks need to be placed preoperatively and many choose to do awake thoracic blocks when possible. The practitioner cannot use the lateral decubitus position after surgery for fear of dislodging the newly placed pectus bar.

Because this surgery is extremely painful, another important preoperative consideration, preferably days to weeks preoperatively, is to alleviate anxiety among the patient and family, and manage expectations about the surgery. A chief method of diminishing anxiety and creating reasonable expectations is through education. Parents and patients, if possible, are expected to attend a mandatory educational class about the surgery and hospital course, or view a simulcast of the class. This helps to create more appropriate expectations and assuage anxiety. Once the preoperative evaluation and preparations are complete, the patient is ready for the operating room.

Intraoperative management is often as follows. The patient is brought into the operating room, and after placement of monitors, a peripheral intravenous (IV) line is placed with the aid of nitrous sedation. After securing IV access, the patient is lightly sedated and assisted to the sitting position in preparation for placement of regional anesthesia, which frequently consists of a thoracic epidural.

Compliance with inserting the epidural catheter awake may be difficult in more immature teenagers and young children. Typically, this is attempted in adults and teenagers, or uncommonly in less anxious children. After local anesthetic is infiltrated subcutaneously, an 18-G Tuohy needle is inserted between the spinous processes of

T5-6 or T6-7, and the epidural space noted by loss of resistance to air or preservative-free saline. Placement of the epidural at higher intervertebral spaces has been noted postoperatively to have a higher rate of failed block; higher rate of Horner syndrome; and higher rate of upper extremity issues, such as weak grip and numbness. Weak grip and numbness, although confirmatory for success of block, may cause distress for the patient and necessitate changes in rate and concentration of epidural solution. The catheter is advanced 3 to 4 cm into the epidural space and secured in place. Further advancement has been noted to result in one-sided and failed blocks. A test dose is administered, and once confirmed negative a sterile dressing is placed around the catheter and the patient is returned to a supine position. If there are problems placing the regional anesthetic in the seated patient because of compliance or positioning issues, it may be more advantageous to induce anesthesia, secure the airway, and then place the epidural in the lateral decubitus position.

In regards to further access and monitoring, a second, preferably large-bore peripheral intravenous line (PIV) is placed in preparation for possible rapid fluid or blood administration. An arterial line is not required unless the patient has significant cardiac or pulmonary derangements requiring continuous blood pressure monitoring or frequent blood gas measurements.

The patient is initially placed in a supine position; however, because the surgeon needs to enter and exit through the midthorax by way of the anterior to midaxillary line, the patient's arms must be placed in anatomic position, palm out, at right angles above their head. To minimize traction injuries of the upper extremity, padding is important, as is keeping the patient's joints at right angles.

There are some major anesthetic concerns intraoperatively, particularly injury to the heart and other mediastinal structures, that have been described with this procedure. This complication can happen at the time of bar placement or later, when the bar is removed. With placement, use of bilateral thoracoscopy aids in the careful dissection around the lungs, mediastinum, and pericardium to pass to the contralateral pleural space.[15] Mediastinal dissection is typically the time when arrhythmias can be an issue. Usually, the volume of the pulse oximetry monitor is increased to help the surgeons recognize moments that the dissection may be imperiling the patient. Auditory cues and heightened focus of the electrocardiogram at this time are expected.

After the bar (or bars) is in place and secured, management of the iatrogenic bilateral pneumothoraces is important. Typically, temporary suctioning of the pleural spaces along with a Valsalva maneuver is used to alleviate the pneumothorax on either side. An intraoperative chest radiograph is used to confirm this.

Avoidance of coughing or straining is preferable to circumvent the development of subcutaneous emphysema, created by forcible expulsion of residual pneumothorax. Obviating this can be achieved by deep extubation or significant narcotics to avoid straining on the endotracheal tube.

Intraoperative mortality from exsanguination caused by cardiac or vascular injury has been described, and although rare, heightened vigilance, adequate IV access, and availability of packed red blood cells are important. When these patients return for pectus bar removal after several years, occasionally the bar has become adherent to the lung or pericardium resulting in a severe, sudden, and catastrophic rupture of a major vessel or heart chamber on removal.[16] It is important to be prepared and establish ample IV access to massively resuscitate and transfuse fluids to these patients should a catastrophe occur.

Other common risks postoperatively include bar displacement, residual pneumothorax, and infection; however, cardiac injury, sternal erosion, arterial pseudoaneurysm, and persistent cardiac arrhythmias are also possible.

Patients undergoing thoracic surgery experience a great amount of postoperative pain, particularly in the older subset because the ribcage has become more rigid and ossified. This may be caused by surgical retraction and dissection of intercostal muscles, and conformational change of an ossified ribcage. These patients have been shown to have better pain control and improved postsurgical ventilation and pulmonary toilet with epidural analgesia.[17–20] However, there are studies that show similar pain control between thoracic epidural and PCA.[21–24] Whichever approach to postoperative pain is chosen, the regimen for pectus excavatum repairs requires a multimodal approach.

Patients and families should be educated preoperatively in regards to the high degree of postoperative pain expected despite being a minimally invasive approach. Classic studies have demonstrated that the knowledgeable patient requires less analgesia in the postoperative period, and at the same time experiences less pain than the less informed patient.[25] The transition from an epidural to oral pain medication can also be challenging and often requires dosing or medication adjustments to establish an optimal regimen. Aggressive physical therapy, particularly ambulation, improves dynamic pain control and may decrease chronic postoperative pain.[25] It is vital for the patient's care team to encourage movement up to the chair and ambulation even before the epidural has been removed.

Patients who have had previous repair of their pectus excavatum with either a modified Ravitch procedure or a Nuss procedure may present with recurrent disease. For patients with recurrent pectus excavatum it is important to know if the patient is having recurrent symptoms. Patients often may present with pain associated with their recurrence, and a return to their original pulmonary symptomatology. Patients with chronic pain as the only feature of their recurrence may continue to have pain after repair.[14]

There are numerous protocols established to manage postoperative pain control after pectus excavatum repairs. Institutions use either a PCA or regional anesthesia, either a thoracic epidural or paravertebral blocks as the main method of controlling immediate postoperative pain.

One such protocol that has been used effectively begins with the placement of a thoracic epidural in the T5-6 or T6-7 interspace followed by a loading dose of local anesthetic (0.2% ropivacaine) up to 10 mL based on weight, given in an incremental fashion. When the loading dose is complete, an epidural infusion is started consisting of local anesthetic plus clonidine. For the local anesthetic in this mixture a higher concentration is often used (eg, 0.15% ropivicaine). The epidural is run until postoperative Day 3 for all pectus repairs.

The multimodal approach to pain management is used and has been shown to be most effective. Intermittent IV narcotics are available to the patient as needed; however, some patients may need a PCA to supplement the epidural analgesia. Other supplemental medications include methocarbamol (Robaxin), 15 mg/kg IV, with a maximum dose of 1000 mg every 8 hours for 3 days followed by transition to oral Robaxin. Diazepam (Valium), 0.05 mg/kg IV every 4 hours as needed, is very effective in the treatment of muscle spasms and postoperative anxiety, and ketorolac (Toradol), 0.5 mg/kg IV with a maximum of 30 mg every 6 hours for 2 days started on postoperative Day 1, is a useful anti-inflammatory agent. IV acetaminophen every 6 hours is started intraoperatively and continued for up to 3 days postoperatively, then transitioned to the oral form as needed.

As the patient begins oral intake, they also begin to be transitioned to oral pain medications. Oxycodone (Oxycontin), 10 mg twice daily, is started on the first postoperative day. This can be titrated upward if needed. Oxycodone, 0.1 to 0.2 mg/kg every 4 hours, is started on the second postoperative day in the morning. The urinary catheter is also removed approximately 4 hours after epidural removal.

All medications are switched to the oral route, and doses and frequency are adjusted as needed to provide optimal patient comfort. The intermitted IV narcotic is kept available for breakthrough pain after epidural removal, because this is a transition when pain scores often increase by one to two points until an optimal oral pain medication regimen has been achieved. Pain medications are continued for 2 weeks postoperatively; older patients may need pain medication coverage for longer. Patients older than the age of 17 years may require narcotic pain medications longer than 2 weeks postoperatively, and patients with excessive pain issues during

---

Box 1
Cincinnati Children's Hospital pectus excavatum postoperative pain protocol

Preoperative preparation
- Manage expectations: despite "minimally invasive" still quite painful
- Pain plan: agree and consent for regional anesthesia if agreed on

Day of surgery (POD#0)
- Epidural placement (T5-7) by anesthesia/pain team
- Epidural solution: ropivacaine, 0.15%–0.2% with clonidine, 1 µg/mL
- IV acetaminophen (Ofirmev), 15 mg/kg IV (Max 1000 mg) every 6 hours ATC × 3 days
- IV methocarbamol (Robaxin), 15 mg/kg IV (Max 1000 mg) every 8 hours ATC × 3 days
- IV diazepam (Valium), 0.05 mg/kg IV every 4–6 hours prn for spasm
- IV opioids, if needed, prn or PCA

Postoperative Day 1 (POD#1)
- Continue epidural analgesia, IV acetaminophen, IV methocarbamol, IV diazepam prn
- Start IV ketorolac (Toradol), 0.5 mg/kg up to 15 mg IV every 6 hours ATC
- Start oxycontin, 10 or 20 mg PO every 12 hours; if needed, make every 8 hours

Postoperative Day 2 (POD#2)
- Start oxycodone, 0.1–0.2 mg/kg PO every 4 hours; schedule as ATC, but may be held for parent-patient refusal, respiratory depression, oversedation (Ramsey 4 to 6)
- Continue epidural analgesia, IV acetaminophen, IV/PO methocarbamol, IV/PO diazepam as needed
- Place order in electronic records to stop epidural at 6 AM on POD#3

Postoperative Day 3 (POD#3)
- Stop epidural at 6 AM and remove on morning pain rounds
- Discontinue urinary catheter 4 hours after stopping epidural (∼10 AM)
- Once epidural is out: continue oxycontin/oxycodone, PO acetaminophen every 6 hours (maximum, 75 mg/kg/d), PO methocarbamol ATC and/or PO diazepam as needed
- Start PO ibuprofen (10 mg/kg/dose, up to 3 times per day)

Postoperative Day 4+ (POD#4+)
- Keep on service and help manage postepidural pain control
- If 17 years+, history of chronic pain, or prolonged need for oral narcotics >2 weeks, have patient follow up in chronic pain clinic to assist in titration off of narcotics

Abbreviations: ATC, around the clock; IV, intravenous; PO, per os (oral); POD, postoperative day.

hospitalization are followed by the chronic pain service until successfully transitioned off pain medications (**Box 1**).

Problems that can be encountered with thoracic epidural analgesia include hypotension, failed epidural, one-sided epidural, upper extremity weakness or tingling, Horner syndrome, inadequate dermatomal coverage requiring a higher epidural rate, and in rare but serious cases an epidural hematoma or an epidural abscess. The epidural site should be checked multiple times daily by the pain management team and nursing staff to assess for signs of infection at the site or dislodgement of the epidural catheter. Fever is also important to follow up, because this can be a sign of epidural infection. Typically, sustained high fever is an indication for epidural removal.

Other forms of regional anesthesia have been described in lieu of placing a thoracic epidural and have been successful in treating postoperative pain control. These include bilateral intercostal nerve blocks, bilateral paravertebral catheters, and wound catheter infusions.

In conclusion, pectus excavatum repairs are a common type of congenital chest wall deformity, and although minimally invasive are categorized as extremely painful procedures. Preoperative evaluation should focus on patient symptoms, cardiopulmonary examination, and radiologic evidence of the magnitude of the defect. Preparation should include patient-parent education, readiness of donor blood products, and establishment of a postoperative pain management plan. Intraoperative vigilance is extremely important during bar placement and dissection because this could be a time of catastrophic events. Postoperatively, thoracic epidurals are the superior form of postoperative pain control, in addition to use of supplemental medications as part of a multimodal analgesic technique.

REFERENCES

1. Ravitch MM. Congenital Deformities of the Chest Wall and their Operative Correction. Philadelphia: W.B. Saunders Company; 1977.
2. Ravitch MM. The operative treatment of pectus excavatum. Ann Surg 1949;129: 429.
3. Nuss D, Kelly RE Jr, Croitoru DP, et al. A 10-year review of a minimally invasive technique for the correction of pectus excavatum. J Pediatr Surg 1998; 33(1):545.
4. Kelly RE Jr, Lawson ML, Paidas CN, et al. Pectus excavatum in a 112-year autopsy series: anatomic findings and the effect on survival. J Pediatr Surg 2005; 40:1275.
5. Westphal FL, Lima LC, Lima Neto JC, et al. Prevalence of pectus carinatum and pectus excavatum in students in the city of Manaus, Brazil. J Bras Pneumol 2009; 35:221.
6. Brochhausen C, Turial S, Muller FK, et al. Pectus excavatum: history, hypotheses and treatment options. Interact Cardiovasc Thorac Surg 2012;14:801.
7. Ellis D, Snyder C, Mann C. The 'redo' chest wall deformity correction. J Pediatr Surg 1997;32:5.
8. Redlinger RE Jr, Kelly RE Jr, Nuss D, et al. One hundred patients with recurrent pectus excavatum repaired via the minimally invasive Nuss technique–effective in most regardless of initial operative approach. J Pediatr Surg 2011;46:1177.
9. Fokin AA, Steuerwald NM, Ahrens WA, et al. Anatomical, histologic, and genetic characteristics of congenital chest wall deformities. Semin Thorac Cardiovasc Surg 2009;21:44.

10. Haller JA Jr, Scherer LR, Turner CS, et al. Evolving management of pectus excavatum based on a single institutional experience of 664 patients. Ann Surg 1989; 209:578.
11. Barua A, Rao VP, Barua B, et al. Patient satisfaction following minimally invasive repair of pectus excavatum: single surgeon experience. J Surg Tech Case Rep 2012;4:86.
12. Croitoru DP, Kelly RE Jr, Goretsky MJ, et al. The minimally invasive Nuss technique for recurrent or failed pectus excavatum repair in 50 patients. J Pediatr Surg 2005;40:181.
13. Antonoff MB, Erickson AE, Hess DJ, et al. When patients choose: comparison of Nuss, Ravitch, and Leonard procedures for primary repair of pectus excavatum. J Pediatr Surg 2009;44:1113.
14. Colombani PM. Preoperative assessment of chest wall deformities. Semin Thorac Cardiovasc Surg 2009;21:58.
15. Guo L, Mei J, Ding F, et al. Modified Nuss procedure in the treatment of recurrent pectus excavatum after open repair. Interact Cardiovasc Thorac Surg 2013;17:258.
16. Cote CJ. A Practice of Anesthesia for Infants and Children. 5th edition. Philadelphia: W.B. Saunders Company; 2009.
17. McBride WJ, Dicker R, Abajian JC, et al. Continuous thoracic epidural infusions for postoperative analgesia after pectus deformity repair. J Pediatr Surg 1996; 31:105.
18. Kavanagh BP, Katz J, Sandler AN. Pain control after thoracic surgery. A review of current techniques. Anesthesiology 1994;81:737.
19. Soliman IE, Apuya JS, Fertal KM, et al. Intravenous versus epidural analgesia after surgical repair of pectus excavatum. Am J Ther 2009;16:398.
20. Weber T, Matzl J, Rokitansky A, et al. Superior postoperative pain relief with thoracic epidural analgesia versus intravenous patient-controlled analgesia after minimally invasive pectus excavatum repair. J Thorac Cardiovasc Surg 2007;134:865.
21. Gasior AC, Weesner KA, Knott EM, et al. Long-term patient perception of pain control experience after participating in a trial between patient-controlled analgesia and epidural after pectus excavatum repair with bar placement. J Surg Res 2013;185(1):12–4.
22. Butkovic D, Kralik S, Matolic M, et al. Postoperative analgesia with intravenous fentanyl PCA vs epidural block after thoracoscopic pectus excavatum repair in children. Br J Anaesth 2007;98:677.
23. St Peter SD, Weesner KA, Sharp RJ, et al. Is epidural anesthesia truly the best pain management strategy after minimally invasive pectus excavatum repair? J Pediatr Surg 2008;43:79.
24. St Peter SD, Weesner KA, Weissend EE, et al. Epidural vs patient-controlled analgesia for postoperative pain after pectus excavatum repair: a prospective, randomized trial. J Pediatr Surg 2012;47:148.
25. Kehlet H, Wilmore DW. Multimodal strategies to improve surgical outcome. Am J Surg 2002;183:630.

Anesthesia for the Child with Cancer

Gregory J. Latham, MD

KEYWORDS

- Cancer • Oncology • Pediatric • Anesthesia • Anterior mediastinal mass
- Anthracycline-induced cardiotoxicity

KEY POINTS

- At present, there are insufficient data regarding the immunomodulatory effects of anesthetic drugs and techniques to support altering the anesthetic plan in adults, let alone children, with cancer undergoing surgery.
- The presence of a clinically significant anterior mediastinal mass is common in children newly diagnosed with lymphoma, as well as leukemia, neuroblastoma, and germ cell tumors.
- Goals for safe provision of anesthesia care in children with anterior mediastinal mass include a meticulous preoperative assessment; discussion with the oncologist, radiologist, and surgeon about whether the procedure is required before treatment of the mass; and cautious administration of anesthesia.
- Treatment-related cardiopulmonary toxicity is common in the acute and chronic settings of childhood cancer; however, most toxicity is subclinical or mild, and thus such children tend to tolerate anesthesia, at least for outpatient procedures, as well as their healthy peers.
- Because cancer and its treatment can affect every organ system of the body, a systems-based approach to the preoperative assessment is a helpful way to ensure a thorough investigation of each potential comorbidity that could affect safe anesthetic management of the child.

INTRODUCTION

Cancer is the second and fourth most common cause of death in children younger than 15 and 20 years of age, respectively.[1,2] More than 23,000 children were newly diagnosed with cancer in the United States in 2009,[3] and the number of Americans living with or having survived childhood cancer in 2006 was nearly 260,000.[4] However, survival from childhood cancer has improved dramatically over the last several

Disclosures: None.
Department of Anesthesiology and Pain Medicine, Seattle Children's Hospital, University of Washington School of Medicine, 4800 Sand Point Way Northeast, MB.11.500.3, Seattle, WA 98105, USA
E-mail address: gregory.latham@seattlechildrens.org

Anesthesiology Clin 32 (2014) 185–213
http://dx.doi.org/10.1016/j.anclin.2013.10.002   **anesthesiology.theclinics.com**

decades, with average 5-year survival rates exceeding 80%.[4,5] This increased survival entails various long-term sequelae of cancer and its therapy in children with ongoing or remissive cancer. In one report, 62% of survivors of childhood cancer reported at least one chronic health condition from cancer, and 28% of patients reported a severe or life-threatening condition.[5] Long-term chronic health conditions can affect nearly every organ system and be pertinent to the anesthetic plan.

The most common cancers in children are different than in adults, and the incidence of specific cancers in children varies not only from those in adults but also between different childhood age groups (**Table 1**). The most common malignancies in children include leukemia, lymphoma, brain tumors, and solid tumors of soft tissue and bone.[3] Other tumors are specific to childhood, including neuroblastoma, retinoblastoma, medulloblastoma, and Wilms tumor.

POTENTIAL COMPLICATIONS OF ANESTHESIA IN THE PEDIATRIC PATIENT WITH CANCER

Children with cancer undergo many surgeries and procedures that require anesthesia during acute phases of the disease, years into remission, or terminal stages of the disease. Inherent to a safe anesthetic plan is consideration of the direct effects of tumor, toxic effects of chemotherapy and radiation therapy, the specifics of the surgical procedure, drug-drug interactions with chemotherapy agents, pain syndromes, and psychological status of the child. However, reports have shown that outpatient anesthetic management of children for radiotherapy, lumbar puncture, and bone marrow aspiration is safe, with a complication rate comparable with similar studies of propofol-based anesthesia in children without cancer.[6,7] However, children with cancer can be very ill, and potential issues arising during anesthetic management include sepsis, multiorgan failure, respiratory insufficiency, thromboembolism, coagulopathy, tumor lysis syndrome, and cardiopulmonary collapse.[8] Therefore, it is imperative for the

Table 1
Incidence of pediatric cancer by age

Type of Cancer	Incidence by Age Group (%)				
	0–4 y	5–9 y	10–14 y	15–19 y	0–19 y
Leukemias	36.1	33.4	21.8	12.4	25.2
Central nervous system tumors	16.6	27.7	19.6	9.5	16.7
Lymphomas	3.9	12.9	20.6	25.1	15.5
Carcinomas and other malignant epithelial tumors	0.9	2.5	8.9	20.9	9.2
Soft tissue sarcomas	5.6	7.5	9.1	8.0	7.4
Germ cell, trophoblastic, and other gonadal tumors	3.3	2.0	5.3	13.9	7.0
Malignant bone tumors	0.6	4.6	11.3	7.7	5.6
Sympathetic nervous system tumors	14.3	2.7	1.2	0.5	5.4
Renal tumors	9.7	5.4	1.1	0.6	4.4
Retinoblastoma	6.3	0.5	0.1	0.0	2.1
Hepatic tumors	2.2	0.4	0.6	0.6	1.1
Other and unspecified malignant neoplasms	0.5	0.3	0.6	0.8	0.6

From Latham GJ, Greenberg RS. Anesthetic considerations for the pediatric oncology patient–part 1: a review of antitumor therapy. Paediatr Anaesth 2010;20(4):296; with permission.

anesthesiologist caring for these children to have an understanding of the multiple effects of the tumor, toxicities of therapy, significant coexisting illnesses, and psychosocial vulnerabilities to best formulate an anesthetic plan that is appropriate for the patient and type of procedure.

EFFECTS OF ANESTHETIC AGENTS ON PERIOPERATIVE IMMUNOMODULATION

Although this is a new area of research, there has been large increase of data over the past decade reporting the impact of multiple perioperative factors on immunomodulation in the patient who has cancer. All of the research thus far has been in tissue cultures or retrospective studies in adults[9] and may or may not be applicable to the common childhood cancers. These data should therefore be interpreted with caution regarding clinical applicability in children.

The host immune system combats progression, spread, and recurrence of cancer. Surgical stress and perhaps some anesthetic agents can suppress the host immune response or directly augment the cancer cells (proliferation, migration, and invasion) and theoretically allow spread or recurrence of cancer.[9,10] Most, but not all, research has shown an association with ketamine, sevoflurane, isoflurane, desflurane, and opiates (predominantly morphine) and harmful immunosuppression or cancer cell augmentation. Propofol has shown mixed results but may prove to be superior compared with volatile anesthetics.[9,10] Nitrous oxide, although shown in vitro to reduce natural killer cell activity, has not been shown in a retrospective adult study to affect cancer recurrence.[9] In addition, regional anesthesia was shown in some but not all studies to lessen immunosuppression during surgery and potentially reduce cancer recurrence in adults, but this prior finding in animal and retrospective data was not confirmed in a more recent prospective trial.[11] Other perioperative factors, such as hypotension, hypothermia, hypoglycemia or hyperglycemia, and blood transfusion are also being investigated.[9]

At present, there is insufficient evidence to support altering the anesthetic plan in adults, let alone children, with cancer undergoing surgery because of any concern about immunomodulation.

A SYSTEMS-BASED APPROACH TO THE TOXICITY OF CANCER AND ANTITUMOR THERAPY
Background

Most childhood cancers are treated by cooperative clinical trial protocols, which may include chemotherapy, radiation therapy, biologic modifiers, and hematopoietic stem cell transplant (HCST). Surgical resection of tumor is warranted with certain types of cancers. Although each of these therapies is designed to eradicate tumor, the effect on healthy tissue is rarely avoidable or benign.

Conventional chemotherapy drugs are designed to be cytotoxic to rapidly dividing cells by various mechanisms. These agents have been the mainstay of cancer treatment in children for decades and have led to remarkable cure rates. However, the toxicity of these agents to healthy tissues can reduce the child's quality of life and cause long-term morbidity and mortality.[12,13] Bone marrow suppression, immunosuppression, myocardial and pulmonary toxicity, and dysfunction of nearly every other organ system are possible. Specific toxicities of chemotherapeutics that are especially pertinent to anesthesia are discussed later, but, as a point of reference, **Table 2** provides an organized list of traditional chemotherapy agents by category, and **Table 3** provides a list of traditional chemotherapeutic agents, molecularly targeted agents, and adjuvant medications used in children, with their corresponding toxicities.

Table 2
Traditional chemotherapeutic agents by class

Alkylating Agents	Antimetabolites	Natural Products	Miscellaneous	Hormonal Agents
Nitrogen mustards	Folic acid analogues	Vinca alkaloids	Anthracenedione	Antiestrogens
Mechlorethamine	Methotrexate	Vinblastine	Mitoxantrone	Estrogens
Cyclophosphamide	Pyrimidine analogues	Vincristine	Substituted urea	Aromatase inhibitors
Ifosfamide	Fluorouracil	Vinorelbine	Hydroxyurea	GNRH analogues
Melphalan	Cytarabine	Vindesine	Methylhydrazine derivative	Antiandrogens
Chlorambucil	Gemcitabine	Epipodophyllotoxins	Procarbazine	
Ethylenimines	Purine analogues	Etoposide	Adrenocortical suppressants	
Thiotepa	6-Mercaptopurine	Teniposide	Mitotane	
Alkyl sulfonates	6-Thioguanine	Enzymes	Aminoglutethimide	
Busulfan	Pentostatin	L-Asparaginase	Estradiol–mustard ester	
Nitrosoureas	Cladribine	Antibiotics	Estramustine	
Carmustine	Fludarabine	Actinomycin D		
Lomustine	Clofarabine	Daunorubicin		
Streptozotocin		Dactinomycin		
Platinum complexes		Doxorubicin		
Cisplatin		Idarubicin		
Carboplatin		Bleomycin		
Oxaliplatin		Mitomycin		
Triazenes		Plicamycin		
Dacarbazine		Camptothecin analogues		
		Topotecan		
		Irinotecan		
		Taxanes		
		Paclitaxel		
		Docetaxel		

Abbreviation: GNRH, gonadotropin-releasing hormone.
From Latham GJ, Greenberg RS. Anesthetic considerations for the pediatric oncology patient–part 1: a review of antitumor therapy. Paediatr Anaesth 2010;20(4):298; with permission.

Although advances in radiation therapy have reduced the morbidity of this therapy, toxicity to healthy tissues occurs. The susceptibility of normal tissues to radiation therapy depends on the total and fractional dose received, the sensitivity of the tissue to the dose of radiation, the volume of tissue irradiated, and time course of treatment.[14] Concurrent treatment with chemotherapeutics also affects toxicity by causing additive tissue damage.[15] **Table 4** lists late effects of radiation therapy that may be present in children with or having survived cancer.

Anterior Mediastinal Mass

Effect of tumor and its treatment
Most children with Hodgkin or non-Hodgkin lymphoma have mediastinal involvement at diagnosis, and half have respiratory symptoms.[16] Other tumors that may present with an anterior mediastinal mass (AMM), albeit much less commonly, include neuroblastoma, germ cell tumors, and acute lymphoblastic leukemia.[17,18]

Anesthetic considerations
The risk of cardiopulmonary collapse under anesthesia is ever present in children with a clinically significant AMM. Although the definitive treatment of an AMM is antitumor therapy, some children may require an anesthetic at presentation. The anesthesiologist, in conjunction with the surgeon and oncologist, must weigh the pros and cons of proceeding with an anesthetic in the setting of symptomatic AMM. Three choices are possible:

- Perform the procedure with local anesthetic if possible
- Administer general anesthesia
- Pretreat the child with chest irradiation or corticosteroids to reduce the mass size

Pretreatment is controversial because of its potential to alter the tumor cell histology if biopsy is required for diagnosis, but a recent study has shown that a histologic diagnosis is still possible in 95% of children treated with up to 5 days of corticosteroids.[19]

Caution should be practiced in the management of any child with an AMM, but certain clinical findings more strongly predict cardiopulmonary compromise under anesthesia, as listed in **Box 1**. Before surgery, the anesthesiologist should review imaging of the chest to gain an understanding of the exact nature and location of obstruction to airways and vascular structures and should have a plan for repositioning the patient should collapse of these structures occur.

Unless an awake fiberoptic intubation is chosen, induction of anesthesia is classically performed gradually with intravenous or inhalational agents, maintaining spontaneous ventilation through the time of intubation.[19–21] Maintenance of spontaneous ventilation and avoidance of paralysis throughout the procedure is prudent to avoid cardiac collapse or collapse of the airway beyond the tip of the endotracheal tube.

Cardiopulmonary collapse can occur rapidly, and treatment must begin immediately; therefore, a plan for resuscitation and the appropriate equipment should be ready at the start of the case. Initial resuscitation of airway compromise includes[20]:

- Increase the inspired oxygen
- Apply continuous positive airway pressure
- Reposition the child into the appropriate lateral or even prone position
- If these maneuvers fail to rescue airway collapse, ventilation through a rigid bronchoscope may be required[22]

If cardiac collapse occurs[20]

- Administer a fluid bolus
- Reposition the patient into the appropriate lateral or even prone position

Table 3
Organ toxicity of chemotherapeutic agents

Drug	Myelotoxicity	Cardiotoxicity	Pulmonary Toxicity	Nephrotoxicity	Hepatotoxicity	Gastrointestinal Toxicity	Neurotoxicity	Other
Alemtuzumab	++	—	—	—	—	+ (N/V/D/M)	—	
Altretamine	++	—	—	—	+ (LFT↑)	++ (N/V)	+	—
Arsenic trioxide	+ (leukocytosis)	++ (prolonged QT interval)	+ (effusion)	—	—	+ (N/V/D)	+/−	Differentiation syndrome
Asparaginase	+ (bleeding)	—	—	—	+ (LFT↑)	+ (pancreatitis)	—	Coagulopathy
5-Azacitidine	+++	—	—	—	+ (LFT↑)	+ (N/V/D)	—	
Bevacizumab	—	++ (HTN, CHF)	—	+ (nephrotic syndrome)	—	+ (N/V/D/M)	+ (asthenia)	
Bleomycin	—	—	+++	+	+	+/−	—	
Bortezomib	+/−	—	—	—	—	+ (N/V/D)	+	Fever common
Busulfan	+++	—	++	—	++ (LFT↑, VOD)	+ (N/V)	+ (seizures)	Electrolyte abnormalities
Capecitabine	++	+ (in adults)	—	—	+ (LFT↑)	++ (D/M)	++	
Carboplatin	+++	—	—	+	—	++	++	
Carmustine	+++	—	+++	+	+ (LFT↑)	+ (N/V)	—	
Cetuximab	—	—	+ (rare)	—	—	—	—	Rash, hypomagnesemia
Chlorambucil	+++	—	++ (rare)	—	—	—	++ (rare)	
Cisplatin	—	—	—	+++	—	++ (N/V)	++	SIADH
Cladribine	+++	—	—	+ (at high doses)	—	—	+ (at high doses)	Tumor lysis syndrome
Clofarabine	+++	—	—	+ (rare)	++ (LFT↑)	++ (N/V)	—	Tumor lysis syndrome

								SIADH
Cyclophosphamide	+++	++ (at high doses)	—	++ (hemorrhagic cystitis)	—	—	—	—
Cytarabine	+++	—	++ (at high doses)	—	+ (LFT↑)	+++ (pancreatitis)	++	Ara-C syndrome
Dacarbazine	+++	—	—	—	—	++ (N/V)	++ (rare)	—
Dactinomycin-D	+++	—	—	—	++ (LFT↑, VOD)	+++ (N/V/D/M)	—	—
Darbepoetin alfa	—	+ (HTN)	—	—	—	—	—	—
Dasatinib	+++	++ (arrhythmias)	—	—	—	++ (N/V/D)	—	Bleeding disorders
Daunorubicin	+++	+++	—	—	—	—	—	Skin disorders
Decitabine	+++	—	+ (cough, edema)	—	+ (LFT↑)	++ (N/V/D)	—	—
Denileukin diftitox	—	++ (Vascular leak syndrome)	—	+ (rare)	+ (rare)	—	+ (rare)	—
Dexamethasone	+ (leukocytosis)	—	—	—	—	—	—	Adrenal suppression
Docetaxel	+++	—	—	—	+ (LFT↑)	—	+ (uncommon)	Fluid retention
Doxorubicin	+++	+++	—	—	—	—	—	Skin disorders
Epirubicin	+++	+++	—	—	—	—	—	Skin rash
Erlotinib	—	—	+++ (ILD; rare)	—	+ (LFT↑)	+ (D)	—	—
Erythropoietin	—	+ (HTN)	—	—	—	—	—	—
Estramustine	—	+++ (very rare)	—	—	—	+++ (N/V)	—	—

(continued on next page)

Table 3
(continued)

Drug	Myelotoxicity	Cardiotoxicity	Pulmonary Toxicity	Nephrotoxicity	Hepatotoxicity	Gastrointestinal Toxicity	Neurotoxicity	Other
Etoposide	+++	—	—	—	+ (rare)	+ (N/V)	+ (rare)	—
Filgrastim	—	—	—	—	—	—	—	Bone pain
Floxuridine	++	++ (rare)	—	—	+++	++ (ulcers)	+ (rare)	—
Fludarabine	+++	—	—	—	—	—	+++ (uncommon)	Autoimmune hemolytic anemia
5-Fluorouracil	+++	++ (rare)	—	—	—	+++ (D/M)	+++ (uncommon)	—
Gefitinib	—	+ (HTN)	+++ (ILD; rare)	—	+ (LFT↑)	—	—	Rash
Gemcitabine	+++	—	+++ (ILD; rare)	+ (hematuria)	+ (LFT↑)	+ (N/V)	+ (rare)	—
Gemtuzumab ozogamicin	+++	—	—	—	++ (LFT↑, VOD)	—	—	—
Hydroxyurea	+++	—	—	—	—	—	—	Skin disorders
Ibritumomab tiuxetan	+++	—	—	—	—	—	+ (asthenia)	Infusion reactions
Idarubicin	+++	+++	—	—	+ (LFT↑)	+ (N/V/D/M)	—	Skin disorders
Ifosfamide	+++	—	+++ (uncommon)	+++ (hemorrhagic cystitis; Fanconi-like syndrome)	+ (LFT↑)	+++ (N/V)	++	SIADH
Imatinib mesylate	+	—	—	—	+ (LFT↑)	+ (D)	—	—

Drug								
Interferon-alpha	++	++ (rare)	—	—	+ (LFT↑)	—	—	Autoimmune symptoms
Interleukin-2	+	++ (vascular leak syndrome)	—	—	+ (LFT↑)	—	+	
Irinotecan	+++	—	—	—	+ (LFT↑)	++ (D)	+ (asthenia)	Electrolyte abnormalities
Lapatinib	+	—	—	—	+ (LFT↑)	++ (N/V/D)	—	
Lenalidomide	++	++	—	—	—	+ (D)	—	Thrombosis
Leucovorin	—	—	—	—	—	+ (N/V)	—	
Lomustine	+++	—	+++ (uncommon)	+++ (uncommon)	—	+ (N/V)	—	Rash
Mechloretha-mine	+++	—	—	—	++	+++ (N/V)	+ (rare)	
Melphalan	+++	—	++ (rare)	—	—	+ (N/V/D/M)	—	SIADH (rare)
Mercapto-purine	+++	—	—	—	+ (LFT↑)	+ (N/V/D/M)	—	Skin disorders
Mesna	—	—	—	—	—	+ (N/V)	—	Rash, arthralgias
Methotrexate	+++	—	+++	++ (uncommon)	—	++ (M/D)	++ (at high doses)	
Mitomycin C	+++	—	+++ (rare)	+++ (HUS – rare)	+++ (VOD – rare)	+ (N/V/M)	—	
Mitoxantrone	+++	+++	—	—	+ (LFT↑)	+ (N/V/D/M)	—	
Nelarabine	+++	—	+ (uncommon)	—	—	+ (N/V/D)	+++ (common)	Edema
Oprelvekin	—	+++	+++ (pleural effusions, dyspnea)	—	—	+ (N/V/D/M)	+	Edema
Oxaliplatin	++	—	+++ (rare)	+++ (rare)	+++ (VOD – rare)	++ (N/V/D)	+++ (common)	Hypersensitivity reactions

(continued on next page)

Table 3
(continued)

Drug	Myelotoxicity	Cardiotoxicity	Pulmonary Toxicity	Nephrotoxicity	Hepatotoxicity	Gastrointestinal Toxicity	Neurotoxicity	Other
Paclitaxel	+++	+ (arrhythmia)	—	—	+ (LFT↑)	+ (N/V/D/M)	+++ (common)	Arthralgias
Panitumumab	—	—	+++ (rare)	—	—	+ (N/V/D)	—	Infusion reactions
Pegaspar-ginase	—	—	—	—	+++ (pancreatitis – uncommon)	—	—	Thrombosis, glucose intolerance
Pegfilgrastim	—	—	—	—	+ (LFT↑)	—	—	Bone pain
Pemetrexed	+++	—	—	—	—	++ (N/V/D/M)	+	Hypersensitivity reactions
Pentostatin	+++	+ (rare)	—	—	+ (LFT↑)	+ (N/V)	+	Hypersensitivity reactions
Prednisone	+ (leukocytosis)	—	—	—	—	—	—	Adrenal suppression
Procarbazine	+++	—	+++ (ILD; rare)	—	—	+ (N/V)	++	Hypersensitivity reactions
Rituximab	+	+ (rare)	—	—	—	—	+	Infusion reactions, tumor lysis syndrome
Sargramostim	—	+ (arrhythmias – uncommon)	—	—	+ (LFT↑)	—	—	Bone pain, infusion reactions
Sorafenib	+	++ (adults – rare)	—	—	+ (LFT↑)	+ (N/V/D)	+	Skin disorders
Streptozocin	+	—	—	+++ (azotemia)	+ (LFT↑)	+++ (N/V)	—	Glucose imbalance

Sunitinib	+++	+ (HTN, ↓LVEF)	—	+ (LFT↑)	++ (N/V/D/M)	—	Bleeding disorder
Temozolomide	+++	—	—	+ (LFT↑)	++ (N/V/D)	—	—
Teniposide	+++	—	—	—	+ (N/V/M)	+	Hypersensitivity reaction
Thalidomide	—	—	—	—	+	+++	Thrombosis, teratogenesis
Thioguanine	+++	—	+ (rare)	+++ (VOD)	+++ (D/M)	+ (rare)	—
Thiotepa	+++	—	—	—	+ (N/V)	—	—
Topotecan	+++	—	+ (hematuria)	+ (LFT↑)	++ (N/V/D)	—	—
Tositumomab	+++	—	—	—	+ (N/V)	—	Infusion reactions
Trastuzumab	—	++ (CHF)	+ (rare)	—	+ (N/V/D)	—	Infusion reactions
Tretinoin (all-trans retinoic acid)	+++ (leukocytosis)	+++ (RAS)	+++ (RAS)	+ (LFT↑)	+ (N/V)	+ (common), +++ (rare)	RAS
Vinblastine	+++	++ (rare)	+++ (rare)	—	++ (N/V/D/M)	+ (common), +++ (rare)	SIADH (rare)
Vincristine	++	++ (rare)	+++ (rare)	—	++ (N/V/D/M)	+++	SIADH (rare)
Vinorelbine	+++	—	—	+ (LFT↑)	++ (N/V/D/M)	+	SIADH (rare)
Vorinostat	+	—	—	—	++ (N/V)	+ (uncommon)	Thrombosis (rare)

Note: data are from pediatric studies whenever possible, but, when pediatric data were incomplete or absent, adult data were included.

Abbreviations: +, mild toxicity; ++, moderate toxicity; +++, severe toxicity or dose-limiting toxicity; Ara-C, arabinofuranosyl cytidine or cytarabine; CHF, congestive heart failure; D, diarrhea; HTN, hypertension; ILD, interstitial lung disease; LFT, liver function test; M, mucositis; N, nausea; RAS, retinoic acid syndrome; SIADH, syndrome of inappropriate antidiuretic hormone; V, vomiting; VOD, veno-occlusive disease.

From Latham GJ, Greenberg RS. Anesthetic considerations for the pediatric oncology patient–part 1: a review of antitumor therapy. Paediatr Anaesth 2010;20(4):299–301; with permission.

Table 4		
Late effects of radiation therapy		
Radiation Field	Late Effects	Risk Factors (if known)
Cranial	Neurocognitive deficits	>18 Gy, IV/IT methotrexate
	Leukoencephalopathy	>18 Gy with IT methotrexate
	Growth hormone deficiency	>18 Gy
	Panhypopituitarism	>40 Gy
	Large vessel stroke	>60 Gy
	Second cancers	Variable
	Dental problems	>10 Gy
	Cataracts	>2–8 Gy single dose, 10–15 Gy fractionated dose
	Ototoxicity	>35–50 Gy
Chest	Cardiac disease:	
	Coronary artery disease	>30 Gy
	Cardiomyopathy	>35 Gy, >25 Gy with anthracyclines
	Valvular disease	>40 Gy
	Pericardial disease	>35 Gy
	Arrhythmias	—
	Thyroid disease:	
	Hypothyroidism	>20 Gy local, >7.5 Gy TBI
	Hyperthyroidism	>20 Gy local, >7.5 Gy TBI
	Thyroid nodules/cancer	Any dose
	Pulmonary disease:	
	Pulmonary fibrosis	>15–20 Gy
	Restrictive lung disease	—
	Obstructive lung disease	—
Abdomen/pelvis	Chronic enteritis	>40 Gy
	Gastrointestinal malignancy	—
	Hepatic fibrosis/cirrhosis	>30 Gy
	Renal insufficiency	>20 Gy
	Bladder disease:	
	Fibrosis	>30 Gy before puberty, >50 after puberty
	Hemorrhagic cystitis	Enhances cyclophosphamide and ifosfamide effect
	Cancer	—
	Gonadal dysfunction:	
	Ovarian failure	4–12 Gy
	Testicular failure	>1–6 Gy
Any radiation	Skin cancer	—
	Musculoskeletal changes:	
	Bone length discrepancy	>20 Gy
	Pathologic fractures	>40 Gy
Total body irradiation	All the effects listed earlier	—

Abbreviations: Gy, gray; IT, intrathecal; IV, intravenous; TBI, total body irradiation.
From Latham GJ, Greenberg RS. Anesthetic considerations for the pediatric oncology patient–part 1: a review of antitumor therapy. Paediatr Anaesth 2010;20(4):302; with permission.

- If these measures fail, immediate sternotomy and elevation of the mass may be life saving

Immediate availability of cardiopulmonary bypass or extracorporeal membrane oxygenation has been described, but the usefulness of these measures as first-line

---

Box 1
Strongest risk factors for acute perioperative cardiac or respiratory complications in patients with an AMM

Clinical signs and symptoms:

  Orthopnea

  Upper body edema (signs of SVCS)

  Stridor

  Wheeze

Diagnostic imaging findings:

  Tracheal, bronchial, or carinal compression

  Great vessel compression, SVC obstruction

  Pulmonary artery outflow obstruction

  Ventricular dysfunction

  Pericardial effusion

Abbreviations: SVC, superior vena cava; SVCS, superior vena cava syndrome.
From Latham GJ, Greenberg RS. Anesthetic considerations for the pediatric oncology patient–part 2: systems-based approach to anesthesia. Paediatr Anaesth 2010;20(5):397; with permission.

---

therapy is questionable because of the degree of global hypoxia that ensues before successful cannulation in many cases.[19]

Oral Cavity and Airway

Effect of tumor and its treatment
Primary tumors of the airway are uncommon in children, and most are benign.[23] However, the impact of chemotherapy and radiation therapy to the airway is common. Mucositis and xerostomia can develop as soon as a week after beginning treatment with many different chemotherapy drugs and as soon as 2 to 4 weeks after radiation to the head and neck.[24,25] Mucositis and more significant ulcerative lesions may occur as part of graft-versus-host disease (GVHD) after hematopoietic stem cell transplant (HSCT). In addition, chronic fibrosis and distortion of the airway is possible after irradiation of the head and neck.[26]

High-dose chemotherapy or total body irradiation (TBI) for HSCT can lead to mucositis that threatens the airway from pseudomembrane formation, supraglottic edema, bleeding, and aspiration of blood and secretions.[27,28] Up to 30% of children who receive HSCT may have a difficult airway.[28] Past irradiation of the neck has been reported to cause difficult airway management, including poor laryngeal mask airway seating and the requirement for a smaller endotracheal tube.[26,29]

Cardiovascular System

Effect of tumor and its treatment
The primary cardiac manifestations of the tumor include AMM and pericardial effusion. Primary tumors of the heart are uncommon and are usually benign.[30]

The anthracycline drugs (doxorubicin, daunorubicin, idarubicin, and epirubicin) are perhaps the most cardiotoxic used in pediatric oncology; however, other drugs are also cardiotoxic. Mitoxantrone should be considered in the same risk stratification as anthracyclines.[31] Cyclophosphamide, fluorouracil, vinca alkaloids, cytarabine, cladribine, asparaginase, paclitaxel, trastuzumab, etoposide, teniposide, and pentostatin have also been reported to cause cardiotoxicity.[32,33]

The effects of chest irradiation on the heart can be significant, and its effects are additive with any administered cardiotoxic chemotherapeutics.[34] It is likely that current dosing protocols using less than 25 to 30 Gy cumulative doses minimize long-term cardiac risk.[35]

Anesthetic considerations

Symptomatic heart failure after anthracycline therapy is uncommon during the childhood years. In one study, echocardiography did not show a significant reduction in cardiac index during anesthesia for central line placement in children treated with anthracyclines versus those who had not.[36] However, the impact during major surgery is unknown. In general, if a child has diminished cardiac function shown by echocardiography, caution should be exercised during the administration of anesthetics with negative inotropic properties, because cardiac failure or arrhythmias can develop at any time after anthracycline therapy.

Unlike anthracyclines, radiation-induced cardiotoxicity can affect any component of the heart, causing pericardial effusions, pericarditis, cardiomyopathy, valvular fibrosis, conduction disturbances, and coronary artery disease.[34,37] Current irradiation protocols use careful blocking and cumulative doses less than 25 to 30 Gy, which seemingly limits the short-term risk of heart disease, but clinically evident, long-term toxicity has been reported at these dosing limits.[34]

Children receiving anthracycline treatment or chest irradiation usually have routine cardiac evaluations. In general, a recent echocardiogram should be available if a patient has received anthracycline therapy or chest radiotherapy and any of the following conditions are met[38]:

- The cumulative dose of anthracycline was greater than 240 mg/m^2
- Any dose of anthracycline was received during infancy
- Chest irradiation was greater than 40 Gy (or >30 Gy with concomitant anthracycline treatment)
- These data are unknown

Pulmonary System

Effect of tumor and its treatment

Primary lung tumors in children are rare, and metastases to the lung are uncommon.[39] Most tumor-related causes of respiratory compromise in the acute setting are therefore indirect effects and include pleural effusion, infiltrate, pulmonary embolus, chylous effusion from obstructed lymphatics, AMM, and hyperleukocytosis-induced pulmonary leukostasis.[40]

Although bleomycin may be the best known and have the highest incidence, many chemotherapeutic agents can cause significant acute and chronic lung toxicity (Table 5). Acute chemotherapy-induced lung toxicity in children may manifest as pneumonitis, pulmonary fibrosis, or noncardiogenic pulmonary edema, all of which can occur after the first dose or months later.[41,42] Pneumonitis has an insidious onset, presenting with nonproductive cough, progressive dyspnea, and rales. Many cases of pneumonitis are subclinical and resolve with cessation of the causative chemotherapeutic, but the course may be irreversible once radiologic changes are evident.[41,43,44]

Chemotherapy-induced lung fibrosis in children has a high incidence of onset acutely during treatment, but fibrosis is also the hallmark of late chemotherapy-induced pulmonary toxicity, with an onset of months to years after treatment.[41,45]

Table 5
Chemotherapy agents and pulmonary toxicity

Drug	Incidence (%)	Onset	Cumulative Dose	Disorders
Bleomycin	Adults: Up to 46	Early (pneumonitis) to late (fibrosis)	Unknown; probably >400 U/m^2	Interstitial pneumonitis; pulmonary fibrosis
Busulfan	Adults: 6 (range, 2.5–43)	Usually late	Unknown in children	Diffuse interstitial fibrosis; bronchopulmonary dysplasia; obstructive bronchiolitis
Carmustine	Up to 53	Early to late	600 mg/m^2	Pulmonary fibrosis
Cyclophosphamide	Unknown	Early to late	Unknown	Interstitial pneumonitis
Lomustine	Adults: up to 63	Early to late	Unknown	Interstitial pneumonitis
Methotrexate	2–33	Early (usually) to late	Unknown	Acute pneumonitis, BOOP, pulmonary fibrosis
Mitomycin	Adults: rare (1.8)	Early	Unknown: probably >15 mg/m^2	Pulmonary fibrosis
Vincristine	Adults: 4	Early	Unknown	ARDS when combined with mitomycin

Abbreviations: ARDS, acute respiratory distress syndrome; BOOP, bronchiolitis obliterans with organizing pneumonia.

From Latham GJ, Greenberg RS. Anesthetic considerations for the pediatric oncology patient–part 2: systems-based approach to anesthesia. Paediatr Anaesth 2010;20(5):401; with permission.

Although most cases are subclinical, severe morbidity and mortality are possible.[45] Bleomycin is the most commonly causative agent of chronic lung toxicity, but others have been implicated (see **Table 5**). Studies of bleomycin-induced pneumonitis in children are scant, but adult studies have reported the incidence to be up 46%, with a mortality of 3%.[46,47]

Radiation-induced pulmonary disease also occurs as a progression from interstitial pneumonitis in the acute phase to pulmonary fibrosis in the late phase,[45] and signs and symptoms are similar to those described earlier. Pulmonary dysfunction after HSCT is likely caused by the combination of aggressive chemotherapy, TBI, and chronic GVHD.[35] Almost 25% of posttransplant children show decrements in pulmonary function testing, but fewer have clinical symptoms.[48,49]

Anesthetic considerations
Bleomycin-induced pulmonary fibrosis can lead to severe restrictive lung disease. Although data are conflicting, most human and animal data suggest that high concentrations of inspired oxygen during or after recent bleomycin therapy might exacerbate pulmonary toxicity and lead to postoperative respiratory distress.[50–53] Despite a lack of definitive data, it is reasonable to recommend adjustment of intraoperative inspired oxygen concentrations to the lowest possible level during and after bleomycin

therapy, as well as judicious use of intraoperative and postoperative fluid administration.[54] In summary, the anesthesiologist must assess the presence of symptomatic pulmonary dysfunction as well as consider the possibility of occult respiratory compromise in the pediatric oncology patient.[54] Overall, 6% of children treated with chemotherapy alone, 20% treated with both chemotherapy and radiation therapy, and 25% after HSCT have symptoms of pulmonary dysfunction or significantly abnormal pulmonary function tests.[38]

Renal System

Effect of tumor and its treatment

Wilms tumor represents most of the primary renal tumors in children, followed by clear cell sarcoma of the kidney, malignant rhabdoid tumor, congenital mesoblastic nephroma, and renal cell carcinoma.[55,56] Nonrenal tumors, typically neuroblastoma, can infiltrate the kidneys or obstruct the urinary tract and renal vasculature, causing acute renal failure (ARF).[57]

Almost all chemotherapy agents can cause nephrotoxicity in high enough doses. Cisplatin, carboplatin, and ifosfamide are the most commonly implicated, but lomustine, carmustine, cyclophosphamide, and high-dose methotrexate are occasionally nephrotoxic.[57,58] Ifosfamide causes chronic glomerular toxicity in up to 30% of patients and subclinical toxicity in up to 90%, but progressive chronic renal failure is uncommon.[59] Fanconi syndrome is of particular concern with ifosfamide and may present up to 18 months after therapy.[59] Cisplatin can produce cumulative nephrotoxicity and hypomagnesemia in children, but lower doses and careful medical management have minimized the incidence of this toxicity in recent years.[60] High-dose methotrexate can lead to severe ARF in 2% of children and represents the need for emergent treatment.[61] Many other supportive drugs used in children with cancer may lead to nephrotoxicity, including amphotericin B, acyclovir, aminoglycosides, and diuretics.[57] The syndrome of inappropriate antidiuretic hormone (SIADH) can be caused by multiple chemotherapeutics as well.

Exposure of one or both kidneys to radiation is common with abdominal irradiation and with TBI before HSCT. Cumulative doses of radiation that cause nephrotoxicity in children are not well known. However, radiation nephritis presents with azotemia, proteinuria, anemia, and hypertension.[62]

Renal toxicity is common after HSCT. The incidence of ARF in children has been reported to be 20% to 40% after HSCT.[63,64] The incidence of chronic renal impairment has been reported to range from 18% to 54% after HSCT.[65,66]

Anesthetic considerations

As with any child with renal impairment, the impact of existing hypertension, electrolyte imbalances, anemia, coagulation, fluid status, need for dialysis, and pharmacokinetics of anesthetic agents must be considered. Nonsteroidal antiinflammatory drugs should be administered with caution, especially in the dehydrated state. Laparotomy for resection of Wilms tumor can result in significant bleeding if the tumor invades the renal vasculature. Cardiopulmonary bypass is rarely required to enable resection of tumor that extends to the right atrium.

Hepatic System

Effect of tumor and its treatment

Primary liver tumors are rare in children, accounting for 1% of childhood cancers. Hepatoblastoma is most common, followed by sarcomas, germ cell tumors, and rhabdoid tumors. In late adolescence, the incidence of hepatocellular carcinoma increases.[67,68] In young children, up to 20% of liver tumors are associated with a genetic syndrome, such as Beckwith-Wiedemann syndrome, that could further affect anesthetic management.[68]

Although many chemotherapeutic agents can cause acute hepatotoxicity that leads to liver function abnormalities, the progression to chronic liver disease in childhood is uncommon. These acute toxicities occur over hours to weeks after a chemotherapeutic dose and are usually reversible. Methotrexate, actinomycin D, 6-mercaptopurine, and 6-thioguanine have been most commonly implicated in childhood acute hepatotoxicity.[54]

Acute radiation-induced hepatotoxicity in children is typically mild and self-limited.[35] The exception is potential development of sinusoidal obstruction syndrome (SOS) after HSCT. SOS can occur days to years after HSCT, and the reported incidence is 11% to 27% after HSCT, with a mortality of 19% to 50%.[69,70] SOS is hallmarked by portal hypertension, liver failure, and failure of other organ systems, especially the kidneys, lungs, and heart.[71] Chronic hepatic fibrosis is possible after abdominal irradiation, but the lower doses in current use (<30–40 Gy) or focal irradiation of just portions of the liver likely limit the risk.[35]

Anesthetic considerations
As for any patient with liver dysfunction, the presence of impaired hepatic biotransformation of drugs and diminished synthetic function of coagulation factors and other proteins must be considered during perioperative management. Furthermore, the risk of exacerbation of hepatocellular damage during anesthesia and surgery must be considered.[54]

Gastrointestinal System

Effect of tumor and its treatment
Primary tumors of the gastrointestinal (GI) tract are rare in children. However, intra-abdominal tumors can cause intestinal obstruction, intussusception, erosive perforation and intra-abdominal hemorrhage, biliary obstruction (rare), and massive hepatomegaly (from end-stage neuroblastoma).[54,72]

Most children undergoing chemotherapy experience episodes of nausea and vomiting. Other GI toxicities of chemotherapeutics include diarrhea, mucositis, neutropenic enterocolitis, and stomatitis, all of which can lead to anorexia, malnutrition, and dehydration.[73]

The rapidly regenerating tissues of the GI tract are sensitive to irradiation, manifesting as inflammation and edema. These changes are usually transient.[74] Chronic GI toxicity is typically not seen with the radiation doses of less than 20 to 30 Gy that are currently used.[35,74]

Anesthetic considerations
Whether a child presents for general anesthesia during active cytotoxic therapy or well after its completion, the risk of delayed gastric emptying and aspiration during induction of anesthesia must be considered. Preoperative use of opiates for pain management may further exacerbate slowing of GI motility. The presence of vomiting, mucositis, enteritis, or bowel obstruction can cause malnutrition, vitamin K deficiency, electrolyte imbalances, and dehydration.[54]

Central Nervous System

Effect of tumor and its treatment
The most common intracranial tumors in children are astrocytomas, ependymomas, primitive neuroectodermal tumors, and gliomas.[2] The direct effect of brain tumors is

variable, depending on type, location, and patient age. Symptoms especially can be nonspecific in young children, including irritability, lethargy, macrocephaly, and vomiting. Acute neurologic deterioration at presentation is possible, including increased intracranial pressure, herniation, seizures, stroke, tumor lysis syndrome, and leukemic meningitis.[18] Primary tumors of the spine are uncommon in children, and spinal cord compression is a rare but potentially severe surgical emergency.[75]

Chemotherapeutics most commonly implicated in neurotoxicity are the platinum agents (cisplatin, carboplatin, oxaliplatin), L-asparaginase, ifosfamide, methotrexate, cytarabine, etoposide, vincristine, and cyclosporin A.[76,77] Acute toxicity, which is often reversible, can include altered mental status, seizures, cerebral infarctions, encephalopathy, ototoxicity, and peripheral nerve dysfunction.[54]

Small doses of brain irradiation (>18 Gy) have been shown to cause neurocognitive changes and leukoencephalopathy, but doses greater than 50 Gy are required to cause severe focal tissue destruction.[74]

Anesthetic considerations
Most pediatric brain tumors require surgical resection. Neurologic deterioration on presentation to the operating room is common, and the anesthesiologist must be prepared to manage alterations in intracranial pressure, risk of aspiration, seizures, impact of antiseizure medications on metabolism of other drugs, and postoperative neurologic assessment.

Endocrine System

Effect of tumor and its treatment
Primary endocrine tumors are rare in children, accounting for less than 5% of childhood cancers.[3] Most childhood endocrine tumors are gonadal germ cell tumors (40%–45%; testicular, ovarian, and extragonadal tumors), followed by thyroid tumors (30%; adenomas and carcinomas) and pituitary tumors (20%; craniopharyngiomas and pituitary adenomas).[54,78] Other endocrine tumors are rare.

Glucocorticoids are an important component of many cancer treatment protocols, and thus adrenal suppression is common. Other traditional chemotherapeutics do not have strong associations with endocrine dysfunction.

However, radiation to the pituitary and hypothalamus can cause significant chronic neuroendocrine dysfunction. Growth hormone and gonadotropin deficiency can occur after radiation therapy that exposes the hypothalamic-pituitary region to cumulative doses as low as 18 to 20 Gy, and the risk of panhypopituitarism increases after doses in excess of 35 to 40 Gy.[79] Hypothyroidism is also common (11%–50% of childhood cancer survivors) after doses of 20 Gy, and onset is typically 2 to 4.5 years after therapy.[80]

Anesthetic considerations
Treatment of children with exogenous corticosteroid therapy can lead to a measurable inability to mount an appropriate stress response for up to a year.[81] Although the need for and benefit of stress dose therapy during anesthesia has been debated, the anesthesiologist should ascertain a history of recent corticosteroid therapy. Because the stress response in children with cancer has been shown to be unpredictable, it has been recommended that stress dose steroids be administered during stressful conditions in the first 1 to 2 months after cessation of glucocorticoids.[82]

Pheochromocytomas are rare in children, and review of the anesthetic management of these children is beyond the scope of this article and well reviewed elsewhere.[83] However, other childhood tumors can be catecholamine secreting (eg, neuroblastoma, ganglioneuroma) or can cause significant hypertension secondary to renal artery compression (eg, neuroblastoma, Wilms tumor).

Hematologic System

Effect of tumor and its treatment

Myelosuppression, which manifests with various degrees of anemia, thrombocytopenia, and neutropenia, is a common direct effect of cancer in children. Anemia is common at diagnosis with neuroblastoma, rhabdomyosarcoma, Hodgkin disease, Ewing sarcoma, or osteosarcoma and with 80% of children with acute lymphoblastic leukemia (ALL).[84,85] Thrombocytopenia is a frequent finding at diagnosis of acute leukemia or solid tumors with marrow infiltration.[86] Neutropenia is usual in children with ALL. In acute myelogenous leukemia (AML), hyperleukocytosis ($>100,000/mm^3$) is present in 20% of patients at diagnosis.[87] Hyperleukocytosis, especially when greater than $200,000/mm^3$ in children, increases blood viscosity and can result in the potentially fatal condition of leukostasis.[87]

Radiation therapy and most chemotherapy agents have the ability to cause acute myelosuppression.[54] Radiation therapy typically does not cause complete myelosuppression unless large volumes or marrow are irradiated, as is the goal with HSCT preconditioning TBI.

Chemotherapy-induced myelosuppression is the most common dose-limiting toxicity of cancer treatment.[12] Leukopenia especially leads to significant morbidity and mortality and is the component of pancytopenia that typically results in dose limitations during treatment. Although use of erythropoietin or recombinant human granulocyte/macrophage colony-stimulating factor for anemia and neutropenia, respectively, is sometimes used in children, the mainstay of treatment is cessation or lowering of cytotoxic treatment and blood transfusions.[54]

Myeloablative preparative regiments for HSCT, by design, cause nearly complete destruction of the host hematopoietic stem cells. Engraftment and hematopoietic recovery occur during the first month after transplantation. This recovery follows a predictable pattern: granulocytes recover first, followed by platelets, lymphocytes, and then erythrocytes. During this period of recovery, the patient is susceptible to infections, bleeding, and symptoms of anemia.[54]

Anesthetic considerations

Neutropenic patients are prone to sepsis, a possibility that must be considered before an anesthetic. Infection precautions are necessary with neutropenic patients, including aseptic technique during invasive procedures, avoidance of drugs or temperature probes per rectum, and protective isolation of the patient.

When considering the perioperative need for red cell transfusion in children with cancer, several factors should be considered. The assessment should include the overall clinical condition of the patient, signs and symptoms of anemia, the patient's ability to tolerate the decreased red cell volume and oxygen carrying capacity, the presence of cardiopulmonary dysfunction, the stress and anticipated blood loss of the surgical procedure, the risk of increased intraoperative hemorrhage caused by a bleeding disorder, and the ability of the patient to tolerate a volume load. Thus, sound clinical judgment and attention to the greater clinical context is warranted in each case.[54]

Although the benefit of transfusion with leukoreduced red cells remains largely untested in pediatric oncology patients, its use is widespread and currently recommended based on some promising prospective study results.[88] Use of irradiated red cells is also recommended to avoid the potentially fatal transfusion-associated GVHD in these immunocompromised patients. Caution must be exercised when transfusing red cells to a patient with hyperleukocytosis because hyperviscosity and leukostasis can occur.[89]

No specific criteria exist for platelet transfusion triggers in children. According to the American Society of Clinical Oncology guideline, a platelet count of 40,000 to 50,000/mL is sufficient before major invasive procedures in patients without concurrent coagulopathies. For minor procedures such as bone marrow biopsies, a platelet count of 20,000/mL is sufficient, but counts of more than 100,000/mL should be present before neurosurgical procedures are performed.[90] A platelet count of 10,000/mL seems to be sufficient for lumbar punctures in children, and even when counts are less than 10,000/mL, data are insufficient to recommend for or against prophylactic platelet transfusion before lumbar puncture to avoid epidural hematoma.[91]

Histocompatible platelets should be use in alloimmunized patients, and use of leukoreduced platelets is recommended in those who have had or will have multiple platelet transfusions to reduce subsequent alloimmunization.[90] If intraoperative bleeding continues despite appropriate platelet transfusion and documented counts, other disorders of hemostasis should be considered, as discussed later.

Children who have recently received HSCT and who require blood transfusion present a unique challenge in determining the appropriate ABO and lesser antigen compatibility for transfusion. Discussion with the patient's hematologist-oncologist and blood bank is warranted to ensure appropriate management.

Coagulation System

Effect of tumor and its treatment
Bleeding disorders caused by the cancer itself are usually multifactorial in cause, including thrombocytopenia, clotting factor deficiencies, circulating anticoagulants, and defects in vascular integrity.

Coagulopathy at the time of diagnosis is common in some types of childhood tumors, especially ALL and AML. Significant disseminated intravascular coagulation can be found at presentation in children with acute promyelocytic leukemia and less commonly with acute monocytic leukemia and T-cell ALL.[92] Children may develop acquired bleeding disorders, including lupus anticoagulant syndrome, acquired von Willebrand syndrome (in up to 8% of children at diagnosis of Wilms tumor), and inhibitors to factor VIII (acquired hemophilia).[92,93]

Treatment-related causes of bleeding are typically multifactorial, including thrombocytopenia caused by cytoreductive chemotherapy and radiotherapy, vitamin K deficiency, hepatic dysfunction, disseminated intravascular coagulation, and infection. The rate of hemorrhagic death in children with cancer is unknown, but it is most commonly reported in children with ALL and AML.[92]

Venous thromboembolism (VTE) is rare in the general pediatric population but is probably more common in children with cancer, especially given the frequent use of long-term indwelling vascular access. The overall incidence of VTE in children with cancer is 8%, a number that likely underreports asymptomatic VTEs, and the incidence is much higher in children with sarcoma or any of the hematologic malignancies.[94]

Anesthetic considerations
In the child with a bleeding diathesis, the anesthesiologist may be required to transfuse fresh frozen plasma (FFP), cryoprecipitate, or factor concentrates. FFP is warranted if the child has documented prolongation of prothrombin or partial thromboplastin time or has surgical bleeding despite normal platelet levels and function.[95] However, FFP is ineffective for reversing the coagulation factor deficiencies induced by L-asparaginase.[96] FFP should be ABO-compatible and leukoreduced.[86] Transfusion of cryoprecipitate and factor concentrates should be guided by laboratory values and possibly in discussion with a hematologist.

Children with ongoing thrombosis may be on chronic anticoagulation, which may be required to be stopped or reversed before surgery. Perioperative consideration of the balance between the risk of thrombosis and anticoagulation-induced bleeding should be discussed with the child's hematologist-oncologist.[54]

OTHER CONSIDERATIONS IN THE CHILD WITH CANCER
Tumor Lysis Syndrome

Tumor lysis syndrome (TLS) is an uncommon but potentially lethal oncologic emergency. TLS is the acute destruction of tumor cells and the subsequent release of cellular components sufficient to overcome the excretory capacity of the body. Resultant ARF can lead to additional organ failure and death. TLS is most common with the hematologic malignancies, especially ALL and Burkitt lymphoma, but can occur with nonhematologic tumors that have a high proliferative rate, large tumor burden, or high sensitivity to cytotoxic therapy.[97] Although TLS can occur spontaneously, especially in children with AML, it most often occurs early in the disease after induction of chemotherapy or during radiation therapy, fever, surgery, or anesthesia.[97] Several reports exist of TLS occurring in children under anesthesia, including 1 fatality.[98]

Children at risk of TLS should receive adequate perioperative hydration to lessen the impact of TLS. Children at high risk should receive aggressive preoperative prophylaxis with hydration, rasburicase, and allopurinol. With such patients, the perioperative plan should be discussed with the child's oncologist before the day of surgery.[99] Dexamethasone is a known trigger of TLS, and the child's oncologist should be consulted before giving intraoperative corticosteroids to a child at risk of TLS.[98]

Retinoic Acid Syndrome

Retinoic acid syndrome (RAS) is seen in 2% to 27% of patients with acute promyelocytic leukemia who receive induction therapy with all-*trans* retinoic acid (ATRA). RAS is fatal in 2% of those who develop it. Primary symptoms are respiratory distress and fever, but weight gain, pulmonary infiltrates, pleural and pericardial effusions, hypotension, cardiac failure, and ARF can occur.[100,101]

Neurocognitive and Psychiatric Changes

Neurocognitive changes are common and continue years after cancer therapy. All components of neurocognitive testing can be abnormal, including executive function and academic achievement.[102] Although the cause is likely multifactorial, intrathecal methotrexate and cranial irradiation seem to lead to the greatest deficits, and thus survivors of central nervous system tumors, head and neck sarcomas, and ALL are at greatest risk.[103]

The response of the child to the diagnosis of cancer and its initial treatment depends on many factors, including the age of the patient, preexisting psychological dysfunction, and support from family and friends. Preschool and young school-aged children are very affected by parental separation, body boundaries, fears of disfigurement, and anticipation of painful procedures during their hospitalization. The coping mechanism at this age is varied, including anxiety, panic, regression, psychosomatic complaints, or stoic acceptance. Children at this age deserve, and often need, an honest discussion of the upcoming procedure to allow them a greater sense of control and understanding of their medical management. However, special preparations are frequently helpful, including role-playing or desensitization of the operating room environment, mask induction, and so forth.[38]

Adolescents diagnosed with or undergoing treatment with cancer are profoundly affected by the impact of their diagnosis. Caught in the transition from childhood to attaining greater independence in life, reliance on and compliance with the medical treatments are often difficult for the adolescent. To the greatest extent possible, these children should be given the opportunity to regain control and be active participants in their care, including cosigning of consents (assent), informed discussion of the procedure and risks, and discussion of the expected effects of the anesthetic and procedure.[38]

Pain

Children with cancer live with significant pain. In a survey of 160 children 10 to 18 years old undergoing cancer treatment, 87% of the inpatients and 75% of the outpatients rated their pain as moderate to severe.[104] Although antitumor therapy–related pain is the most common cause of pain in children with cancer, children reported in a survey that the single greatest painful episode during their cancer treatment was a medical procedure or surgery. The only variable that led to reduced pain scores from painful medical procedures was the use of general anesthesia during lumbar punctures and bone marrow biopsies.[38,105]

Therefore, anesthesiologists who care for these children likely have a key role in being able to reduce what has been reported as the most severe pain during cancer treatment. Several general anesthetic techniques can be administered for these brief but painful procedures. Although mask anesthesia with or without intravenous access can be used, these children usually have central access. Therefore, total intravenous anesthetic techniques with supplemental oxygen are commonly used for lumbar punctures and bone marrow biopsies, including propofol, propofol and ketamine, propofol and opiate (fentanyl, alfentanil, or remifentanil), or midazolam and ketamine.[38]

Children with cancer who experience chronic pain benefit from a multimodal approach to perioperative analgesia. Opioid tolerance must be assessed and appropriately managed when providing perioperative opiates. Regional anesthesia can be advantageous, but additional risks exist in children with cancer. The primary concern is the presence of an inherent coagulopathy or therapeutic anticoagulation and the risk of bleeding with a regional procedure, especially an epidural hematoma. Chemotherapy-induced neuropathy may be considered a relative contraindication to regional anesthesia. Therefore, a preoperative neurologic evaluation and special discussion of potential risks and benefits of regional anesthesia are warranted.[106] Overall, discussion between anesthesia, oncology, surgery, and pain service providers is recommended to formulate the optimal perioperative analgesic plan for children with cancer undergoing major surgery.

PREOPERATIVE LABORATORY EVALUATION

As is true for children without cancer, there is insufficient evidence to recommend any routine preoperative laboratory testing in children with cancer. The decision to obtain tests should be guided by the history, physical examination, concurrent illnesses, known abnormalities, and whether such testing will augment safe perioperative management of the child.

Evidence-based guidelines are not available to guide the decision of whether a complete blood count is needed or how recent a test is needed before surgery in children. Determination of the need for a complete blood count should include the condition of the patient, presence of comorbidities, proposed surgical procedure and potential blood loss, potential thrombocytopenia, attendant risk of prolonged bleeding, and known or suspected anemia.[38]

- Children at risk for anemia include[38]:
  - New diagnosis of leukemia (50%–80% incidence) or lymphoma
  - Recent chemotherapy, radiation therapy, or HSCT
  - Children with cancer and age less than 6 months
- Children at risk for hyperleukocytosis include any new diagnosis of leukemia (>20% incidence)
- Children at risk for leukopenia and neutropenia include any child receiving aggressive chemotherapy or irradiation
- Children at risk for thrombocytopenia include[38]:
  - New diagnosis of leukemia
  - Any child receiving aggressive chemotherapy or irradiation
  - Disseminated intravascular coagulation
  - Splenomegaly

The need for preoperative coagulation testing is not well defined in this patient population. If the platelet count is sufficient for the type of surgery and there is no clinical evidence of bleeding, then testing is probably not required. Testing may be considered for children with conditions that are known to cause a coagulopathy, including[38]:

- Sepsis
- Vitamin K deficiency or malnutrition
- Hyperleukocytosis
- L-Asparaginase treatment
- Diagnosis of T-cell acute lymphoblastic leukemia, myelomonocytic leukemia, or acute promyelocytic leukemia

Electrolyte testing should also be driven by the history and physical examination. Conditions that can lead to electrolyte derangements include[38]:

- SIADH
- Hypercalcemia (bone tumors and neuroblastoma)
- Intracranial disorder with altered level of consciousness
- Dehydration or malnutrition
- Aggressive hydration
- Renal dysfunction
- Recent TLS (hyperkalemia, hyperphosphatemia, hypocalcemia)

SUMMARY

Childhood cancers pose a wide array of challenges for the anesthesiologist caring for children. The unique interplay among the direct effects of the tumor, complex pharmacologic management, and potentially extensive physiologic derangements mandates a firm knowledge of each of these components to best formulate an anesthetic plan that is appropriate for the individual patient and type of procedure. The considerations described in this article also provide many opportunities for collaboration between the anesthesiologist, oncologist, and surgeon to optimize perioperative outcomes for children with these disorders.

REFERENCES

1. Jemal A, Siegel R, Ward E, et al. Cancer statistics, 2009. CA Cancer J Clin 2009; 59(4):225–49.
2. Ries LA, Percy CL, Bunin GR. Introduction. In: Ries LA, Smith MA, Gurney JG, et al, editors. Cancer incidence and survival among children and

adolescents: United States SEER Program 1975-1995. Bethesda (MD): National Cancer Institute SEER Program; 1999. p. 1 NIH Pub. No. 99-4649 ed.

3. US Cancer Statistics Working Group. United States cancer statistics: 1999–2009 incidence and mortality Web-based report. Atlanta (GA): US Department of Health and Human Services, Centers for Disease Control and Prevention and National Cancer Institute; 2013. Available at: www.cdc.gov/uscs. Accessed June 5, 2013.

4. Horner MJ, Ries LA, Krapcho M. SEER cancer statistics review, 1975-2006. Bethesda (MD): National Cancer Institute; 2009. Available at: http://seer.cancer.gov/csr/1975_2006/. Accessed June 5, 2013.

5. Oeffinger KC, Mertens AC, Sklar CA, et al. Chronic health conditions in adult survivors of childhood cancer. N Engl J Med 2006;355(15):1572–82.

6. Meneses CF, de Freitas JC, Castro CG Jr, et al. Safety of general anesthesia for lumbar puncture and bone marrow aspirate/biopsy in pediatric oncology patients. J Pediatr Hematol Oncol 2009;31(7):465–70.

7. Anghelescu DL, Burgoyne LL, Liu W, et al. Safe anesthesia for radiotherapy in pediatric oncology: St. Jude Children's Research Hospital Experience, 2004-2006. Int J Radiat Oncol Biol Phys 2008;71(2):491–7.

8. Latham GJ, Greenberg RS. Anesthetic considerations for the pediatric oncology patient–part 1: a review of antitumor therapy. Paediatr Anaesth 2010;20(4):295–304.

9. Heaney A, Buggy DJ. Can anaesthetic and analgesic techniques affect cancer recurrence or metastasis? Br J Anaesth 2012;109(Suppl 1):i17–28.

10. Tavare AN, Perry NJ, Benzonana LL, et al. Cancer recurrence after surgery: direct and indirect effects of anesthetic agents. Int J Cancer 2012;130(6):1237–50.

11. Myles PS, Peyton P, Silbert B, et al. Perioperative epidural analgesia for major abdominal surgery for cancer and recurrence-free survival: randomised trial. BMJ 2011;342:d1491.

12. Adamson PC, Balis FM, Berg S, et al. General principles of chemotherapy. In: Pizzo PA, Poplack DG, editors. Principles and practice of pediatric oncology. 5th edition. Philadelphia: Lippincott Williams & Wilkins; 2006. p. 290.

13. Lowenthal RM, Eaton K. Toxicity of chemotherapy. Hematol Oncol Clin North Am 1996;10(4):967–90.

14. Oeffinger KC, Hudson MM. Long-term complications following childhood and adolescent cancer: foundations for providing risk-based health care for survivors. CA Cancer J Clin 2004;54(4):208–36.

15. Tarbell NJ, Yock T, Kooy H. Principles of radiation oncology. In: Pizzo PA, Poplack DG, editors. Principles and practice of pediatric oncology. 5th edition. Philadelphia: Lippincott Williams & Wilkins; 2006. p. 421.

16. King DR, Patrick LE, Ginn-Pease ME, et al. Pulmonary function is compromised in children with mediastinal lymphoma. J Pediatr Surg 1997;32(2):294–9 [discussion: 299–300].

17. Wright CD. Mediastinal tumors and cysts in the pediatric population. Thorac Surg Clin 2009;19(1):47–61, vi.

18. Rheingold SR, Lange BJ. Oncologic emergencies. In: Pizzo PA, Poplack DG, editors. Principles and practice of pediatric oncology. 5th edition. Philadelphia: Lippincott Williams & Wilkins; 2006. p. 1202.

19. Hack HA, Wright NB, Wynn RF. The anaesthetic management of children with anterior mediastinal masses. Anaesthesia 2008;63(8):837–46.

20. Slinger P, Karsli C. Management of the patient with a large anterior mediastinal mass: recurring myths. Curr Opin Anaesthesiol 2007;20(1):1–3.

21. Vas L, Naregal F, Naik V. Anaesthetic management of an infant with anterior mediastinal mass. Paediatr Anaesth 1999;9(5):439–43.
22. Hammer GB. Anaesthetic management for the child with a mediastinal mass. Paediatr Anaesth 2004;14(1):95–7.
23. Trobs RB, Mader E, Friedrich T, et al. Oral tumors and tumor-like lesions in infants and children. Pediatr Surg Int 2003;19(9–10):639–45.
24. Raber-Durlacher JE, Barasch A, Peterson DE, et al. Oral complications and management considerations in patients treated with high-dose chemotherapy. Support Cancer Ther 2004;1(4):219–29.
25. Tartaglino LM, Rao VM, Markiewicz DA. Imaging of radiation changes in the head and neck. Semin Roentgenol 1994;29(1):81–91.
26. Delbridge L, Sutherland J, Somerville H, et al. Thyroid surgery and anaesthesia following head and neck irradiation for childhood malignancy. Aust N Z J Surg 2000;70(7):490–2.
27. Chaimberg KH, Cravero JP. Mucositis and airway obstruction in a pediatric patient. Anesth Analg 2004;99(1):59.
28. Drew B, Peters C, Rimell F. Upper airway complications in children after bone marrow transplantation. Laryngoscope 2000;110(9):1446–51.
29. Giraud O, Bourgain JL, Marandas P, et al. Limits of laryngeal mask airway in patients after cervical or oral radiotherapy. Can J Anaesth 1997;44(12):1237–41.
30. Burke A, Virmani R. Pediatric heart tumors. Cardiovasc Pathol 2008;17(4):193–8.
31. van Dalen EC, van der Pal HJ, Bakker PJ, et al. Cumulative incidence and risk factors of mitoxantrone-induced cardiotoxicity in children: a systematic review. Eur J Cancer 2004;40(5):643–52.
32. Simbre VC, Duffy SA, Dadlani GH, et al. Cardiotoxicity of cancer chemotherapy: implications for children. Paediatr Drugs 2005;7(3):187–202.
33. Huettemann E, Sakka SG. Anaesthesia and anti-cancer chemotherapeutic drugs. Curr Opin Anaesthesiol 2005;18(3):307–14.
34. Adams MJ, Lipshultz SE, Schwartz C, et al. Radiation-associated cardiovascular disease: manifestations and management. Semin Radiat Oncol 2003;13(3):346–56.
35. National Cancer Institute. PDQ® late effects of treatment for childhood cancer. Bethesda (MD): National Cancer Institute; 2013. Available at: http://cancer.gov/cancertopics/pdq/treatment/lateeffects/HealthProfessional. Accessed June 5, 2013.
36. Huettemann E, Junker T, Chatzinikolaou KP, et al. The influence of anthracycline therapy on cardiac function during anesthesia. Anesth Analg 2004;98(4):941–7.
37. Berry GJ, Jorden M. Pathology of radiation and anthracycline cardiotoxicity. Pediatr Blood Cancer 2005;44(7):630–7.
38. Latham GJ, Greenberg RS. Anesthetic considerations for the pediatric oncology patient–part 3: pain, cognitive dysfunction, and preoperative evaluation. Paediatr Anaesth 2010;20(6):479–89.
39. McCahon E. Lung tumours in children. Paediatr Respir Rev 2006;7(3):191–6.
40. Meyer S, Reinhard H, Gottschling S, et al. Pulmonary dysfunction in pediatric oncology patients. Pediatr Hematol Oncol 2004;21(2):175–95.
41. Abid SH, Malhotra V, Perry MC. Radiation-induced and chemotherapy-induced pulmonary injury. Curr Opin Oncol 2001;13(4):242–8.
42. Fauroux B, Meyer-Milsztain A, Boccon-Gibod L, et al. Cytotoxic drug-induced pulmonary disease in infants and children. Pediatr Pulmonol 1994;18(6):347–55.

43. Limper AH. Chemotherapy-induced lung disease. Clin Chest Med 2004;25(1): 53–64.
44. Klein DS, Wilds PR. Pulmonary toxicity of antineoplastic agents: anaesthetic and postoperative implications. Can Anaesth Soc J 1983;30(4):399–405.
45. Mertens AC, Yasui Y, Liu Y, et al. Pulmonary complications in survivors of childhood and adolescent cancer. A report from the Childhood Cancer Survivor Study. Cancer 2002;95(11):2431–41.
46. Sleijfer S. Bleomycin-induced pneumonitis. Chest 2001;120(2):617–24.
47. Carver JR, Shapiro CL, Ng A, et al. American Society of Clinical Oncology clinical evidence review on the ongoing care of adult cancer survivors: cardiac and pulmonary late effects. J Clin Oncol 2007;25(25):3991–4008.
48. Cerveri I, Fulgoni P, Giorgiani G, et al. Lung function abnormalities after bone marrow transplantation in children: has the trend recently changed? Chest 2001;120(6):1900–6.
49. Marras TK, Szalai JP, Chan CK, et al. Pulmonary function abnormalities after allogeneic marrow transplantation: a systematic review and assessment of an existing predictive instrument. Bone Marrow Transplant 2002;30(9):599–607.
50. Ingrassia TS 3rd, Ryu JH, Trastek VF, et al. Oxygen-exacerbated bleomycin pulmonary toxicity. Mayo Clin Proc 1991;66(2):173–8.
51. Luis M, Ayuso A, Martinez G, et al. Intraoperative respiratory failure in a patient after treatment with bleomycin: previous and current intraoperative exposure to 50% oxygen. Eur J Anaesthesiol 1999;16(1):66–8.
52. Hay JG, Haslam PL, Dewar A, et al. Development of acute lung injury after the combination of intravenous bleomycin and exposure to hyperoxia in rats. Thorax 1987;42(5):374–82.
53. Jules-Elysee K, White DA. Bleomycin-induced pulmonary toxicity. Clin Chest Med 1990;11(1):1–20.
54. Latham GJ, Greenberg RS. Anesthetic considerations for the pediatric oncology patient–part 2: systems-based approach to anesthesia. Paediatr Anaesth 2010; 20(5):396–420.
55. Ahmed HU, Arya M, Levitt G, et al. Part I: Primary malignant non-Wilms' renal tumours in children. Lancet Oncol 2007;8(8):730–7.
56. Shamberger RC. Pediatric renal tumors. Semin Surg Oncol 1999;16(2):105–20.
57. Rossi R, Kleta R, Ehrich JH. Renal involvement in children with malignancies. Pediatr Nephrol 1999;13(2):153–62.
58. Dome JS, Perlman EJ, Ritchey ML, et al. Renal tumors. In: Pizzo PA, Poplack DG, editors. Principles and practice of pediatric oncology. 5th edition. Philadelphia: Lippincott Williams & Wilkins; 2006. p. 905.
59. Skinner R. Chronic ifosfamide nephrotoxicity in children. Med Pediatr Oncol 2003;41(3):190–7.
60. Stohr W, Paulides M, Bielack S, et al. Nephrotoxicity of cisplatin and carboplatin in sarcoma patients: a report from the late effects surveillance system. Pediatr Blood Cancer 2007;48(2):140–7.
61. Widemann BC, Adamson PC. Understanding and managing methotrexate nephrotoxicity. Oncologist 2006;11(6):694–703.
62. Smith GR, Thomas PR, Ritchey M, et al. Long-term renal function in patients with irradiated bilateral Wilms tumor. National Wilms' Tumor Study Group. Am J Clin Oncol 1998;21(1):58–63.
63. Esiashvili N, Chiang KY, Hasselle MD, et al. Renal toxicity in children undergoing total body irradiation for bone marrow transplant. Radiother Oncol 2009;90(2): 242–6.

64. Hazar V, Gungor O, Guven AG, et al. Renal function after hematopoietic stem cell transplantation in children. Pediatr Blood Cancer 2009;53(2):197–202.
65. Frisk P, Bratteby LE, Carlson K, et al. Renal function after autologous bone marrow transplantation in children: a long-term prospective study. Bone Marrow Transplant 2002;29(2):129–36.
66. Gronroos MH, Bolme P, Winiarski J, et al. Long-term renal function following bone marrow transplantation. Bone Marrow Transplant 2007;39(11):717–23.
67. Finegold MJ, Egler RA, Goss JA, et al. Liver tumors: pediatric population. Liver Transpl 2008;14(11):1545–56.
68. Litten JB, Tomlinson GE. Liver tumors in children. Oncologist 2008;13(7):812–20.
69. Cesaro S, Pillon M, Talenti E, et al. A prospective survey on incidence, risk factors and therapy of hepatic veno-occlusive disease in children after hematopoietic stem cell transplantation. Haematologica 2005;90(10):1396–404.
70. Hasegawa S, Horibe K, Kawabe T, et al. Veno-occlusive disease of the liver after allogeneic bone marrow transplantation in children with hematologic malignancies: incidence, onset time and risk factors. Bone Marrow Transplant 1998;22(12):1191–7.
71. Bearman SI. The syndrome of hepatic veno-occlusive disease after marrow transplantation. Blood 1995;85(11):3005–20.
72. Kaste SC, Rodriguez-Galindo C, Furman WL. Imaging pediatric oncologic emergencies of the abdomen. AJR Am J Roentgenol 1999;173(3):729–36.
73. Berde CB, Billett AL, Collins JJ. Symptom management in supportive care. In: Pizzo PA, Poplack DG, editors. Principles and practice of pediatric oncology. 5th edition. Philadelphia: Lippincott Williams & Wilkins; 2006. p. 1348.
74. FitzGerald TJ, Aronowitz J, Giulia Cicchetti M, et al. The effect of radiation therapy on normal tissue function. Hematol Oncol Clin North Am 2006;20(1):141–63.
75. Binning M, Klimo P Jr, Gluf W, et al. Spinal tumors in children. Neurosurg Clin N Am 2007;18(4):631–58.
76. Reddy AT, Witek K. Neurologic complications of chemotherapy for children with cancer. Curr Neurol Neurosci Rep 2003;3(2):137–42.
77. Hildebrand J. Neurological complications of cancer chemotherapy. Curr Opin Oncol 2006;18(4):321–4.
78. Koch CA, Pacak K, Chrousos GP. Endocrine tumors. In: Pizzo PA, Poplack DG, editors. Principles and practice of pediatric oncology. 5th edition. Philadelphia: Lippincott Williams & Wilkins; 2006. p. 1139.
79. Hata M, Ogino I, Aida N, et al. Prophylactic cranial irradiation of acute lymphoblastic leukemia in childhood: outcomes of late effects on pituitary function and growth in long-term survivors. Int J Cancer 2001;96(Suppl):117–24.
80. Madanat LM, Lahteenmaki PM, Hurme S, et al. Hypothyroidism among pediatric cancer patients: a nationwide, registry-based study. Int J Cancer 2008;122(8):1868–72.
81. Jabbour SA. Steroids and the surgical patient. Med Clin North Am 2001;85(5):1311–7.
82. Einaudi S, Bertorello N, Masera N, et al. Adrenal axis function after high-dose steroid therapy for childhood acute lymphoblastic leukemia. Pediatr Blood Cancer 2008;50(3):537–41.
83. Hack HA. The perioperative management of children with phaeochromocytoma. Paediatr Anaesth 2000;10(5):463–76.
84. Hockenberry MJ, Hinds PS, Barrera P, et al. Incidence of anemia in children with solid tumors or Hodgkin disease. J Pediatr Hematol Oncol 2002;24(1):35–7.

85. Margolin JF, Steuber CP, Poplack DG. Acute lymphoblastic leukemia. In: Pizzo PA, Poplack DG, editors. Principles and practice of pediatric oncology. 5th edition. Philadelphia: Lippincott Williams & Wilkins; 2006. p. 538.

86. Hastings CA, Lubin BH, Feusner J. Hematologic supportive care for children with cancer. In: Pizzo PA, Poplack DG, editors. Principles and practice of pediatric oncology. 5th edition. Philadelphia: Lippincott Williams & Wilkins; 2006. p. 1231.

87. Golub TR, Arceci RJ. Acute myelogenous leukemia. In: Pizzo PA, Poplack DG, editors. Principles and practice of pediatric oncology. 5th edition. Philadelphia: Lippincott Williams & Wilkins; 2006. p. 591.

88. Rios JA, Korones DN, Heal JM, et al. WBC-reduced blood transfusions and clinical outcome in children with acute lymphoid leukemia. Transfusion 2001;41(7): 873–7.

89. Harris AL. Leukostasis associated with blood transfusion in acute myeloid leukaemia. Br Med J 1978;1(6121):1169–71.

90. Schiffer CA, Anderson KC, Bennett CL, et al. Platelet transfusion for patients with cancer: clinical practice guidelines of the American Society of Clinical Oncology. J Clin Oncol 2001;19(5):1519–38.

91. Howard SC, Gajjar A, Ribeiro RC, et al. Safety of lumbar puncture for children with acute lymphoblastic leukemia and thrombocytopenia. JAMA 2000; 284(17):2222–4.

92. Athale UH, Chan AK. Hemorrhagic complications in pediatric hematologic malignancies. Semin Thromb Hemost 2007;33(4):408–15.

93. Coppes MJ, Zandvoort SW, Sparling CR, et al. Acquired von Willebrand disease in Wilms' tumor patients. J Clin Oncol 1992;10(3):422–7.

94. Athale U, Siciliano S, Thabane L, et al. Epidemiology and clinical risk factors predisposing to thromboembolism in children with cancer. Pediatr Blood Cancer 2008;51(6):792–7.

95. Roseff SD, Luban NL, Manno CS. Guidelines for assessing appropriateness of pediatric transfusion. Transfusion 2002;42(11):1398–413.

96. Nowak-Gottl U, Rath B, Binder M, et al. Inefficacy of fresh frozen plasma in the treatment of L-asparaginase-induced coagulation factor deficiencies during ALL induction therapy. Haematologica 1995;80(5):451–3.

97. Del Toro G, Morris E, Cairo MS. Tumor lysis syndrome: pathophysiology, definition, and alternative treatment approaches. Clin Adv Hematol Oncol 2005;3(1): 54–61.

98. McDonnell C, Barlow R, Campisi P, et al. Fatal peri-operative acute tumour lysis syndrome precipitated by dexamethasone. Anaesthesia 2008;63(6):652–5.

99. Coiffier B, Altman A, Pui CH, et al. Guidelines for the management of pediatric and adult tumor lysis syndrome: an evidence-based review. J Clin Oncol 2008; 26(16):2767–78.

100. Patatanian E, Thompson DF. Retinoic acid syndrome: a review. J Clin Pharm Ther 2008;33(4):331–8.

101. De Botton S, Dombret H, Sanz M, et al. Incidence, clinical features, and outcome of all trans-retinoic acid syndrome in 413 cases of newly diagnosed acute promyelocytic leukemia. The European APL Group. Blood 1998;92(8): 2712–8.

102. Harila MJ, Winqvist S, Lanning M, et al. Progressive neurocognitive impairment in young adult survivors of childhood acute lymphoblastic leukemia. Pediatr Blood Cancer 2009;53(2):156–61.

103. Nathan PC, Patel SK, Dilley K, et al. Guidelines for identification of, advocacy for, and intervention in neurocognitive problems in survivors of childhood cancer: a

report from the Children's Oncology Group. Arch Pediatr Adolesc Med 2007; 161(8):798–806.

104. Collins JJ, Byrnes ME, Dunkel IJ, et al. The measurement of symptoms in children with cancer. J Pain Symptom Manage 2000;19(5):363–77.

105. Zernikow B, Meyerhoff U, Michel E, et al. Pain in pediatric oncology–children's and parents' perspectives. Eur J Pain 2005;9(4):395–406.

106. Hebl JR, Horlocker TT, Pritchard DJ. Diffuse brachial plexopathy after interscalene blockade in a patient receiving cisplatin chemotherapy: the pharmacologic double crush syndrome. Anesth Analg 2001;92(1):249–51.

Anesthesia for Craniofacial Surgery in Infancy

Paul A. Stricker, MD*, John E. Fiadjoe, MD

KEYWORDS

- Craniofacial surgery • Craniosynostosis • Pediatrics • Transfusion • Endoscopic

KEY POINTS

- Complex cranial vault reconstruction remains a significant challenge for anesthetic management.
- Primary concerns include blood loss and its management.
- Evolution of procedures to treat craniosynostosis has resulted in improvements in perioperative morbidity with less blood loss and shorter operations and length of hospital stays.
- An understanding of the procedures performed to treat craniosynostosis is necessary to provide optimal anesthetic management.

INTRODUCTION

Craniosynostosis is a disorder of skull development that occurs as a result of the premature fusion of one or more cranial sutures, occurring with an incidence of approximately 1 in 2000 live births. The observed deformity relates to which sutures are affected, with characteristic deformities associated with specific suture involvement (**Fig. 1**). Although the relationship between craniofacial dysmorphism and fusion of the cranial sutures was observed earlier, Virchow (1851)[1] was the first to formally describe many of the more common specific abnormalities, and in particular, he was the first to describe the arrest of skull growth that occurs in a direction perpendicular to the affected suture.

Craniosynostosis most commonly presents as an isolated abnormality but can present as a component of an identified syndrome or genetic disorder (15%–40% of cases (**Table 1**)). Ongoing research will likely reveal genetic causes of cases currently thought to be isolated or idiopathic. In most infants, the abnormality is congenital and diagnosed within the first few months of life, whereas some infants may present later. The diagnosis is most commonly made based on the phenotype of skull deformation.

Department of Anesthesiology and Critical Care, Children's Hospital of Philadelphia and the Perelman School of Medicine at the University of Pennsylvania, 34th Street and Civic Center Boulevard, Philadelphia, PA 19104, USA
* Corresponding author.
E-mail address: strickerp@email.chop.edu

Anesthesiology Clin 32 (2014) 215–235
http://dx.doi.org/10.1016/j.anclin.2013.10.007   anesthesiology.theclinics.com
1932-2275/14/$ – see front matter © 2014 Elsevier Inc. All rights reserved.

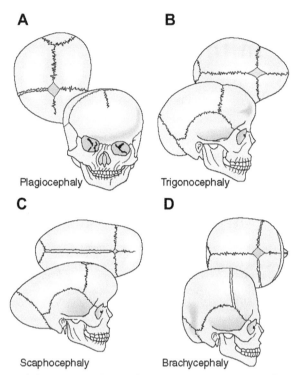

Fig. 1. Depictions of characteristic skull deformities associated with different forms of craniosynostosis. (*A*) Plagiocephaly caused by unicoronal synostosis (approximately 20%–25% of craniosynostosis). (*B*) Trigonocephaly caused by metopic synostosis accounts (approximately 5%–15% of craniosynostosis). (*C*) Scaphocephaly caused by sagittal synostosis, the most common form of nonsyndromic craniosynostosis (40%–55% of synostosis). (*D*) Bicoronal synostosis is less common and more likely associated with syndromic craniosynostosis. (*From* Seruya M, Magge S, Keating R. Diagnosis and surgical options for craniosynostosis. In: Ellenbogen RG, Abdulrauf S, Sekhar L, editors. Principles of neurologic surgery. 3rd edition. St Louis (MO): Saunders; 2012. p. 138; with permission.)

Subsequent CT scanning and 3-D reconstruction allow for accurate diagnosis of specific suture involvement and can be used for surgical planning (**Fig. 2**). Untreated craniosynostosis can lead to elevated intracranial pressure (ICP) and disturbances in intellectual and neurologic development. Syndromic craniosynostosis is more commonly associated with multiple suture involvement and is also more often associated with increased ICP. Children with syndromic craniosynostosis also require multiple operations throughout infancy and childhood.

From both a cosmetic and neurodevelopmental perspective, optimal outcomes are achieved when these procedures are performed before a year of age, and earlier surgical intervention may translate to a less extensive operation. Surgical treatment of craniofacial dysmorphism associated with craniosynostosis was principally pioneered by Dr Paul Tessier. Dr Tessier presented his initial work in 1967 and went on to train the first generation of craniomaxillofacial surgeons. As a result, Dr Tessier is widely regarded as the father of modern craniofacial surgery. The development of these surgical techniques has led to dramatic improvements in cosmetic, neurodevelopmental, and psychosocial outcomes in children afflicted by these conditions.[2,3]

Table 1
Selected craniosysnostosis syndromes

Disorder	Genetic Mutation Locus	Inheritance Pattern	Incidence	Associated Features
Apert syndrome (acrocephalosyndactyly)	FGFR2 (chromosome 10)	Most cases sporadic de novo mutations, autosomal dominant, affects males/females equally	~1 in 65,000	Midface hypoplasia, maxillary retrusion, proptosis, hypertelorism, syndactly, cleft palate. Can be associated with intellectual disability but intelligence can be normal.
Crouzon syndrome	FGFR2 (chromosome 10)	Autosomal dominant, de novo mutations, affects males/females equally	~1 in 60,000	Midface hypoplasia, maxillary retrusion, proptosis, hypertelorism, strabismus, beaked nose, often normal intelligence.
Pfeiffer syndrome	FGFR 1 (chromosome 8), FGFR2 (chromosome 10)	Autosomal dominant, de novo mutations, affects males/females equally	~1 in 100,000	Midface hypoplasia, maxillary retrusion, nasopharyngeal stenosis, proptosis, hypertelorism, strabismus, beaked nose, hearing loss, partial syndacylty, cartilaginous tracheal sleeve, broad thumbs and great toes, often normal intelligence.
Saethre-Chotzen syndrome (acrocephalosyndacytly type III)	TWIST (chromosome 7)	Majority familial autosomal dominant, de novo mutations possible, phenotype can be mild, affects males/females equally	~1 in 25,000–50,000	Short stature, hypertelorism, facial asymmetry, hearing loss, low frontal hairline, ptosis, mild partial syndactyly, usually normal intelligence.
Muenke syndrome (FGFR3-related craniosynostosis)	FGFR3 (chromosome 4)	Autosomal dominant, 61% de novo mutations, affects males/females equally	~0.8–1 in 10,000	Unicoronal or bicoronal synsostosis, ptosis, hypertelorism, high-arched palate, facial asymmetry, abnormalities of phalanges without syndactyly, developmental delay in approximately one-third of cases.

Data from Refs.[77–83]

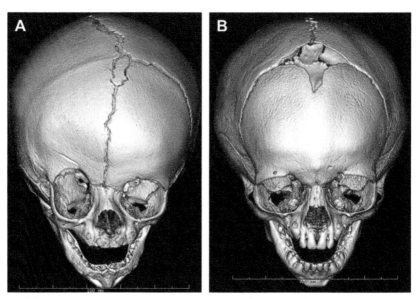

Fig. 2. (*A*) Preoperative 3-D CT reconstruction image from an infant with right unicoronal synostosis. Note ipsilateral orbital retrusion and contralateral frontal bossing. (*B*) Preoperative 3-D CT reconstruction image of an infant with metopic synostosis.

Together with the development of these extensive procedures have come significant challenges for anesthetic management. Early reports revealed major perioperative complications, including massive hemorrhage, airway complications, infection, and death.[4–6] These morbidities persist in the current era (although at lower rates), with complications relating to massive blood loss of greatest concern to anesthesiologists.[7–11]

The psychosocial implications of untreated craniosynostosis are tremendous. Throughout history, and even today, children with significant craniofacial deformities have been ostracized and excluded from society. Consequently, normalization of skull shape, although "cosmetic," has a tremendous and lasting impact on a child. This review explores some of the current procedures performed in this population and approaches to anesthetic management.

CURRENT SURGICAL APPROACHES TO CRANIOSYNOSTOSIS

As with any complex procedure, a firm understanding of the surgical procedure performed is necessary to provide optimal anesthetic management. A description of the most common procedure types follows, with attention to elements relevant to anesthesiologists.

Open Strip Craniectomy and the Modified Pi Procedure

Craniectomy to treat craniosynostosis was described as early as 1890 and 1892 by Lannelongue and Lane.[12–14] Simple strip craniectomies in which the cranial stenotic suture is excised alone do not result in good cosmetic outcomes and are rarely performed. Instead, for the most common deformity of isolated sagittal synostosis, the modified pi procedure or a variant thereof is performed (**Fig. 3**).[15] Although traditional anesthetic management of intracranial procedures involves invasive arterial pressure

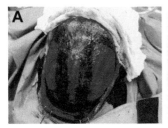
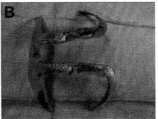
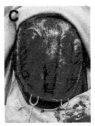

Fig. 3. Modified pi procedure. This procedure involves a scalp incision with exposure of the stenotic suture and adjacent calvarium. (*A*) Shows the exposed cranial vault with the areas of bone to be excised adjacent to the stenotic suture marked with methylene blue. (*B*) Shows the bone that has been removed (note the resemblance to the Greek letter pi). (*C*) Shows the cranium after these osteotomies. (*From* Seruya M, Magge S, Keating R. Diagnosis and surgical options for craniosynostosis. In: Ellenbogen RG, Abdulrauf S, Sekhar L, editors. Principles of neurologic surgery. 3rd edition. St Louis (MO): Saunders; 2012. p. 149; with permission.)

monitoring, some anesthesiologists manage these cases without an arterial catheter.[16] Adequate venous access is vital; 22-gauge or larger catheters are preferred for blood administration. Careful attention must be paid to proper positioning of these small infants. Other concerns relevant to children in this age group should be addressed, including selection of the appropriate endotracheal tube size and attention to blood glucose levels. Small size and blood volume coupled with the timing of these operations at the physiologic hemoglobin nadir puts these infants at high risk of needing transfusion, and most are transfused.

Endoscopic Strip Craniectomy and Postoperative Helmet Therapy

In 1996–1998, Jimenez and Barone[14] described the novel approach of excision of the stenotic sagittal suture followed by parietal barrel-stave osteotomies through two small incisions using an endoscope. For sagittal synostosis, a small incision is made over the anterior fontanelle and over the lambdoid. The scalp is then dissected off the cranium in a subgaleal plane over the stenotic suture and extended parietally. Under endoscopic visualization, the dura is dissected off the underside of the cranium over the same area. The stenotic suture is then excised using bone cutting scissors, followed by performance of parietal barrel stave osteotomies. The incisions are then closed and the child is fitted postoperatively for a cranial molding helmet.

The principal advantage of the endoscopic approach is the use of smaller incisions and minimization of blood loss, often allowing for transfusion to be avoided.[17] In addition, shorter hospital stays are realized, with many infants discharged on the first postoperative day.[18] Most importantly, satisfactory cosmetic results compared with traditional modified pi procedure are achieved.

After endoscopic surgery, infants wear cranial molding orthotics (helmets) for approximately 6 months to promote normalization of skull shape with subsequent brain growth and skull development (**Fig. 4**). These endoscopic procedures are most often performed to treat isolated sagittal synostosis in infants under 6 months but they can also be performed in infants with other suture involvement.[19] Although blood loss is typically minimal and transfusion can often be avoided, there is potential for inadvertent dural venous sinus entry or emissary vein disruption and significant hemorrhage. These children should, therefore, have preoperative laboratory testing that includes a hemoglobin/hematocrit measurement and a specimen for blood typing and cross-matching.

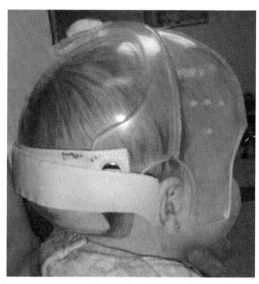

Fig. 4. Infant wearing a custom cranial molding helmet after endoscopic strip craniectomy. (*From* Kaufman BA, Muszynski CA, Matthews A, et al. The circle of sagittal synostosis surgery. Semin Pediatr Neurol 2004;11:243–8; with permission.)

Preparation for hemorrhage should include two peripheral intravenous catheters, and packed red blood cells (PRBCs) should be immediately available.

Spring-Mediated Cranioplasty

Although endoscopic strip craniectomy has the benefits of very low transfusion rates, small incisions, and short hospital stays, the principal drawback is the need for months of postoperative helmet therapy. In the mid-1980s, the concept of using springs to promote skull expansion was developed in an animal model[20] and later applied to infants with isolated sagittal synostosis by Lauritzen and colleagues in 1998.[21] Subsequent reports on larger series of children revealed good surgical results with low perioperative morbidity.[22,23] These procedures involve a scalp incision followed by surgical exposure of the length of the involved suture followed by simple strip craniectomy. Springs calibrated to deliver a specific force are then inserted between the cut edges of bone (**Fig. 5**) or into drill holes lateral to the osteotomy and the incision is closed. The forces applied by the springs result in cranial expansion perpendicular to the excised suture and normalization of skull shape with subsequent growth.

Similar to endoscopic strip craniectomy, spring-mediated cranioplasties are most commonly performed for isolated sagittal synostosis, and often can be done without the need for transfusion. Patients are ideally under 6 months of age. These children return for a second operation approximately 6 months after the initial surgery to have the springs removed. The need for a second operation is the principal disadvantage of this procedure. Anesthetic management is similar to that for endoscopic strip craniectomy. These infants can often be discharged home on postoperative day 1. Similar to endoscopic procedures, shorter hospital stays and shorter operating times, together with less intraoperative blood loss and very low transfusion rates, have been reported.[24]

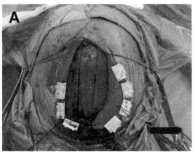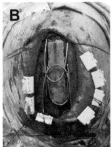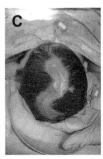

Fig. 5. Spring-mediated cranioplasty. (*A*) View showing surgical exposure and cranium after strip craniectomy of sagittal suture. (*B*) View of springs in place with excised cranial bone strip beneath springs. (*C*) Patient prepped at follow-up operation for spring removal. Note normal skull shape with correction of scaphocephaly.

Complex Cranial Vault Reconstruction

Infants with nonsagittal synostosis, infants with sagittal synostosis with a late presentation, and infants with syndromic craniosynostosis all have significant cranial vault deformities for which optimal surgical results are achieved with complex cranial vault reconstruction. These procedures are typically performed in older infants between 6 and 12 months of age. Some children who previously underwent treatment of sagittal synostosis may have residual cranial deformity that requires a subsequent operation. Children with syndromic craniosynostosis usually require multiple operations as they grow. In addition to concerns about the effects of untreated craniosynostosis and elevated ICP, complete reossification of the cranial vault defects that are created during these procedures is more likely the younger the child is at the time of operation; the potential for residual postoperative bony defects increases as the age of the child increases after 1 year of age (**Fig. 6**). Complex cranial reconstructions include total calvarial reconstruction, fronto-orbital advancement, and posterior cranial vault reconstruction.

Total calvarial reconstruction

At some centers, total calvarial reconstructions are performed. For this procedure, infants are typically placed in the modified prone or sphinx position, where the child is prone but with the head and neck extended. As its name suggests, it is an extensive procedure and its association with problematic complications has led the approach to be abandoned at many centers in favor of sequential operations separated by an interval of several months (eg, fronto-orbital advancement followed by posterior cranial vault reconstruction). Complications include massive hemorrhage and venous air embolism from the elevated head position. The sphinx position may also cause venous outflow obstruction that promotes both edema and bleeding.

Fronto-orbital advancement and reconstruction

Fronto-orbital advancement and reconstruction are performed for infants with metopic, unicoronal, bicoronal, and multiple-suture craniosynostosis. These procedures are done in the supine position and involve a wide bicoronal incision followed by a frontal craniotomy and removal of the orbital bandeau (**Figs. 7** and **8**). The excised bones are then cut, shaped, repositioned, bent, and replaced using wires or reabsorbable plates and screws to achieve the desired result depending on the preoperative deformity (**Fig. 9**).

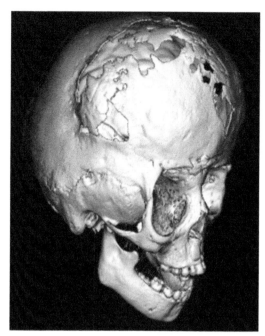

Fig. 6. Preoperative 3-D CT reconstruction showing residual bony defects in the skull in a child with syndromic craniosynostosis who has undergone prior craniofacial surgery. A ventriculoperitoneal shunt is also present.

Epinephrine solutions (with or without local anesthetic) are often infiltrated in the scalp to promote hemostasis. Other techniques include application of scalp clips and temporary locking scalp sutures that are placed anterior and posterior to the incision that have a tourniquet effect on the scalp. Although bleeding can occur during scalp dissection and exposure of the calvarium (particularly if the dissection is in the subperiosteal plane rather than subgaleal plane), the period of greatest risk for bleeding (and air embolism) is during the frontal craniotomy and during the osteotomies for removal of the orbital bandeau. Once the osteotomies have been completed and hemostasis obtained, the potential for catastrophic hemorrhage generally subsides.

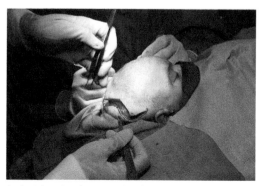

Fig. 7. Bicoronal scalp incision for fronto-orbital advancement. The incision is made zigzag rather than straight so the scar is later hidden by hair.

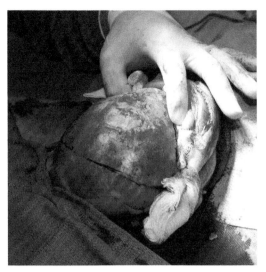

Fig. 8. Intraoperative view after scalp dissection and exposure of the calvarium in the same infant in **Fig. 7** with metopic synostosis. The prominent metopic ridge can be seen between the surgeon's fingers.

When a surgeon is operating near the orbits, the oculocardiac reflex may be triggered and bradycardia observed. This usually requires no treatment because there are typically no worrisome invasive blood pressure changes. If necessary, simply having the surgeon release pressure stops the reflex. Occasionally, the reflex is problematic and an anticholinergic may be administered to allow the surgeon to continue operating in this area.

Posterior cranial vault reconstruction
Posterior cranial vault reconstructions are performed in infants with late presentation sagittal synostosis, children with residual deformity from sagittal synostosis treated in

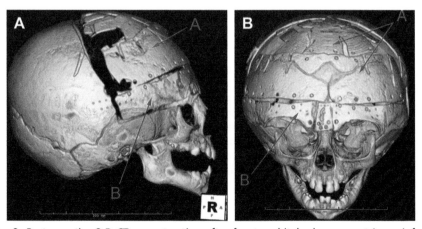

Fig. 9. Postoperative 3-D CT reconstruction after fronto-orbital advancement in an infant with metopic synostosis. The reconstructed cranial bones from the bifrontal craniotomy are labeled A and the reconstructed orbital bandeau is labeled B.

early infancy, and children with syndromic craniosynostosis. These procedures are done in the prone position, and a bicoronal incision is made as in fronto-orbital advancements. After scalp dissection for cranial exposure, a neurosurgeon removes a posterior cranial bone flap. Barrel stave osteotomies are performed laterally and inferiorly along the edges of the craniotomy to allow for release and expansion of the cranial vault. The bone flap is then cut, shaped, repositioned, and replaced and anchored with wires or reabsorbable plates and screws. Concerns for anesthesiologists are similar to those for fronto-orbital advancement, with additional concerns related to prone positioning.

PREOPERATIVE PREPARATION

In addition to surgical planning, infants and children undergoing these procedures require a thorough medical evaluation as well as laboratory testing prior to surgery. Most infants presenting with nonsyndromic forms of craniosynostosis are otherwise healthy and require little preoperative preparation beyond appropriate laboratory testing. Preoperative laboratory testing for all children should include a complete blood cell count (hemoglobin, hematocrit, and platelet count) and a specimen for type and screen (at a minimum); in most cases, in particular, open procedures, cross-matching of blood is necessary.

Even those procedures associated with low rates of transfusion carry a risk of unanticipated hemorrhage, and appropriate preparation is warranted. This is especially true of younger infants undergoing these procedures, who are able to tolerate only small volumes of blood loss. A coagulation profile is routinely ordered at many centers (prothrombin time [PT]/international normalized ratio [INR], partial thromboplastin time [PTT]). The cost-effectiveness and value of preoperative coagulation testing can be questioned. One argument in favor of such testing is that these infants have little history for identifying a bleeding tendency.

Infants with syndromic craniosynostosis may have associated abnormalities that affect the perioperative period. For example, midface hypoplasia and retrusion may cause obstructive sleep apnea and postoperative airway obstruction such that postoperative tracheal intubation and mechanical ventilation may be indicated. Children with severe airway obstruction may require or may present with a tracheostomy.

SPECIFIC INTRAOPERATIVE CONCERNS
Hemorrhage

The most recent report from the Pediatric Perioperative Cardiac Arrest Registry demonstrated the most common cardiovascular cause of cardiac arrest in children was hypovolemia, often from hemorrhage during procedures involving a craniotomy.[25] Complex cranial vault reconstructions involve large scalp incisions followed by large craniotomies. Large surgical areas and cranial bone cuts result in large surface areas for bleeding to occur. Infants undergoing open cranial remodeling procedures commonly sustain blood losses in excess of the circulating blood volume,[11,26,27] and blood losses up to 5 times the circulating blood volume have been described.[27] In addition to steady blood loss that occurs during the procedure, precipitous hemorrhage can also occur with inadvertent dural venous sinus tears or disruption of large emissary veins.

Venous Air Embolism

Having a surgical incision, in particular, cut edges of the cranial table at a level above the heart, creates a risk of venous air embolism. The incidence of venous air embolism during these cases is high (83%); however, a vast majority of these episodes are clinically silent (Doppler tone changes only) and not associated with hemodynamic compromise.[28] Venous air embolism can also occur during endoscopic procedures; however, the incidence seems much lower (8%) and is infrequently associated with hemodynamic instability.[29]

Intracranial Hypertension

Children may present with evidence of elevated ICP, diagnosed by ophthalmic examination or CT scan or inferred from nonspecific findings, such as headaches in older children. Elevated ICP is common in syndromic craniosynostosis with multiple suture involvement (47%). Increased ICP may be also present in as many as 14% of infants with isolated single-suture synostosis.[30] Despite these incidence rates, a majority of these children present as outpatients and, in the absence of overt symptoms, an inhaled induction of anesthesia can usually be performed while other principles of management of ICP are otherwise adhered to.

Hypothermia

Intraoperatively, the large surface area of an infant's head coupled with its high perfusion, together with anesthetic effects and administration of large volumes of cool intravenous fluids, can result in hypothermia. With the proper measures in place, hypothermia can be prevented, but it requires attention by the team. Active warming techniques include forced air convection blankets, circulating warm water mattresses, overhead radiant lights, and fluid warmers. Even mild hypothermia (less than 36°C) impairs coagulation enzyme function and is associated with increased bleeding and transfusion[31]; therefore, it is imperative that management be directed to prevent it.

Positioning and Eye Protection

Many craniofacial procedures are lengthy and careful attention to proper patient positioning is important. During cranial vault reconstruction procedures in the supine position, surgeons may prefer that the eyes not be taped closed because the eyes are within the surgical field. Ophthalmic ointment should be applied and careful attention paid to the vulnerable eyes by all members of the team. Ophthalmic ointment should be periodically reapplied. Children with syndromic forms of craniosynostosis can have proptosis so severe that full eyelid closure is difficult. In these cases, the surgeons may perform tarsorrhaphies. Infants undergoing procedures in the prone position are placed in a horseshoe headrest. The head must be positioned and the headrest configured to ensure there is no pressure on the orbits or other pressure points. Satisfactory positioning should be periodically reassessed throughout the operation.

INTRAOPERATIVE MANAGEMENT
Induction, Airway Management, and Anesthetic Maintenance

An inhaled induction of anesthesia is most commonly performed. Children with signs or symptoms of significant ICP elevation may benefit from an intravenous anesthetic induction. Administration of a muscle relaxant facilitates laryngoscopy, tracheal intubation, and vascular access and prevents coughing and movement during positioning. Orotracheal intubation using a standard tracheal tube is preferred. Some anesthesiologists place a nasotracheal tube for infants in the prone position because they think it is more secure. Although an oral RAE tube can be placed, the preformed bend can make intraoperative tracheal suctioning difficult, and selecting the proper tube for both length (location of the preformed bend) and diameter may be particularly challenging in younger infants. In general, RAE tubes are unnecessary and not worth the extra trouble. Anesthesia is typically maintained with an inhaled anesthetic in air and oxygen. Because of the risk of venous air embolism, nitrous oxide is avoided as is spontaneous/negative pressure ventilation. Opioids are administered by bolus or by infusion; some anesthesiologists supplement the anesthetic with a dexmedetomidine infusion.

Peripheral Venous Access

All infants should have at least 2 peripheral intravenous lines when possible, preferably 22 gauge or larger. Blood products should be administered through large bore peripheral intravenous lines rather than through a central line, because peripheral administration allows potentially high potassium content as well as citrate to mix and be diluted before it returns to the heart.

Arterial Catheter

Invasive arterial pressure monitoring is generally recommended for intracranial procedures because it allows for the immediate detection of hypotension and for frequent blood sampling. An arterial catheter also allows for postoperative blood sampling.

Central Venous Catheter

Some centers routinely insert central venous catheters for children undergoing complex cranial vault reconstruction procedures to measure central venous pressure to guide fluid and transfusion management, whereas most reserve their use in these procedures for children in whom adequate peripheral access is difficult to obtain.[16]

Precordial Doppler

A precordial Doppler can be used for the detection of venous air embolism. This monitor is a simple and effective noninvasive monitor for air embolus detection. Because this monitor is so sensitive and because most episodes are clinically silent, however, the majority of anesthesiologists do not use a precordial Doppler.[16,28]

MANAGEMENT OF MASSIVE HEMORRHAGE

Complications of massive hemorrhage not only relate to the immediate concerns of hypovolemia but also the sequelae of imperfect replacement with crystalloids, colloids, and blood components. These sequelae include metabolic acidosis, dilutional coagulopathy, thrombocytopenia, hyperkalemia (from high potassium content of stored PRBCs), hypocalcemia (citrate toxicity), and hypothermia.

Rapid administration of PRBCs with prolonged storage, particularly in the setting of hypovolemia, can result in hyperkalemic cardiac arrest.[25,32] The potassium concentration in a unit of PRBCs increases in a linear fashion with time. Irradiation of blood drastically accelerates the transmembrane leakage of potassium from stored red blood cells.[33] In a recent advisory statement the Wake up Safe group recommends using PRBCs less than 7 days from collection or PRBCs that have been washed and resuspended in saline to minimize the risk of hyperkalemia in scenarios where massive hemorrhage is antcipated.[34]

When blood loss is replaced with crystalloid and PRBCs, coagulopathy resulting from dilution of soluble clotting factors develops after approximately 1.2 blood volumes have been lost, and fresh frozen plasma (FFP) transfusion is indicated.[35] In a recent assessment of the authors' practice, where median and average blood losses have been in excess of a blood volume, replacement with crystalloid and PRBCs was associated with a high incidence (24%) of postoperative dilutional coagulopathy.[11]

Over that time period, intraoperative FFP was administered once coagulopathy was identified either by laboratory or clinical evidence, consistent with current American Society of Anesthesiologists practice guidelines.[11] In response to the findings in this review, the authors implemented a practice in which FFP is administered prophylactically together with PRBCs in a 1:1 ratio (1 unit of FFP:1 unit of PRBCs). Implementation of this practice resulted in near elimination of postoperative dilutional coagulopathy.[36] The number of blood donor exposures was minimized by using FFP from the same blood donors from whom the PRBC units were obtained.

Another option for blood loss replacement is whole blood. Replacement with whole blood provides coagulation proteins in addition to red blood cells. Beyond the simplicity of replacing blood loss with whole blood, whole blood has the advantage of replacing red blood cell loss and coagulation factors without the need for additional blood donor exposures that would be required using traditional component therapy. Also, refrigerated whole blood contains platelets. Although platelets contained in refrigerated whole blood are cleared rapidly from the circulation after transfusion, they have intact coagulation function as assessed by in vitro testing and may be able to participate in coagulation after transfusion.[37] Refrigerated whole blood retains coagulation activity, as measured in vitro testing, within normal limits for up to 14 days of storage.[38] Unfortunately, the availability of whole blood is often limited.

Another technique to be considered in the setting of replacement of significant blood loss is administration of fibrinogen concentrate. In a variety of settings, decreased perioperative blood loss has been correlated with higher fibrinogen levels.[39,40] Haas and colleagues[41] demonstrated that fibrinogen replacement using fibrinogen concentrate was effective in maintaining normal hemostatic function in infants undergoing craniofacial surgery, without the need for FFP transfusion. Fibrinogen concentrate is a lyophilized, purified, pasteurized product that has several advantages, including pathogen inactivation and elimination of infectious disease transmission risk, ability to be stored for prolonged periods before reconstitution and administration, and the ability for precise dosing. High cost may be a disadvantage, although preventing transfusion of other hemostatic blood products may outweigh this.

The off-label use of recombinant activated factor VII has been described as a rescue measure in a variety of settings with massive hemorrhage, including craniofacial surgery.[42] Acidosis, hypothermia, thrombocytopenia, and hypofibrinogenemia all impair the efficacy of recombinant factor VIIa and should be corrected to maximize efficacy. Off-label use of recombinant activated factor VII has been associated with significant thrombotic complications; therefore, its use should be reserved for life-threatening situations in which all other methods of achieving hemostasis have failed.

ASSESSMENT OF INTRAVASCULAR VOLUME STATUS

One of the greatest challenges of complex cranial vault reconstruction and open craniectomy procedures is the accurate identification of blood loss and its timely replacement. It is often impossible to accurately estimate ongoing losses because blood seeps into and underneath surgical drapes, mixes with irrigation fluid, or is otherwise difficult to account for in surgical sponges (**Fig. 10**).

Intravascular volume status is assessed most commonly through invasive arterial pressure measurement in combination with invasive arterial pressure waveform assessment. There is a body of evidence supporting the efficacy of using changes in variability in pulse pressure/systolic pressure with positive pressure ventilation

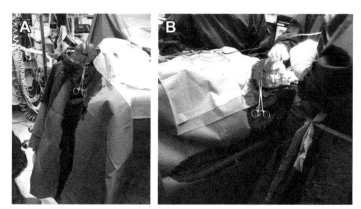

Fig. 10. Intraoperative photographs from the right (*A*) and left (*B*) sides of the same infant showing blood loss soaked into drapes. Accurate quantification of losses is not possible.

as a tool to direct fluid management in adults. There are conflicting data, however, supporting the applicability of this technique to infants and children.[43] Qualitative waveform assessment has traditionally been done; more recently, software and equipment have become available that can perform continuous automated quantitative measurement of these parameters. The utility of these devices in infants remains largely unexplored.

Some anesthesiologists use central venous pressure monitoring in addition to these methods (discussed previously) for guiding fluid and transfusion therapy. In adults, central venous pressure performs poorly compared with other measures for predicting fluid responsiveness.[44] The authors' results showed that the implementation of central venous pressure monitoring in infants undergoing complex craniofacial reconstruction was not associated with a reduction in the incidence or duration of hypotension.[45] The authors also found that changes in heart rate (tachycardia) are not a valuable indicator of hypovolemia in infants undergoing complex craniofacial surgery.[46]

Ultimately, constant vigilance remains the best tool for successful assessment of intravascular volume status and prevention of hypovolemia, and in practice all available clinical data are combined to guide fluid administration. This includes direct observation of the surgical field and directing close attention to the invasive blood pressure and waveform, central venous pressure (if monitored), response to fluid challenges, urine output, hemoglobin measurements, and blood gas assessments.

STRATEGIES FOR MINIMIZATION OF BLOOD LOSS AND TRANSFUSION

Although anesthesiologists have made notable efforts to reduce blood loss and transfusion, overall the reductions achieved with these approaches are modest. The greatest reductions have resulted from innovations in surgical technique (eg, endoscopic strip craniectomy and spring-mediated cranioplasty). A wide variety of nonsurgical techniques to minimize blood loss and transfusion in this population have been studied, including antifibrinolytic administration,[47–49] cell salvage,[27,50–53] acute normovolemic hemodilution,[54,55] preoperative erythropoietin,[55–58] reinfusion of shed blood,[27] administration of fibrinogen concentrates,[41] and prophylactic administration of FFP.[59] Each of these carries its own risks, evidence of efficacy, and costs.

When transfusion minimization strategies are considered, it is important to evaluate what the achieved reduction means in terms of patient risk. One of the key multipliers of transfusion risk is the number of unique blood donor exposures. Each additional blood donor exposure from a new unit of PRBCs results in additive risks for infectious disease transmission and alloimmunization. For this reason, if the volume of transfusion is reduced from 200 mL to 100 mL, there is no benefit for a patient because the number of blood donor exposures has not been reduced.

Transfusion Protocols

Implementation of standardized transfusion protocols is a simple, inexpensive, and effective strategy to safely minimize transfusion. Moreover, there is a body of scientific evidence demonstrating efficacy. Standardized transfusion thresholds have been shown to reduce red blood cell transfusion without an increased incidence of adverse events in adult patients without cardiac disease,[60] in critically ill children,[61] and in pediatric postoperative patients.[62,63] The use of transfusion protocols has been recommended in pediatric craniofacial surgery.[64,65] At the authors' institution, the implementation of a postoperative transfusion protocol for both hemostatic blood products (FFP, platelets, and cryoprecipitate) and PRBCs (**Box 1**) resulted in a 60% overall reduction in postoperative transfusion.[66] For these reasons, transfusion protocols should be a first-line approach to safe transfusion minimization in this population.

Administration of Antifibrinolytic Agents

The antifibrinolytic drug, tranexamic acid, has been shown effective in reducing blood loss and perioperative transfusion in children undergoing craniofacial surgery.[18,48] There are also data demonstrating the efficacy of aprotinin[47]; however, this drug is no longer available. Efficacy data in this population are currently not available for aminocaproic acid (another antifibrinolytic with the same mechanism of action as tranexamic acid), although there are data in adults suggesting comparable efficacy of the two drugs.[67–71]

Administration of antifibrinolytics is an attractive strategy because they are simple to administer, inexpensive, and there seems to be a low incidence of adverse events. The results of one study showed that tranexamic acid was efficacious despite the lack of a measurable difference in fibrinolytic activity on thromboelastography.[49]

Cell Salvage

Intraoperative cell salvage is a technique that may allow for reduction of transfusion in infant craniofacial surgery. There is one randomized trial supporting the efficacy of cell

---

Box 1
Postoperative transfusion protocol used at the Children's Hospital of Philadelphia

Indications for hemostatic blood product transfusion:

Platelet count <100,000

Fibrinogen <100 mg/dL

PT >18.7

PTT >45.7

INR >1.5

Indications for PRBC transfusion:

Hemoglobin <7.5 g/dL

Hemodynamic instability with ongoing blood loss

saver in combination with preoperative erythropoietin in children undergoing cranial vault reconstruction.[72] Other published evidence includes mostly retrospective data.[27,52,53,65,73]

Implementation of cell salvage may require changes in draping and attention to technique to maximize blood recovery. Special cell salvage machines are available that can be used in infants. These machines require small initial volumes for processing and are subsequently able to process blood as it is recovered. The principal drawbacks of cell salvage are the equipment costs and the attention (and possibly additional personnel) needed to operate the machine.

Administration of Preoperative Erythropoietin and Acute Preoperative Normovolemic Hemodilution

The use of preoperative recombinant erythropoietin has been described as part of a strategy to minimize transfusion in pediatric craniofacial surgery[55–57]; however, its current use seems infrequent and limited to select patients.[16] When administered, this technique is often combined with acute preoperative normovolemic hemodilution and other techniques to maximize efficacy. An evaluation of acute preoperative normovolemic hemodilution using a mathematical model suggests that the blood savings achieved with this method alone are modest at best.[74]

High cost and the need for multiple preoperative visits for injections and hemoglobin surveillance are significant drawbacks of this therapy. Moreover, recent adult data showing associations of recombinant erythropoietin with increased risk for stroke, hypertension, vascular access thrombosis, and probably increased risk for death, serious cardiovascular events, and end-stage renal disease[75] have led the Food and Drug Administration to apply a black box warning to these drugs in the United States. For these reasons, use in pediatric craniofacial surgery remains limited.

Transfusion-free Perioperative Course in Infants Undergoing Complex Cranial Reconstruction

Despite the literature replete with descriptions of significant bleeding and transfusion, low transfusion rates in children undergoing complex cranial vault reconstruction are possible. One group was able to achieve low transfusion rates in using simple surgical techniques for achieving intraoperative hemostasis and accepting a low postoperative hemoglobin value (7.0 g/dL).[64] Another group has achieved low transfusion rates using preoperative erythropoietin combined with preoperative autologous donation, intraoperative hemodilution, and cell salvage.[50] A recent practice survey corroborates these reports, with some centers self-reporting achieving a transfusion-free perioperative course in some of these children.[16]

POSTOPERATIVE CARE

At the authors' hospital, all children who have had a craniotomy as part of their procedure are admitted to the ICU postoperatively. The duration of ICU stay varies between institutions, but in many cases these children can be transferred to the general ward on postoperative day 1. At some centers, children are admitted to the general ward after endoscopic procedures and spring-mediated cranioplasties.

Postoperative pain is usually not severe, and intermittent opioids together with acetaminophen provide satisfactory postoperative analgesia. Nearly all infants are extubated in the operating room at the completion of surgery. Infants who may require postoperative intubation and mechanical ventilation include infants in the prone position for lengthy procedures with significant facial swelling and infants with syndromic craniosynostosis who have significant preoperative obstructive sleep apnea.

As discussed previously, transfusion protocols should be in place to guide transfusion therapy in the postoperative period. Postoperative hyponatremia is common (31% in one study) although direct complications from hyponatremia seem uncommon.[76] Other postoperative concerns include cerebrospinal fluid leaks and infection.[84]

SUMMARY

Normalization of skull shape from craniofacial surgery in infancy has a major and lasting impact on the life of a child. These operations involve risks, with the potential for major intraoperative hemorrhage the primary concern for anesthesiologists. Optimal anesthetic management involves preparation for blood loss replacement, proper positioning, and attention to the fundamentals of anesthetic management of infants.

Various methods have been used to reduce the amount of blood transfused in this population. Simple techniques, such as meticulous surgical attention to hemostasis, administration of antifibrinolytic agents, and implementation of transfusion thresholds, are probably the most cost-effective ways to safely minimize transfusion requirements. The greatest reductions in both perioperative transfusion and morbidity have been achieved through innovations in surgical techniques, such as with the development of endoscopic strip craniectomy and spring-mediated cranioplasty procedures.

REFERENCES

1. Virchow R. Uever den Cretinismus, namenlich in Franken, und uer pathologische Schadelformen. Verh Phys Med Ges Wurzburg 1851;2:230.
2. Tessier P. The definitive plastic surgical treatment of the severe facial deformities of craniofacial dysostosis. Crouzon's and Apert's diseases. Plast Reconstr Surg 1971;48:419–42.
3. Waterhouse N. The history of craniofacial surgery. Facial Plast Surg 1993;9: 143–50.
4. Whitaker LA, Munro IR, Salyer KE, et al. Combined report of problems and complications in 793 craniofacial operations. Plast Reconstr Surg 1979;64:198–203.
5. Whitaker LA, Munro IR, Jackson IT, et al. Problems in craniofacial surgery. J Maxillofac Surg 1976;4:131–6.
6. Munro IR, Sabatier RE. An analysis of 12 years of craniomaxillofacial surgery in Toronto. Plast Reconstr Surg 1985;76:29–35.
7. Kearney RA, Rosales JK, Howes WJ. Craniosynostosis: an assessment of blood loss and transfusion practices. Can J Anaesth 1989;36:473–7.
8. Tuncbilek G, Vargel I, Erdem A, et al. Blood loss and transfusion rates during repair of craniofacial deformities. J Craniofac Surg 2005;16:59–62.
9. Buntain SG, Pabari M. Massive transfusion and hyperkalemic cardiac arrest in craniofacial surgery in a child. Anaesth Intensive Care 1999;27:530–3.
10. Faberowski LW, Black S, Mickle JP. Blood loss and transfusion practice in the perioperative management of craniosynostosis repair. J Neurosurg Anesthesiol 1999;11:167–72.
11. Stricker PA, Shaw TL, Desouza DG, et al. Blood loss, replacement, and associated morbidity in infants and children undergoing craniofacial surgery. Paediatr Anaesth 2010;20:150–9.
12. Lannelongue M. De la craniectomie dans la microcephalie. Compt Rend Seances Acad Sci 1890;50:1382–5.

13. Lane L. Pioneer craniectomy for relief of mental imbecility due to premature sutural closure and microcephalus. JAMA 1892;18:49–50.
14. Jimenez DF, Barone CM. Endoscopic craniectomy for early surgical correction of sagittal craniosynostosis. J Neurosurg 1998;88:77–81.
15. Guimaraes-Ferreira J, Gewalli F, David L, et al. Sagittal synostosis: II. Cranial morphology and growth after the modified pi-plasty. Scand J Plast Reconstr Surg Hand Surg 2006;40:200–9.
16. Stricker PA, Cladis FP, Fiadjoe JE, et al. Perioperative management of children undergoing craniofacial reconstruction surgery: a practice survey. Paediatr Anaesth 2011;21:1026–35.
17. Jimenez DF, Barone CM, Cartwright CC, et al. Early management of craniosynostosis using endoscopic-assisted strip craniectomies and cranial orthotic molding therapy. Pediatrics 2002;110:97–104.
18. Meier PM, Goobie SM, DiNardo JA, et al. Endoscopic strip craniectomy in early infancy: the initial five years of anesthesia experience. Anesth Analg 2011;112:407–14.
19. Jimenez DF, Barone CM. Multiple-suture nonsyndromic craniosynostosis: early and effective management using endoscopic techniques. J Neurosurg Pediatr 2010;5:223–31.
20. Persing JA, Babler WJ, Nagorsky MJ, et al. Skull expansion in experimental craniosynostosis. Plast Reconstr Surg 1986;78:594–603.
21. Lauritzen C, Sugawara Y, Kocabalkan O, et al. Spring mediated dynamic craniofacial reshaping. Case report. Scand J Plast Reconstr Surg Hand Surg 1998;32:331–8.
22. Lauritzen CG, Davis C, Ivarsson A, et al. The evolving role of springs in craniofacial surgery: the first 100 clinical cases. Plast Reconstr Surg 2008;121:545–54.
23. David LR, Plikaitis CM, Couture D, et al. Outcome analysis of our first 75 spring-assisted surgeries for scaphocephaly. J Craniofac Surg 2010;21:3–9.
24. Taylor JA, Maugans TA. Comparison of spring-mediated cranioplasty to minimally invasive strip craniectomy and barrel staving for early treatment of sagittal craniosynostosis. J Craniofac Surg 2011;22:1225–9.
25. Bhananker SM, Ramamoorthy C, Geiduschek JM, et al. Anesthesia-related cardiac arrest in children: update from the Pediatric Perioperative Cardiac Arrest Registry. Anesth Analg 2007;105:344–50.
26. White N, Marcus R, Dover S, et al. Predictors of blood loss in front-orbital advancement and remodeling. J Craniofac Surg 2009;20:378–81.
27. Orliaguet GA, Bruyere M, Meyer PG, et al. Comparison of perioperative blood salvage and postoperative reinfusion of drained blood during surgical correction of craniosynostosis in infants. Paediatr Anaesth 2003;13:797–804.
28. Faberowski LW, Black S, Mickle JP. Incidence of venous air embolism during craniectomy for craniosynostosis repair. Anesthesiology 2000;92:20–3.
29. Tobias JD, Johnson JO, Jimenez DF, et al. Venous air embolism during endoscopic strip craniectomy for repair of craniosynostosis in infants. Anesthesiology 2001;95:340–2.
30. Renier D, Sainte-Rose C, Marchac D, et al. Intracranial pressure in craniostenosis. J Neurosurg 1982;57:370–7.
31. Rajagopalan S, Mascha E, Na J, et al. The effects of mild perioperative hypothermia on blood loss and transfusion requirement. Anesthesiology 2008;108:71–7.
32. Brown KA, Bissonnette B, McIntyre B. Hyperkalaemia during rapid blood transfusion and hypovolaemic cardiac arrest in children. Can J Anaesth 1990;37:747–54.

33. Brugnara C, Churchill WH. Effect of irradiation on red cell cation content and transport. Transfusion 1992;32:246–52.
34. WakeUpSafe. 2011. Available at: http://www.wakeupsafe.org/Hyperkalemia_statement.pdf. Accessed June 1, 2013.
35. Hiippala ST, Myllyla GJ, Vahtera EM. Hemostatic factors and replacement of major blood loss with plasma-poor red cell concentrates. Anesth Analg 1995; 81:360–5.
36. Stricker PA, Fiadjoe JE, Davis AR, et al. Reconstituted blood reduces blood donor exposures in children undergoing craniofacial reconstruction surgery. Paediatr Anaesth 2011;21:54–61.
37. Kaufman RM. Uncommon cold: could 4 degrees C storage improve platelet function? Transfusion 2005;45:1407–12.
38. Jobes D, Wolfe Y, O'Neill D, et al. Toward a definition of "fresh" whole blood: an in vitro characterization of coagulation properties in refrigerated whole blood for transfusion. Transfusion 2011;51:43–51.
39. Fries D, Martini WZ. Role of fibrinogen in trauma-induced coagulopathy. Br J Anaesth 2010;105:116–21.
40. Karlsson M, Ternstrom L, Hyllner M, et al. Plasma fibrinogen level, bleeding, and transfusion after on-pump coronary artery bypass grafting surgery: a prospective observational study. Transfusion 2008;48:2152–8.
41. Haas T, Fries D, Velik-Salchner C, et al. Fibrinogen in craniosynostosis surgery. Anesth Analg 2008;106:725–31 [table of contents].
42. Stricker PA, Petersen C, Fiadjoe JE, et al. Successful treatment of intractable hemorrhage with recombinant factor VIIa during cranial vault reconstruction in an infant. Paediatr Anaesth 2009;19:806–7.
43. Pereira de Souza Neto E, Grousson S, Duflo F, et al. Predicting fluid responsiveness in mechanically ventilated children under general anaesthesia using dynamic parameters and transthoracic echocardiography. Br J Anaesth 2011; 106:856–64.
44. Marik PE, Cavallazzi R, Vasu T, et al. Dynamic changes in arterial waveform derived variables and fluid responsiveness in mechanically ventilated patients: a systematic review of the literature. Crit Care Med 2009;37:2642–7.
45. Stricker PA, Lin EE, Fiadjoe JE, et al. Evaluation of central venous pressure monitoring in children undergoing craniofacial reconstruction surgery. Anesth Analg 2013;116:411–9.
46. Stricker PA, Lin EE, Fiadjoe JE, et al. Absence of tachycardia during hypotension in children undergoing craniofacial reconstruction surgery. Anesth Analg 2012;115:139–46.
47. D'Errico CC, Munro HM, Buchman SR, et al. Efficacy of aprotinin in children undergoing craniofacial surgery. J Neurosurg 2003;99:287–90.
48. Dadure C, Sauter M, Bringuier S, et al. Intraoperative tranexamic acid reduces blood transfusion in children undergoing craniosynostosis surgery: a randomized double-blind study. Anesthesiology 2011;114:856–61.
49. Goobie SM, Meier PM, Pereira LM, et al. Efficacy of tranexamic acid in pediatric craniosynostosis surgery: a double-blind, placebo-controlled trial. Anesthesiology 2011;114:862–71.
50. Velardi F, Di Chirico A, Di Rocco C. Blood salvage in craniosynostosis surgery. Childs Nerv Syst 1999;15:695–710.
51. Deva AK, Hopper RA, Landecker A, et al. The use of intraoperative autotransfusion during cranial vault remodeling for craniosynostosis. Plast Reconstr Surg 2002;109:58–63.

52. Dahmani S, Orliaguet GA, Meyer PG, et al. Perioperative blood salvage during surgical correction of craniosynostosis in infants. Br J Anaesth 2000;85:550–5.

53. Fearon JA. Reducing allogenic blood transfusions during pediatric cranial vault surgical procedures: a prospective analysis of blood recycling. Plast Reconstr Surg 2004;113:1126–30.

54. Hans P, Collin V, Bonhomme V, et al. Evaluation of acute normovolemic hemodilution for surgical repair of craniosynostosis. J Neurosurg Anesthesiol 2000;12: 33–6.

55. Meneghini L, Zadra N, Aneloni V, et al. Erythropoeitin therapy and acute preoperative normovolaemic haemodilution in infants undergoing craniosynostosis surgery. Paediatr Anaesth 2003;13:392–6.

56. Fearon JA, Weinthal J. The use of recombinant erythropoietin in the reduction of blood transfusion rates in craniosynostosis repair in infants and children. Plast Reconstr Surg 2002;109:2190–6.

57. Helfaer MA, Carson BS, James CS, et al. Increased hematocrit and decreased transfusion requirements in children given erythropoietin before undergoing craniofacial surgery. J Neurosurg 1998;88:704–8.

58. Meara JG, Smith EM, Harshbarger RJ, et al. Blood-conservation techniques in craniofacial surgery. Ann Plast Surg 2005;54:525–9.

59. Hildebrandt B, Machotta A, Riess H, et al. Intraoperative fresh-frozen plasma versus human albumin in craniofacial surgery- a pilot study comparing coagulation profiles in infants younger than 12 months. Thromb Haemost 2007;98: 172–7.

60. Hill SR, Carless PA, Henry DA, et al. Transfusion thresholds and other strategies for guiding allogeneic red blood cell transfusion. Cochrane Database Syst Rev 2002;(2):CD002042.

61. Lacroix J, Hebert PC, Hutchison JS, et al. Transfusion strategies for patients in pediatric intensive care units. N Engl J Med 2007;356:1609–19.

62. Rouette J, Trottier H, Ducruet T, et al. Red blood cell transfusion threshold in postsurgical pediatric intensive care patients: a randomized clinical trial. Ann Surg 2010;251:421–7.

63. Willems A, Harrington K, Lacroix J, et al. Comparison of two red-cell transfusion strategies after pediatric cardiac surgery: a subgroup analysis. Crit Care Med 2010;38:649–56.

64. Steinbok P, Heran N, Hicdonmez T, et al. Minimizing blood transfusions in the surgical correction of metopic craniosynostosis. Childs Nerv Syst 2004;20: 445–52.

65. Duncan C, Richardson D, May P, et al. Reducing blood loss in synostosis surgery: the Liverpool experience. J Craniofac Surg 2008;19:1424–30.

66. Stricker PA, Fiadjoe JE, Kilbaugh TJ, et al. Effect of transfusion guidelines on postoperative transfusion in children undergoing craniofacial reconstruction surgery. Pediatr Crit Care Med 2012;13:e357–62.

67. Tzortzopoulou A, Cepeda MS, Schumann R, et al. Antifibrinolytic agents for reducing blood loss in scoliosis surgery in children. Cochrane Database Syst Rev 2008;(3):CD006883.

68. Henry DA, Carless PA, Moxey AJ, et al. Anti-fibrinolytic use for minimising perioperative allogeneic blood transfusion. Cochrane Database Syst Rev 2011;(1):CD001886.

69. Chauhan S, Das SN, Bisoi A, et al. Comparison of epsilon aminocaproic acid and tranexamic acid in pediatric cardiac surgery. J Cardiothorac Vasc Anesth 2004;18:141–3.

70. Chauhan S, Gharde P, Bisoi A, et al. A comparison of aminocaproic acid and tranexamic acid in adult cardiac surgery. Ann Card Anaesth 2004;7:40–3.
71. Martin K, Gertler R, Sterner A, et al. Comparison of blood-sparing efficacy of epsilon-aminocaproic acid and tranexamic acid in newborns undergoing cardiac surgery. Thorac Cardiovasc Surg 2011;59:276–80.
72. Krajewski K, Ashley RK, Pung N, et al. Successful blood conservation during craniosynostotic correction with dual therapy using procrit and cell saver. J Craniofac Surg 2008;19:101–5.
73. Jimenez DF, Barone CM. Intraoperative autologous blood transfusion in the surgical correction of craniosynostosis. Neurosurgery 1995;37:1075–9.
74. Feldman JM, Roth JV, Bjoraker DG. Maximum blood savings by acute normovolemic hemodilution. Anesth Analg 1995;80:108–13.
75. Palmer SC, Navaneethan SD, Craig JC, et al. Meta-analysis: erythropoiesis-stimulating agents in patients with chronic kidney disease. Ann Intern Med 2010;153:23–33.
76. Cladis FP, Bykowski M, Schmitt E, et al. Postoperative hyponatremia following calvarial vault remodeling in craniosynostosis. Paediatr Anaesth 2011;21:1020–5.
77. Fearon JA. Treatment of the hands and feet in Apert syndrome: an evolution in management. Plast Reconstr Surg 2003;112:1–12 [discussion: 3–9].
78. Fearon JA, Podner C. Apert syndrome: evaluation of a treatment algorithm. Plast Reconstr Surg 2013;131:132–42.
79. Cohen MM Jr, Kreiborg S. Birth prevalence studies of the Crouzon syndrome: comparison of direct and indirect methods. Clin Genet 1992;41:12–5.
80. Hoefkens MF, Vermeij-Keers C, Vaandrager JM. Crouzon syndrome: phenotypic signs and symptoms of the postnatally expressed subtype. J Craniofac Surg 2004;15:233–40 [discussion: 41–2].
81. Greig AV, Wagner J, Warren SM, et al. Pfeiffer syndrome: analysis of a clinical series and development of a classification system. J Craniofac Surg 2013;24:204–15.
82. Clauser L, Galie M, Hassanipour A, et al. Saethre-Chotzen syndrome: review of the literature and report of a case. J Craniofac Surg 2000;11:480–6.
83. Sabatino G, Di Rocco F, Zampino G, et al. Muenke syndrome. Childs Nerv Syst 2004;20:297–301.
84. Kaufman BA, Muszynski CA, Matthews A, et al. The circle of sagittal synostosis surgery. Semin Pediatr Neurol 2004;11:243–8.

Pediatric Obstructive Sleep Apnea

Deborah A. Schwengel, MD[a,b,*], Nicholas M. Dalesio, MD[a],
Tracey L. Stierer, MD[c,d]

KEYWORDS

- Obstructive sleep apnea • OSAS • Pediatric • Adenotonsillectomy

KEY POINTS

- Obstructive sleep apnea syndrome (OSAS) is a disorder of airway obstruction with multisystem implications and associated complications.
- OSAS affects children from infancy to adulthood and is responsible for behavioral, cognitive, and growth impairment as well as cardiovascular and perioperative respiratory morbidity and mortality.
- OSAS is associated commonly with comorbid conditions, including obesity and asthma.
- Adenotonsillectomy is the most commonly used treatment option for OSAS in childhood, but efforts are underway to identify medical treatment options.

INTRODUCTION

Obstructive sleep apnea (OSA) is a public health problem that affects approximately 1% to 6% of all children,[1,2] up to 59% of obese children,[3–5] 2% to 24% of adults, and 70% of bariatric surgery patients.[6] The incidence increases with age; the disorder is responsible for billions of dollars of direct and indirect health care costs[7] in the form of motor vehicle crashes; medical conditions, including cardiovascular disease, metabolic syndrome, diabetes, and cerebrovascular disease; as well as perioperative morbidity and mortality. The presence of OSA syndrome (OSAS) also has implications for job and school performance and has been associated with potentially life-long cognitive impairment as well as sudden death. Treatment programs for those identified with OSAS may improve functional outcomes, reduce health care costs, and contribute to longevity.[7,8]

[a] Division of Pediatric Anesthesiology, Department of Anesthesiology and Critical Care Medicine, Johns Hopkins University School of Medicine, Baltimore, MD, USA; [b] Department of Pediatrics, Johns Hopkins University School of Medicine, Baltimore, MD, USA; [c] Department of Anesthesiology and Critical Care Medicine, Johns Hopkins University School of Medicine, Baltimore, MD, USA; [d] Department of Otolaryngology-Head and Neck Surgery, Johns Hopkins University School of Medicine, 601 N. Caroline Street, 6th Floor, Baltimore, MD 21287, USA
* Corresponding author. Bloomberg 6222, 1800 Orleans Street, Baltimore, MD 21287-4904.
E-mail address: dschwen1@jhmi.edu

Anesthesiology Clin 32 (2014) 237–261
http://dx.doi.org/10.1016/j.anclin.2013.10.012
1932-2275/14/$ – see front matter © 2014 Elsevier Inc. All rights reserved.

Once thought to be an isolated disorder of pharyngeal muscular mechanical dysfunction leading to partial or complete intermittent airway obstruction, we now know that OSAS is much more complicated and should be thought of as a syndrome with multisystem implications including the central nervous, cardiovascular, metabolic, and immune systems. Although some of its potential causative mechanisms are understood, the inciting cause is often unclear. Newer information about the implications of sleep hygiene and inflammation are especially relevant to the obesity phenotype in OSA but does not delineate which comes first, hence, the chicken versus the egg phenomenon. OSAS, also known as *sleep apnea hypopnea syndrome*, is characterized by symptoms such as snoring, frequent nighttime awakenings, daytime sleepiness, irritability, and depression in adults and behavioral disorders and poor school performance in children. Sobering is the evidence of long-term and possibly permanent cognitive impairment in patients of all ages, but particularly in younger pediatric patients and older adult patients; they may demonstrate deficits in executive function and lower IQ scores.[9] Because the sequelae of OSAS are thought to be a function of recurrent hypoxic injury and chronic sleep deprivation, prompt treatment of the disorder seems imperative. The recommended treatment modalities differ by age, cause, and comorbid conditions.

There are typically 4 main phenotypes that characterize OSAS, shown in **Fig. 1**. Although some patients may have contributions of more than one cause, it has become abundantly clear that the obesity phenotype now exceeds the other phenotypes fourfold.[10]

As anesthesiologists, we are challenged with recognizing the patients at risk of perioperative complications of OSAS. Perioperative morbidity and mortality in patients with OSAS have been well described,[11-14] although evidence of an association with the severity of disease and specific adverse events is lacking. The presence of a known diagnosis of OSAS carries implications for the anesthetic technique and disposition planning; however, the decision dialogue is hampered by inconsistencies in attitude regarding the need for formal testing and postoperative monitoring requirements. The minority of patients presenting for otolaryngologic and general surgical procedures have undergone polysomnography (PSG), the gold standard diagnostic test. Expensive, inconvenient, and not universally available, PSG is infrequently performed

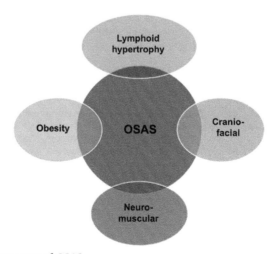

Fig. 1. The 4 phenotypes of OSAS.

in children unless required by the surgeon before intervention for surgical treatment of OSAS. In addition, testing algorithms and interpretation of the resulting data are not consistent among all facilities. Furthermore, pediatric patients may present a challenge to some sleep centers that routinely test adult patients because these facilities may not be set up to accommodate children. Although pediatric OSAS has traditionally been considered to be a disorder predominately affecting preschool to early school-aged children, the age range of patients with the syndrome extends from infancy to young adulthood. Three distinct groups of patients exist based on age: infants younger than 2 years, children aged between 2 and 8 years, and children older than 8 years or those with disease characteristics that more closely resemble those of adult patients with OSAS. There is some crossover in age ranges between the groups; the characteristics of patients in the groups are shown in **Table 1**.

The goals of this article are to review the diagnostic criteria, sleep science, pathophysiology, treatment, and perioperative management of children with OSAS.

DIAGNOSIS

The early identification and diagnosis of infants or children with OSAS is challenging at best. Focused surveillance and clear communication between the patients' caregivers and health care providers are required to distinguish patients who might be at risk for a sleep-related breathing disorder from patients with primary snoring. Recently published guidelines recommend the screening of every child for snoring and sleep

Table 1
Characteristics of 3 different types of pediatric OSAS

	Infants	Children	Teens
Age range (y)	0–2	2–8	8–21
Description	Congenital, craniofacial, or prematurity	Lymphoid hypertrophy dominance	Teen or obese children with features similar to adult OSA
Prevailing causes (comorbid conditions may exacerbate all groups)	Congenital, craniofacial[121] genetic, neuromuscular, prematurity	Enlarged tonsils and/or adenoids, genetic, craniofacial	Obesity, genetic, craniofacial
Presentation	Snoring, failure to thrive, recurrent respiratory infections, developmental delay[122]	Snoring, small, normal or overweight for age, behavioral problems, impaired school performance, enuresis	Snoring, daytime somnolence, impaired school performance, hypertension, males >females, increasing age, African American
Treatment	Observation, adenoidectomy, AT, CPAP, other medical management, tracheotomy, other craniofacial surgeries[114–116,123]	AT	AT, CPAP, weight loss

Abbreviations: AT, adenotonsillectomy; CPAP, continuous positive airway pressure.

apnea–related signs and symptoms.[15] Unfortunately, compliance with these guidelines is poor in both primary care settings and in preoperative otolaryngologic and non-otolaryngologic populations.[16] Suspicion for OSAS may be high in children with predisposing or associated conditions, such as those listed in **Box 1**, or in infants with severe forms of the disease who may present after witnessed episodes of apnea, cyanosis, or failure to thrive. In addition, unlike adults with OSAS who may exhibit daytime somnolence, children with OSAS are more likely to present with behavioral and cognitive disorders, including hyperactivity, attention-deficit disorder, poor school performance, and nocturnal enuresis. Frequently, these children are found to be mouth breathers and assume bizarre positions during sleep, optimizing their airway patency by hyperextending their neck. Additional physical characteristics that may lead the primary care provider to suspect sleep-disordered breathing include maxillofacial abnormalities, such as retrognathia, high-arched palate, narrow intermolar distance, and adenotonsillar hypertrophy.

Overnight PSG performed in a laboratory is the gold standard for the diagnosis of OSAS in pediatric as well as adult patients. However, the test is expensive, time consuming, and labor intensive. Furthermore, it is neither possible nor pragmatic to refer every child in whom there is concern for OSAS for a PSG. Over the last quarter of a century, multiple questionnaires have been developed and studied in order to find an easy-to-use tool to screen for pediatric OSAS. These questionnaires exhibit varying degrees of performance depending on the population to which they are administered, and they tend to be relatively sensitive but not very specific. In a systematic literature review, Brietzke and colleagues[17] identified 12 articles that evaluated the ability of a clinical history and physical examination to accurately identify patients with OSAS. They concluded, based on the existing evidence, that history and clinical evaluation were inadequate to accurately diagnose OSAS when compared with PSG. Some individuals use overnight oximetry as a screening tool for OSAS based on the depth and duration of desaturation. Oximetry is a simple and available resource, but it does not qualify as a diagnostic tool. Compared with PSG, it has limited sensitivity and specificity. It can identify some children with significant nocturnal hypoxemia, but a negative result requires PSG; there is poor positive predictive value with the occurrence of postoperative respiratory complications.[15,18,19]

The various physiologic parameters of the pediatric PSG are similar to those measured in adult patients; however, in accordance with the American Academy of Sleep Medicine (AASM), the scoring criteria are specific for infants and children. A full montage pediatric PSG recording includes the parameters shown in **Table 2**.

According to the 2012 AASM scoring manual, the criteria for events during sleep for infants and children can be used for children who are less than 18 years of age, but individual sleep specialists can choose to score children who are 13 years of age or older using adult criteria. **Table 3** shows pediatric scoring rules for apnea and hypopnea. The severity of OSAS can be categorized by the apnea/hypopnea index (AHI) as shown in **Table 4**.

Test-retest validity exists for PSG as a diagnostic tool for OSAS.[20] However, linking the diagnosis and severity grading of OSAS to perioperative outcomes is an important research question. Previous studies have shown increased postoperative respiratory morbidity in patients having 10 or more obstructive events each hour, and a high baseline AHI is linked to persistent OSAS following adenotonsillectomy (AT).[21–24] Few pediatric patients come to surgery having had a PSG, thus necessitating additional investigation to determine which patients are at the highest risk of perioperative morbidity and mortality.

Box 1
Some congenital and medical conditions associated with OSAS

Maxillofacial associations

  Apert

  Crouzon

  Pfeiffer

  Pierre-Robin

  Treacher Collins

  Goldenhar (hemifacial microsomia)

  Choanal atresia/stenosis

  Hallermann–Streiff syndrome

  Klippel–Feil syndrome

  Osteopetrosis

  Sickle cell disease

  Cleft syndromes

Soft tissue associations

  Obesity

  Cystic hygroma

  Papillomatosis (oropharyngeal)

  Prader–Willi syndrome

  Mucopolysaccharidosis

  Beckwith–Wiedemann syndrome

  Pharyngeal flap surgery

  Down syndrome

  Cleft syndromes

Neuromuscular associations

  Cerebral palsy

  Hypothyroidism

  Achondroplasia

  Patients with cleft palate after repair

  Down syndrome

Inflammatory associations

  Asthma[47]

  Metabolic syndrome

  Sickle cell disease[125]

Data from Refs.[47,65–69,72,121,124,125]

Table 2
Recommended monitoring parameters of PSG

Device	Purpose
Oronasal thermistor	Detection of apnea/hypopnea
Nasal pressure transducer	Detection of airflow/hypopnea
Capnometry (optional)	Detection of hypercarbia
Thoracoabdominal respiratory plethysmography	Detection of chest/abdominal wall activity
Electroencephalography	Determination of sleep stage, arousal, identification of seizure activity
Pulse oximeter	Detection of oxyhemoglobin desaturation
Cutaneous carbon dioxide detector (optional)	Diagnosis of hypercarbia
Electrocardiogram	Detection of dysrhythmia
Electromyography (chin & legs)	Identification of REM sleep and leg movement disorders
Electrooculogram	Identification of stage of sleep
Video	To ascertain activity and body position
Acoustic sensor/microphone (optional)	Documentation of snoring/airflow

Abbreviation: REM, rapid eye movement.

PEDIATRIC AIRWAY PHYSIOLOGY

The upper airway is a vital component of the respiratory system, compromised of highly complex neurologic, muscular, and boney structures that interact to maintain a patent conduit to the lungs. As in adults, the upper airway of children follows the concepts of a Starling resistor model (explained below), although neuromechanical control and airway response mechanisms differ slightly in children. Alterations in consciousness, as seen in stages of sleep and anesthesia, in addition to anatomic, genetic, and neuromuscular factors can predispose patients to airway obstruction or complete occlusion. Other causes for airway collapse during sleep include inflammatory responses, both systemic and local within the upper airway. In the following, the authors describe the upper airway physiology and the causes of OSA as it pertains to children.

The upper airway has been described as a simple collapsible tube or Starling resistor, despite the intricate multisystem involvement for patency regulation.[25,26]

Table 3
The apnea/hypopnea index score is the average of apneic and hypopneic episodes per hour

Terminology	Definition
Apnea	Any 1 of the following can apply: • 90% decrease in airflow that lasts 2 breaths caused by obstruction • >20 s associated with an arousal • >3% oxygen desaturation with no respiratory effort (central apnea)
Hypopnea	All of the following must apply: • Nasal pressure decrease of >30% of baselines • Duration of >30% decrease in signal lasts for >2 breaths • >3% oxygen desaturation from baseline

Table 4
Definition criteria for mild, moderate, and severe OSAS

Severity	AHI Score	Descriptors	Oxygen Saturation Nadir (%)
Mild	1–5	SpO2 <90% for 2%–5 % of sleep time	>92
Moderate	5–9	SpO2 <90% for 5%–10% of total sleep time	—
Severe	≥10	SpO2 <90% for >10% of total sleep time	<80

Children with OSAS often have carbon dioxide retention. The peak values for end-tidal carbon dioxide concentration in the expired air ($ETCO_2$) and the percent of time spent with $ETCO_2$ of more than 50 mm Hg may be good markers to determine the severity of patients' sleep-disordered breathing. Postoperative admission is recommended for patients with a peak $ETCO_2$ of more than 60 mm Hg.[15]

The Starling resistor model can be described as having rigid proximal and distal ends with a collapsible region in between. This collapsible region is exposed to surrounding tissue pressures, leading to collapse at high pressures. The term used for the point at which the pharynx collapses is called the *critical pressure* (P_{CRIT}). For the collapsible segment to remain open, both the upstream and the downstream pressures must be higher than the P_{CRIT}. To create *complete occlusion*, the pressure upstream and downstream to the collapsible segment must be lower than the P_{CRIT}, as seen with inspiratory airflow limitation (ie, caused by adenotonsillar hypertrophy). *Flow-limited (hypopneic) breathing*, however, maintains some airflow through the collapsible segment. During inspiratory flow limitation, airflow reaches a maximal level during inspiration as long as upstream pressures remain higher than the P_{CRIT}. This pattern occurs during severe snoring whereby airflow oscillates during the closing and reopening of the upper airway.

PATHOPHYSIOLOGY OF PEDIATRIC SLEEP APNEA

The pathophysiology of pediatric OSAS is usually different than that of adults. OSAS in the adult population is frequently associated with obesity and an increased mechanical load to the airway. Children have airways that are resistant to collapse, with those suffering from OSAS manifesting predominantly with hypopneic breathing as opposed to frank apnea. They have few apneic events during flow-limited breathing and have increased arousal threshold compared with children without OSAS. Unlike in adults, apneic events (when they do occur) are sleep-stage specific, occurring predominantly during rapid-eye-movement (REM) sleep. In addition to hypoxemia, hypercarbia is a dominant characteristic in children with OSA caused by prolonged hypoventilation and is uncommonly seen in adult patients with OSA.

Anatomic Obstruction

Adenotonsillar hypertrophy is a predominant characteristic of airway obstruction in pediatric OSAS. As normal children age, adenotonsillar tissue enlarges at a faster rate than other airway structures. Adenotonsillar tissues are largest in relation to the underlying airway between 3 and 6 years of age, which is the age range at which the OSAS incidence peaks in children.[27,28] During anesthesia, it has been shown that the location of airway obstruction in children with OSAS occurs at the level of the tonsils and adenoids compared with airways of normal children that collapse at the level of the soft palate.[29] Adenotonsillar size, however, does not directly correlate to the severity of OSAS. Other anatomic abnormalities, such as those associated with craniofacial disorders, physically obstruct the upper airway. As many as 50% of patients with craniofacial abnormalities also suffer from OSAS. Many of these morphometric variations decrease the physical space within the posterior oropharynx, the site that is most associated with obstructive breathing.[30,31] However, not all children with anatomic airway obstruction develop OSAS, indicating that other factors must be necessary to acquire sleep-disordered breathing.

Neuromechanical Dysfunction

Neuromechanical control of the upper airway plays a vital role in maintaining airway patency. Mechanoreceptors and chemoreceptors, in addition to central neurologic centers, control the ventilatory drive and airway patency muscles (genioglossus, intrinsic palatal, posterior cricoarytenoid, and pharyngeal constrictor muscles). Output from these neuromuscular centers is influenced by changes in airway pressure, airflow, carbon dioxide, and oxygen tensions. Normal children have been found to have less collapsible airways during sleep, despite anatomically smaller airway structures. Upper airway muscular tone is partially preserved, maintaining patency despite increases in subatmospheric pressure.[31] Airway pressure responses can be measured by determining patients' P_{CRIT}, which is performed by intermittent negative pressure drops induced via a nasal mask or face mask. Children with OSAS have been found to have higher P_{CRIT} values when compared with children without OSAS. After AT, however, P_{CRIT} values of patients with OSAS do not return to that of controls. These results suggest dysfunction in the neuromuscular response to changes in airway pressures in patients with OSAS despite the removal of an anatomic airway obstruction.[32] Responses to carbon dioxide and oxygen are predominantly unchanged in children with OSAS. In normal children, muscular tone of the airway can *increase* when exposed to hypercarbic and hypoxic environments. The administration of carbon dioxide increases airflow by decreasing upper airway resistance; the response remains intact in children with OSAS compared with controls, suggesting that some neuromechanical pathways continue to be active and resist airway collapse.[33,34] But patients with OSAS have a decreased arousal threshold when exposed to hypercarbia; only approximately one-third of patients have a cortical arousal after an obstructive apnea during REM sleep.[33,35] By not awakening during obstructive breathing, patients continue prolonged hypopneic breathing and increase their exposure to hypoxia and hypercarbia. Nevertheless, carbon dioxide levels have been shown to be different in children with OSA during wakefulness and under anesthesia. In awake and anesthetized patients, a direct correlation to OSAS severity and resting carbon dioxide concentration has been shown.[36,37] It is postulated that insufficient gas exchange explains the signs and symptoms of inattentiveness, enuresis, and opioid sensitivity that are common in children with OSAS.

Anatomic and Neuromuscular Dysfunction

Disease processes, such as Down syndrome and obesity, contribute to upper airway obstruction via a multitude of physiologic changes. Patients with Down syndrome are at risk of airway obstruction because of their many predisposing physical characteristics, including midface hypoplasia, glossoptosis, small upper airways, mandibular hypoplasia, and obesity. In addition, these patients suffer from generalized hypotonia that leads to neuromuscular dysfunction, predisposing patients to airway collapse. Obesity increases P_{CRIT}, primarily through an increased anatomic load on the pharyngeal airway structures. Neurohumoral defects are also noted in obese patients with OSAS. Leptin, a satiety factor produced by adipose tissue, alters ventilatory responses and regulates body fat composition. Resistance to leptin has been shown in patients with OSAS.[38]

Genetic Causes

Genetics and inflammation also play important roles in the pathophysiology of pediatric OSAS. Children of African American decent are thought to be at a greater risk for OSAS than the Caucasian or Hispanic pediatric population.[39] Although family cohort studies demonstrate the role of genetics in OSAS, it is unclear whether ventilatory drive, anatomic features, or both are the sources of dysfunction. Research identifying genetic causes of children with OSAS is currently in its infancy; however, studies have identified genetic polymorphisms associated with the disorder.[40] The Apolipoprotein E (ApoE)-e4 allele of the ApoE gene alters membrane stability and has been associated with children with OSAS who manifest with decreased neurocognitive performance.[41] Children with excessive daytime sleepiness are more likely to have single nucleotide polymorphisms in the tumor necrosis factor (TNF)-alpha–308G gene, where TNF-alpha is an important proinflammatory cytokine and enhancer of slow-wave sleep. Genetic variations in the reduced form of nicotinamide adenine dinucleotide phosphate oxidase complex, an enzyme active in oxidative stress linked to stroke, hypertension, and heart disease, have been linked to children with OSAS who have cognitive dysfunction.[42] Although genetic polymorphisms have been linked to OSAS, the complex interplay between genic variations leading to phenotypic characteristics has yet to be described.

Inflammation

Inflammation, both local and systemic, has been associated with OSAS. Adenotonsillar hypertrophy is a common predisposing factor for OSAS; however, the cause of the lymphoid tissue enlargement is unknown. Some hypothesize that environmental or genetic factors initiate an inflammatory response leading to tonsillar hypertrophy, whereas others think enlarged adenotonsillar tissue triggers an inflammatory response. Regardless, there is ample evidence to show that inflammatory markers are associated with pediatric OSAS.[43–46] Glucocorticoid receptor and leukotriene expression have been reported in the adenotonsillar tissue of children with OSAS, likely playing a role in hypertrophy of the lymphoid tissue. Chronic upper airway inflammatory disorders, including sinusitis, allergic rhinitis, and asthma, coexist in patients with OSAS, with increased production of proinflammatory cytokines, such as interleukin (IL)-6, IL-1alpha, and TNF-alpha.[40] Asthma is commonly associated with OSAS and is thought to perpetuate a positive feedback loop of inflammation, nasal obstruction, and airway collapse (**Fig. 2**).[47] From this inflammatory response, urinary biomarker concentrations, including cysteinyl leukotrienes and lipocalin-type prostaglandin D synthase, have been found to correlate to the severity of sleep-disordered breathing in children. This finding suggests a possible role for the assessment of the severity of OSAS through the measurement of urinary inflammatory markers.[45,48,49]

Sleep and Anesthesia

Sleep and anesthesia share similar neurophysiologic pathways; however, there are distinct characteristics that separate the two states. Sleep is a natural state of unconsciousness that is governed by homeostatic drive and circadian patterns, consisting of various stages of brain activity. Anesthesia is a drug-induced state of fairly constant brain activity, with arousal only after the drug has been eliminated.

Anesthesia and sleep both decrease ventilatory drive and neuromuscular activity of airway patency musculature. Patients do not obstruct during periods of wakefulness,

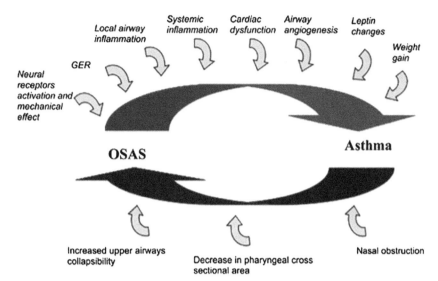

Fig. 2. Interrelationship between asthma and sleep apnea. GER, gastroesophageal reflux. (*From* Alkhalil M, Schulman E, Getsy J. Obstructive sleep apnea syndrome and asthma: what are the links? J Clin Sleep Med 2009;5(1):72; with permission.)

suggesting decreases in consciousness increase the propensity for airway collapse. Children with OSAS have increased Electromyogram, genioglossus muscle (EMG_{GG}) activity during wakefulness as well as a greater decrease in EMG_{GG} activity at the onset of sleep compared with normal children. This fact suggests that airway patency is more dependent on neuromuscular control of pharyngeal dilator muscles in OSAS children, reinforced by studies showing a greater decrease in airway diameter compared with controls after local anesthetic is applied to the airway.[50,51] With increasing concentrations of anesthetic agents, such as propofol, benzodiazepines, and inhalational anesthetics, the pediatric airway decreases in cross-sectional area.[52–56] Children with OSAS are more sensitive than normal children to these agents, having airway collapse at higher airway pressures.[57] Analgesic medications produce a decrease in ventilatory and pharyngeal neuromotor drive to the upper airway. In addition to these effects, opioid sensitivity has been observed in children with severe OSAS thought to be secondary to the upregulation of opioid receptors in the brainstem from recurrent hypoxic episodes.[58–60] In contrast, dexmedetomidine, a centrally acting alpha-2 agonist, has sedative properties that work directly at the locus coeruleus, or sleep center. The sedation produced by dexmedetomidine is similar to natural non-REM sleep, does not produce significant respiratory depression, and is associated with fewer oxygen desaturation episodes when compared with propofol or midazolam, which exert their effects primarily by GABAergic mechanisms. These beneficial effects related to the preservation of the respiratory drive are more pronounced in children with severe OSAS.[61,62]

TREATMENT

AT remains the mainstay of treatment of OSAS in children. In a national trial of 464 children with OSAS, patients were randomized to tonsillectomy versus watchful waiting. The primary outcome of the study was to detect differences in cognition. There were no differences in executive function or attention between the groups; however, there were reduced symptoms of OSAS and improved AHI, behavior, and quality of life, thus providing evidence of the beneficial effects of AT.[63] Infants, obese children, syndromic children, and those with severe OSAS should be considered at risk for treatment failure or incomplete response to tonsillectomy. Nevertheless, AT may provide some relief by decreasing severity and can be offered in conjunction with other therapies, such as various forms of positive airway pressure (PAP) and control of comorbidities, such as asthma. Children with mild OSAS or children with mild residual OSAS following AT may be considered candidates for a 6-week trial of inhaled steroids.[64] Some children with OSAS have maxillofacial abnormalities that may be treatable with orthodontic therapies. Orofacial narrowing, malocclusion, and mandibular retrognathia are abnormalities associated with OSAS.[65,66]

All patients with craniofacial syndromes should be suspected of having OSAS. Children with cleft syndromes have a high prevalence of OSAS and should be assessed with PSG.[67–69] Children with abnormalities of anatomy or muscle tone may require therapies, including craniofacial or pharyngeal surgeries or potentially tracheostomy. Tissue-reduction surgeries have been used in patients with obstructive tissues other than the tonsils and adenoids to create more room in the oropharyngeal or nasopharyngeal spaces. Craniofacial surgeries may include mandibular or maxillary advancement procedures. Although they are more invasive procedures with longer recovery times, these surgical interventions may be considered to improve OSAS in patients with disorders shown in **Box 1**, especially if AT has already been tried and some degree of OSAS persists.[70–72]

Teens and older children with OSAS may share phenotypic features of adult OSAS and, therefore, may benefit from treatments similar to those offered to adult patients. In 2009, a task force designated by the AASM developed evidence-based clinical guidelines for the long-term management of adults with OSAS.[73] The treatment of patients with a diagnosis of OSAS requires a multidisciplinary approach and robust patient/care-giver education with regard to physiology and treatment options. Once the severity of disease has been established, there are behavioral, surgical, dental, and medical treatment options. However, continuous PAP (CPAP) is the treatment of choice for patients with moderate to severe disease. Although CPAP therapy has been shown to be highly effective in the treatment of OSAS, adult compliance with the use of the device has been reported to be very poor.[74]

Secondary behavioral treatments include weight-loss counseling, position therapy or side sleeping, avoidance of factors that worsen the disease, use of oral dental devices, and practice of proper sleep hygiene. Surgical options include single and multilevel procedures, such as tracheostomy, maxillomandibular advancement, uvulopalatopharyngoplasty, radiofrequency ablation, palatal implants, or a combination of these options, all of which are outside of the scope of this article. However, in pediatric populations, as well as adults, success rates and potential complications should be discussed during contemplation of the surgical treatment of OSAS. Obese patients may be treated with AT but have a higher chance of residual disease. In a meta-analysis, Costa and Mitchell[75] reported that 88% of obese patients were not cured by AT, although their OSAS was significantly improved.

PERIOPERATIVE MANAGEMENT
Preoperative Management, Assessment, and Disposition Planning

Preoperative assessment of patients should be done with disposition planning in mind. Doing so permits the full discussion of plans and risks with patients, their parents, surgeons, and nurses. Pediatric patients with OSAS commonly present for AT, adenoidectomy, or tonsillectomy but certainly may undergo other types of surgeries. The suggestion of sleep-disordered breathing is obvious in AT patients but may go unrecognized in patients having nonotolaryngologic surgeries. Unfortunately, a minority of patients receive PSG testing preoperatively, even in the AT population.[76] As a result, the anesthesiologist must screen patients for OSAS and consider whether it is safe to discharge them to an unmonitored setting after surgery, particularly if opioids will be used for pain management. Consequently, it is incumbent on the anesthesia provider to preoperatively screen all surgical patients for signs and symptoms of obstructive sleep apnea. The problem is that even extensively developed OSAS screening questionnaires have variable specificity, sensitivity, and/or negative predictive value depending on the population being studied; most surveys are too long to be useful on the morning of surgery.[77–79] Although the literature is clear that this type of evidence of OSAS is imprecise and such tools have not been studied for the purpose of determining perioperative risk, their use raises awareness. Snoring is a nonspecific sign but is often used as a starting question. The questions listed in **Fig. 3** scored with a Likert scale have been recently shown to have some validity as components of a short questionnaire for primary care providers; a score of 2.72 or more indicated a high risk for the presence of OSAS.[80] No matter the tool used, it is imperative that surgeons and anesthesiologists communicate effectively about the safety of discharge and discuss whether postoperative monitoring is needed. Postoperative respiratory complications have been reported extensively in pediatric AT patients and may occur in as many as 36% of these patients, particularly those with severe OSAS, younger age (aged <3 years), and medical comorbidities.[81–86] Although critical complications are not common, adverse events may be severe, including death and permanent neurologic injury.[11–14,87]

The preoperative physical examination should include all of the elements of a standard preoperative assessment but should also include any notable facial features of the child and their overall body habitus. Guilleminault and colleagues[66] have reported on the contributions of facial development and interaction of long, narrow facial features, high-arched palate, and retromandibular positioning as risk features of OSAS, especially in conjunction with enlarged tonsils. Mouth breathing, poor handling of oral secretions, reduced muscle tone, and a large tongue, such as in patients with Down syndrome, are other physical features suggestive of risk. The Mallampati score has not consistently been shown to be predictive of OSAS in adult patients[88] and has not been well studied in pediatric patients.

Preoperative laboratory tests or imaging should be considered in the context of the surgical procedure, the known severity of OSAS, and comorbidities. Patients with severe OSAS are at risk of cardiovascular complications of their disease, and obese patients have an increased risk of metabolic syndrome. Multiple studies have shown that children without clinical evidence of cardiovascular effects of OSAS may have echocardiographic evidence of wall motion abnormalities, diastolic dysfunction, ventricular hypertrophy, or elevated pulmonary artery pressures; in most children, these findings reverse with effective treatment.[89] Severe and long-standing OSAS can lead to cor pulmonale or cardiac failure. Therefore, an echocardiogram is recommended if a child with severe OSAS is suspected to have cardiac involvement as indicated by systemic hypertension; right ventricular dysfunction; or frequent, severe desaturations (<70%).[72] Chest radiographs, electrocardiograms, and blood gases are not recommended.

The metabolic syndrome can occur in normal patients but is most common in patients with obesity and/or OSAS, and the likelihood of its presence increases as

Does your child snore when asleep?

Never	Rarely	Once per week	Twice per week	3-4 times per week	Almost always
0	1	2	3	4	5

How loudly does your child snore?

Quietly	Medium	Loudly	Very Loudly	Extremely Loudly
0	1	2	3	4

Does your child struggle to breathe when asleep?

Never	Rarely	Once per week	Twice per week	3-4 times per week	Almost always
0	1	2	3	4	5

Have you witnessed an apnea during sleep?

Never	Rarely	Once per week	Twice per week	3-4 times per week	Almost always
0	1	2	3	4	5

Do you shake your child to breathe?

Never	Rarely	Once per week	Twice per week	3-4 times per week	Almost always
0	1	2	3	4	5

Do you have concerns about your child's breathing when asleep?

Never	Rarely	Once per week	Twice per week	3-4 times per week	Almost Always
0	1	2	3	4	5

Fig. 3. A short screening tool using severity discrimination scores. (*Data from* Spruyt K, Gozal D. Screening of pediatric sleep-disordered breathing: a proposed unbiased discriminative set of questions using clinical severity scales. Chest 2012;142(6):1508–15; and Kadmon G, Shapiro CM, Chung SA, et al. Validation of a pediatric obstructive sleep apnea screening tool. Int J Pediatr Otorhinolaryngol 2013;77(9):1461–4.)

the severity of OSAS increases; up to 10% of children and 20% of adults have been estimated to be affected.[90] Women with polycystic ovary syndrome are at particular risk.[91] There is also evidence that daytime somnolence is a sign that especially indicates the inflammatory pathophysiology involved in the metabolic syndrome, obesity, and OSAS.[91] Metabolic syndrome is characterized by metabolically active visceral fat (typically in patients with central obesity), fatty liver, insulin resistance, hypertension, and dyslipidemia. These derangements, especially in association with each other, are thought to be associated with increased morbidity in the form of cardiovascular and neurovascular pathological conditions and/or mortality.[91,92] Specific perioperative risk data are scarce, and the current recommendations only support the management of the individual metabolic and cardiovascular derangements, such as glucose control and blood pressure control. There are some data to suggest that statin therapies may reduce the perioperative risk.[93] It is, therefore, prudent to consider obtaining lipid and hepatic panels in addition to serum glucose in patients at risk for metabolic syndrome.

Consideration should also be given to providing a referral to a pulmonologist for patients with severe OSAS. Children with signs of cardiovascular complications or likely persistence of OSAS following surgery (**Box 2**) should be referred for consideration of perioperative PAP therapies (CPAP or bilevel PAP [BiPAP]). Although data suggests that perioperative CPAP therapy may reduce postoperative adverse outcomes, investigations examining the utility of preoperative CPAP therapy in newly diagnosed patients with OSAS have been inconclusive.[94] **Table 5** summarizes the preoperative testing options.

ANESTHETIC TECHNIQUES

There is little evidence to support the benefit of any single anesthetic technique for patients with OSAS. Most anesthetic agents reduce pharyngeal tone, diminish the ventilatory response to carbon dioxide,[95] and impair or abolish patients' ability to rescue

---

Box 2
Risk of persistent OSAS following tonsillectomy

Genetic or congenitally related

  Family history of OSAS

  Genetic or chromosomal disorders

  Neuromuscular disorders

  Nasal or maxillofacial disorders

  Age <2 years

Comorbidity related

  Obesity

  Asthma

  History of prematurity

  Infiltrative soft tissue disorders of the airway

  Upper respiratory infection within 4 weeks of surgery

Severity related

  Severe OSA

  Systemic hypertension

  Cor pulmonale

  Growth impairment caused by chronic obstructed breathing

Data from Refs.[15,72,105,126,127]

Table 5
Preoperative testing for patients with known or suspected OSAS

Test	Indication
PSG	To diagnose OSAS and determine severity
Echocardiography	To establish evidence of cardiovascular risk, any of the following are present: • Systemic hypertension • Evidence of right ventricular dysfunction • Frequent, severe oxygen desaturation (<70%)
Blood chemistries: liver function tests, lipid panel, glucose	If suspected metabolic syndrome
Other	As dictated by the surgical procedure or presence of comorbidities

themselves from obstructive apnea during sleep. One exception is dexmedetomidine, which does not produce significant respiratory depression and may be particularly useful in children with severe OSAS.[61,62] Historically used as a staple for postoperative analgesia, opioids have been shown to produce more profound respiratory depression in children, with smaller doses in patients with severe OSAS.[37,60,96] Regional anesthesia or other opioid-sparing management plans may be helpful; but pure regional techniques are often not possible in pediatric patients or appropriate for some surgical procedures, including AT. If opioids are necessary for pain management, they should be administered judiciously and patients monitored appropriately for complications. Sedatives should likewise be used with caution and with an appropriate monitoring plan.

Nonsteroidal antiinflammatory agents (NSAIDS), acetaminophen, and adjuvant pain medications have been used to treat postoperative pain in patients for AT surgery and other surgeries. However, there continues to be a debate about whether NSAIDS can be safely used in AT surgery because of the risk of post-tonsillar hemorrhage (PTH). It is clear that aspirin and aspirin-containing products should not be used in the perioperative care of tonsillectomy patients,[97] and it is prudent to avoid ketorolac until hemostasis is achieved. Ibuprofen products have been used extensively for postoperative care, and a recent meta-analysis suggests no increased risk of PTH and no significant differences between individual nonaspirin NSAIDS.[98]

Dexamethasone, well known to reduce nausea and vomiting, may have a role in the effective treatment of postoperative pain. Raghavendran and colleagues[99] have reported the management of pain in tonsillectomy patients with severe OSAS using a dose of 0.3 mg/kg of dexamethasone (maximum of 10 mg). In 2008, dexamethasone was implicated as a cause of increased PTH in doses of 0.5 mg/kg or greater.[100] More recently, observations of dexamethasone use have not been linked to bleeding[101]; a meta-analysis of dexamethasone use in AT did not show an overall association with PTH, but it could not exclude the possibility of a bleeding association with specific doses. Studies comparing doses of 0.4 to 0.6 mg/kg with placebo did demonstrate increased odds of bleeding.[102] Consequently, it may be prudent to avoid high doses of dexamethasone; high doses are not needed to reduce vomiting.[103] A dose-finding study of the effects of dexamethasone related to analgesic effect is needed.

Airway management has the potential for difficulty in cases of craniofacial narrowing or anomalies, especially with the addition of soft tissue enlargement. Studies both support and refute the prediction of difficult airway management in patients with OSAS. Preparations should be made for difficulties with mask ventilation or endotracheal intubation. Helpful mask ventilation strategies include elevation of the head of the bed, lateral positioning, jaw thrust maneuver, CPAP, and oral or nasal airway placement.[104] When an inhalational induction is performed, care must be used to avoid placing an airway while patients still react to stimulation or laryngospasm may occur. Persistent respiratory efforts against an obstructed airway from laryngospasm or pharyngeal airway obstruction can result in negative pressure pulmonary edema.[72,105] In patients with a high risk of airway obstruction during induction, intravenous induction may be considered to facilitate rapid instrumentation of the airway. This induction may be done for patients with documented or suspected severe OSAS. Most patients presenting for AT with enlarged tonsils but no craniofacial defects have airways that can usually easily be managed with an oral airway, and endotracheal intubation is generally straightforward.

The laryngeal mask airway (LMA) is preferred by some anesthesiologists during AT surgeries but must be accepted by the operating surgeon. Lalwani and colleagues[106] reported that the use of LMA in AT is associated with a higher incidence of airway obstruction on insertion or when the gag is placed by the surgeon. The overall complication rate in the LMA group was 14.2% versus 7.7% in the endotracheal tube group, but the total case time was less in the LMA group. LMA failure was 6.8% and was associated with younger patients, controlled ventilation, and the surgeon. The LMA may also be used as an adjunct to the management of a difficult airway.

On completion of the anesthetic in patients with OSAS, it is the opinion of these authors that patients should be allowed to emerge from general anesthesia before extubation of the airway because of the lingering effect of anesthetics on the airway muscle tone. In addition, regular respiratory effort and adequate strength should be demonstrated. However, the authors do acknowledge that some anesthesiologists choose to extubate the trachea when patients are still deeply anesthetized and breathing spontaneously.

POSTOPERATIVE MANAGEMENT

Opioids remain a major treatment option for perioperative pain management; but patients with documented or suspected severe OSAS are at an increased risk of postoperative respiratory complications, and their opioid doses should be reduced.[99] These patients have central alteration of their opioid receptors associated with severe intermitted nocturnal hypoxemia; this change leads to vulnerability of these patients when opioids are administered in the perioperative period.[60,96] The options are, therefore, to monitor postoperatively, discharge without opioid therapy, or discharge with opioid therapy and the knowledge of mild or moderate OSAS severity. Codeine, hydrocodone, and oxycodone liquid formulations are available for pediatric patients. Some drugs are typically dispensed as combination drugs with acetaminophen, although single-drug formulations are available. Combination drugs do not allow the flexibility of dosing that is necessary to avoid toxicity of either of the drug components and, therefore, should generally not be used. Codeine should be avoided because of the genetic heterogeneity associated with its metabolism. Codeine is a prodrug metabolized by the cytochrome P450 CYP2D system to morphine, the active drug. Both slow and ultrarapid metabolizers exist in the population; slow metabolizers have little to no pain relief, and ultrarapid metabolizers may experience unpredictable toxic morphine levels. This toxicity has been implicated as the cause of death in several children treated postoperatively with codeine.[107] In 2013, the Federal Drug Administration issued a warning with regard to the hazard of the use of codeine in children. Oxycodone, hydrocodone, and tramadol are also metabolized by the CYP2D system;

caution is also required with their use, particularly in AT patients with severe OSAS. Around-the-clock dosing with opioids in the perioperative outpatient setting is extremely dangerous. Many deaths related to opioids are reported in children; 18% of deaths and 5% of hypoxic brain injuries have been related to opioids.[107] The Cincinnati Children's Hospital has adopted a nonopioid analgesic regimen in their tonsillectomy patients. The protocol is for use in patients younger than 6 years and includes around-the-clock acetaminophen (maximum 75 mg/kg/d), dexamethasone once a day for 3 days, and ibuprofen as needed beginning on day 2 and limited to 2 doses per day.[107]

The American Society of Anesthesiology's guidelines recommends that patients at risk for OSAS remain in the postanesthesia care unit (PACU) 3 hours longer than their non-OSA counterparts; if patients exhibit any signs of obstruction, their stay should be extended for an additional 7 hours.[108] This recommendation is a consensus of opinion statement, not based on evidence; but it has been demonstrated that patients may experience morbidity many hours after PACU discharge even when the PACU stay has been uncomplicated.[85,109,110]

Protocols between institutions vary widely with regard to the admission of patients following AT, and no consensus exists about which patients should be admitted to an intensive care unit (ICU).[111,112] Nevertheless, there is evidence that patients with documented or suspected severe OSAS should be kept overnight. Children younger than 3 years[78,113] and those with comorbidities should be admitted, and children requiring opioids for pain management should be considered for admission.[11] More specific perioperative guidelines are lacking, and it must be stated that being older than 3 years is not evidence of safety for discharge. Fatal respiratory events following tonsillectomy occur with twice the occurrence rate in children than adults, and the younger children have greater risk.[87,99] Infants with OSAS are a special group of patients who are more likely to have craniofacial disorders, neuromuscular disorders, or prematurity. In addition, they are less likely to be effectively treated by AT and are more likely to warrant ICU admissions for oxygen and/or CPAP administration.[114–116] A proposed algorithm of disposition planning is shown in **Fig. 4.**

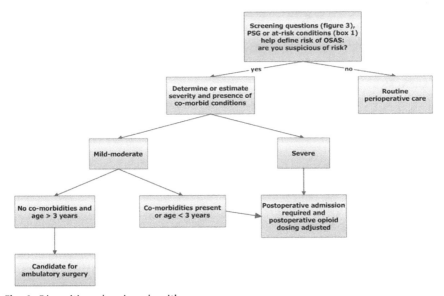

Fig. 4. Disposition planning algorithm.

The duration of stay in the hospital if admitted depends on the surgical procedure but also on the risk of postoperative respiratory complications. The effects of anesthetics and pain medications continue into the postoperative period and may be complicated by the physiologic effects of surgical stress and pain. Postoperative sleep disruption and REM rebound may make patients with OSAS vulnerable to respiratory complications for several days.[117,118]

SUMMARY

OSAS is a multisystem disorder with a complex of inciting factors that lead to a pathophysiology that is still not completely understood. It is clear that OSAS is not purely a mechanical disorder that can always be cured by removing the tonsils. In children, normal growth and lymphoidal hypertrophy mismatch is often implicated as causative; but maxillofacial, neuromuscular, and genetic factors are involved too. Obese children may have large tonsils and adenoids but clearly have contributing fat pads and inflammatory factors. Tonsillectomy is still the most common treatment in children with OSAS; but more often, we are recognizing residual disease after AT. As the understanding of OSAS improves, medical treatments may become more prominent, especially in children with a risk of residual disease after AT. Pharmacologic therapies are being explored and may add significantly to the resolution of inflammation and metabolic syndrome.[119,120] Treatment should be pursued for children with OSAS; permanent cognitive impairment and cardiovascular and neurovascular disease are possible consequences of no treatment.

Perioperative management of children with OSAS remains controversial and challenging because many patients come to surgery without an assessment of disease severity, leaving the anesthesiologist to wonder if it is safe to discharge patients to an unmonitored environment. This situation is especially challenging if opioids are needed for pain management. Mortality and respiratory morbidity in the perioperative period is a concerning risk. All anesthesiologists should screen patients for OSAS. Although questionnaires and screening tools are not perfect, they may be all that is available on the day of surgery. The authors recommend the routine use of a preoperative screening tool on all patients presenting for surgery or procedural sedation. Patients with known or suspected significant OSAS, comorbidities, young age, or obesity should be considered for postoperative monitoring with continuous pulse oximetry or possibly in an ICU setting for at least one night and perhaps longer.

REFERENCES

1. Bixler EO, Vgontzas AN, Lin HM, et al. Sleep disordered breathing in children in a general population sample: prevalence and risk factors. Sleep 2009;32(6): 731–6.
2. Li AM, So HK, Au CT, et al. Epidemiology of obstructive sleep apnoea syndrome in Chinese children: a two-phase community study. Thorax 2010;65(11):991–7.
3. Arens R, Sin S, Nandalike K, et al. Upper airway structure and body fat composition in obese children with obstructive sleep apnea syndrome. Am J Respir Crit Care Med 2011;183(6):782–7.
4. Supriyatno B, Said M, Hermani B, et al. Risk factors of obstructive sleep apnea syndrome in obese early adolescents: a prediction model using scoring system. Acta Med Indones 2010;42(3):152–7.
5. Verhulst SL, Van Gaal L, De Backer W, et al. The prevalence, anatomical correlates and treatment of sleep-disordered breathing in obese children and adolescents. Sleep Med Rev 2008;12(5):339–46.

6. Vasu TS, Grewal R, Doghramji K. Obstructive sleep apnea syndrome and peri-operative complications: a systematic review of the literature. J Clin Sleep Med 2012;8(2):199–207.

7. Leger D, Bayon V, Laaban JP, et al. Impact of sleep apnea on economics. Sleep Med Rev 2012;16(5):455–62.

8. Hoffman B, Wingenbach DD, Kagey AN, et al. The long-term health plan and disability cost benefit of obstructive sleep apnea treatment in a commercial motor vehicle driver population. J Occup Environ Med 2010;52(5):473–7.

9. Grigg-Damberger M, Ralls F. Cognitive dysfunction and obstructive sleep apnea: from cradle to tomb. Curr Opin Pulm Med 2012;18(6):580–7.

10. Arens R, Muzumdar H. Childhood obesity and obstructive sleep apnea syndrome. J Appl Physiol 2010;108(2):436–44.

11. Brown KA. Outcome, risk, and error and the child with obstructive sleep apnea. Paediatr Anaesth 2011;21(7):771–80.

12. Cote CJ, Posner KL, Domino KB. Death or neurologic injury after tonsillectomy in children with a focus on obstructive sleep apnea: Houston, we have a problem! Anesth Analg 2013. [Epub ahead of print].

13. Goldman JL, Baugh RF, Davies L, et al. Mortality and major morbidity after ton-sillectomy: etiologic factors and strategies for prevention. Laryngoscope 2013; 123(10):2544–53.

14. Jennum P, Ibsen R, Kjellberg J. Morbidity and mortality in children with obstruc-tive sleep apnoea: a controlled national study. Thorax 2013;68(10):949–54.

15. Marcus CL, Brooks LJ, Draper KA, et al. Diagnosis and management of child-hood obstructive sleep apnea syndrome. Pediatrics 2012;130(3):e714–55.

16. Erichsen D, Godoy C, Granse F, et al. Screening for sleep disorders in pediatric primary care: are we there yet? Clin Pediatr (Phila) 2012;51(12):1125–9.

17. Brietzke SE, Katz ES, Roberson DW. Can history and physical examination reli-ably diagnose pediatric obstructive sleep apnea/hypopnea syndrome? A sys-tematic review of the literature. Otolaryngol Head Neck Surg 2004;131(6): 827–32.

18. Brouillette RT, Morielli A, Leimanis A, et al. Nocturnal pulse oximetry as an abbreviated testing modality for pediatric obstructive sleep apnea. Pediatrics 2000;105(2):405–12.

19. Nixon GM, Kermack AS, Davis GM, et al. Planning adenotonsillectomy in chil-dren with obstructive sleep apnea: the role of overnight oximetry. Pediatrics 2004;113(1 Pt 1):e19–25.

20. Aurora RN, Zak RS, Karippot A, et al. Practice parameters for the respiratory in-dications for polysomnography in children. Sleep 2011;34(3):379–88.

21. Tauman R, Gulliver TE, Krishna J, et al. Persistence of obstructive sleep apnea syndrome in children after adenotonsillectomy. J Pediatr 2006;149(6):803–8.

22. Ye J, Liu H, Zhang GH, et al. Outcome of adenotonsillectomy for obstructive sleep apnea syndrome in children. Ann Otol Rhinol Laryngol 2010;119(8):506–13.

23. Mitchell RB. Adenotonsillectomy for obstructive sleep apnea in children: outcome evaluated by pre- and postoperative polysomnography. Laryngoscope 2007;117(10):1844–54.

24. Mitchell RB, Kelly J. Outcome of adenotonsillectomy for obstructive sleep apnea in obese and normal-weight children. Otolaryngol Head Neck Surg 2007;137(1): 43–8.

25. Schwartz AR, Smith PL, Wise RA, et al. Induction of upper airway occlusion in sleeping individuals with subatmospheric nasal pressure. J Appl Physiol 1988;64(2):535–42.

26. Schwartz AR, Smith PL, Wise RA, et al. Effect of positive nasal pressure on upper airway pressure-flow relationships. J Appl Physiol 1989;66(4):1626–34.

27. Jeans WD, Fernando DC, Maw AR, et al. A longitudinal study of the growth of the nasopharynx and its contents in normal children. Br J Radiol 1981; 54(638):117–21.

28. Marcus CL. Pathophysiology of childhood obstructive sleep apnea: current concepts. Respir Physiol 2000;119(2–3):143–54.

29. Isono S, Shimada A, Utsugi M, et al. Comparison of static mechanical properties of the passive pharynx between normal children and children with sleep-disordered breathing. Am J Respir Crit Care Med 1998;157(4 Pt 1):1204–12.

30. Isono S, Remmers JE, Tanaka A, et al. Anatomy of pharynx in patients with obstructive sleep apnea and in normal subjects. J Appl Physiol 1997;82(4): 1319–26.

31. Isono S. Developmental changes of pharyngeal airway patency: implications for pediatric anesthesia. Paediatr Anaesth 2006;16(2):109–22.

32. Marcus CL, Katz ES, Lutz J, et al. Upper airway dynamic responses in children with the obstructive sleep apnea syndrome. Pediatr Res 2005;57(1):99–107.

33. Marcus CL, Lutz J, Carroll JL, et al. Arousal and ventilatory responses during sleep in children with obstructive sleep apnea. J Appl Physiol 1998;84(6): 1926–36.

34. Marcus CL, McColley SA, Carroll JL, et al. Upper airway collapsibility in children with obstructive sleep apnea syndrome. J Appl Physiol 1994;77(2):918–24.

35. McNamara F, Issa FG, Sullivan CE. Arousal pattern following central and obstructive breathing abnormalities in infants and children. J Appl Physiol 1996;81(6):2651–7.

36. Fregosi RF, Quan SF, Jackson AC, et al. Ventilatory drive and the apnea-hypopnea index in six-to-twelve year old children. BMC Pulm Med 2004;4:4.

37. Waters KA, McBrien F, Stewart P, et al. Effects of OSA, inhalational anesthesia, and fentanyl on the airway and ventilation of children. J Appl Physiol 2002;92(5): 1987–94.

38. Ip MS, Lam KS, Ho C, et al. Serum leptin and vascular risk factors in obstructive sleep apnea. Chest 2000;118(3):580–6.

39. Lumeng JC, Chervin RD. Epidemiology of pediatric obstructive sleep apnea. Proc Am Thorac Soc 2008;5(2):242–52.

40. Kheirandish-Gozal L, Gozal D. Genotype-phenotype interactions in pediatric obstructive sleep apnea. Respir Physiol Neurobiol 2013;189(2):338–43.

41. Gozal D, Capdevila OS, Kheirandish-Gozal L, et al. APOE epsilon 4 allele, cognitive dysfunction, and obstructive sleep apnea in children. Neurology 2007;69(3):243–9.

42. Gozal D, Khalyfa A, Capdevila OS, et al. Cognitive function in prepubertal children with obstructive sleep apnea: a modifying role for NADPH oxidase p22 subunit gene polymorphisms? Antioxid Redox Signal 2012;16(2):171–7.

43. Gozal D, Capdevila OS, Kheirandish-Gozal L. Metabolic alterations and systemic inflammation in obstructive sleep apnea among nonobese and obese prepubertal children. Am J Respir Crit Care Med 2008;177(10):1142–9.

44. Goldbart AD, Krishna J, Li RC, et al. Inflammatory mediators in exhaled breath condensate of children with obstructive sleep apnea syndrome. Chest 2006; 130(1):143–8.

45. Kaditis AG, Alexopoulos E, Chaidas K, et al. Urine concentrations of cysteinyl leukotrienes in children with obstructive sleep-disordered breathing. Chest 2009;135(6):1496–501.

46. Li AM, Hung E, Tsang T, et al. Induced sputum inflammatory measures correlate with disease severity in children with obstructive sleep apnoea. Thorax 2007; 62(1):75–9.
47. Alkhalil M, Schulman E, Getsy J. Obstructive sleep apnea syndrome and asthma: what are the links? J Clin Sleep Med 2009;5(1):71–8.
48. Kheirandish-Gozal L, McManus CJ, Kellermann GH, et al. Urinary neurotransmitters are selectively altered in children with obstructive sleep apnea and predict cognitive morbidity. Chest 2013;143(6):1576–83.
49. Chihara Y, Chin K, Aritake K, et al. A urine biomarker for severe OSA patients: lipocaline-type prostaglandin D synthase. Eur Respir J 2012. [Epub ahead of print].
50. Katz ES, White DP. Genioglossus activity in children with obstructive sleep apnea during wakefulness and sleep onset. Am J Respir Crit Care Med 2003; 168(6):664–70.
51. Gozal D, Burnside MM. Increased upper airway collapsibility in children with obstructive sleep apnea during wakefulness. Am J Respir Crit Care Med 2004;169(2):163–7.
52. Eastwood PR, Szollosi I, Platt PR, et al. Collapsibility of the upper airway during anesthesia with isoflurane. Anesthesiology 2002;97(4):786–93.
53. Eastwood PR, Platt PR, Shepherd K, et al. Collapsibility of the upper airway at different concentrations of propofol anesthesia. Anesthesiology 2005;103(3): 470–7.
54. Eikermann M, Malhotra A, Fassbender P, et al. Differential effects of isoflurane and propofol on upper airway dilator muscle activity and breathing. Anesthesiology 2008;108(5):897–906.
55. Litman RS, McDonough JM, Marcus CL, et al. Upper airway collapsibility in anesthetized children. Anesth Analg 2006;102(3):750–4.
56. Montravers P, Dureuil B, Desmonts JM. Effects of i.v. midazolam on upper airway resistance. Br J Anaesth 1992;68(1):27–31.
57. Eastwood PR, Szollosi I, Platt PR, et al. Comparison of upper airway collapse during general anaesthesia and sleep. Lancet 2002;359(9313):1207–9.
58. Moss IR, Brown KA, Laferriere A. Recurrent hypoxia in rats during development increases subsequent respiratory sensitivity to fentanyl. Anesthesiology 2006; 105(4):715–8.
59. Brown KA. Intermittent hypoxia and the practice of anesthesia. Anesthesiology 2009;110(4):922–7.
60. Brown KA, Laferriere A, Lakheeram I, et al. Recurrent hypoxemia in children is associated with increased analgesic sensitivity to opiates. Anesthesiology 2006; 105(4):665–9.
61. Mahmoud M, Gunter J, Donnelly LF, et al. A comparison of dexmedetomidine with propofol for magnetic resonance imaging sleep studies in children. Anesth Analg 2009;109(3):745–53.
62. Mahmoud M, Radhakrishman R, Gunter J, et al. Effect of increasing depth of dexmedetomidine anesthesia on upper airway morphology in children. Paediatr Anaesth 2010;20(6):506–15.
63. Marcus CL, Moore RH, Rosen CL, et al. A randomized trial of adenotonsillectomy for childhood sleep apnea. N Engl J Med 2013;368(25):2366–76.
64. Tapia IE, Marcus CL. Newer treatment modalities for pediatric obstructive sleep apnea. Paediatr Respir Rev 2013;14(3):199–203.
65. Sauer C, Schluter B, Hinz R, et al. Childhood obstructive sleep apnea syndrome: an interdisciplinary approach: a prospective epidemiological study of 4,318 five-and-a-half-year-old children. J Orofac Orthop 2012;73(5):342–58.

66. Guilleminault C, Pelayo R, Leger D, et al. Recognition of sleep-disordered breathing in children. Pediatrics 1996;98(5):871–82.
67. MacLean JE, Fitzsimons D, Fitzgerald DA, et al. The spectrum of sleep-disordered breathing symptoms and respiratory events in infants with cleft lip and/or palate. Arch Dis Child 2012;97(12):1058–63.
68. Muntz HR. Management of sleep apnea in the cleft population. Curr Opin Otolaryngol Head Neck Surg 2012;20(6):518–21.
69. Smith D, Abdullah SE, Moores A, et al. Post-operative respiratory distress following primary cleft palate repair. J Laryngol Otol 2013;127(1):65–6.
70. Maturo SC, Mair EA. Submucosal minimally invasive lingual excision: an effective, novel surgery for pediatric tongue base reduction. Ann Otol Rhinol Laryngol 2006;115(8):624–30.
71. Sundaram S, Bridgman SA, Lim J, et al. Surgery for obstructive sleep apnoea. Cochrane Database Syst Rev 2005;(4):CD001004.
72. Schwengel DA, Sterni LM, Tunkel DE, et al. Perioperative management of children with obstructive sleep apnea. Anesth Analg 2009;109(1):60–75.
73. Epstein LJ, Kristo D, Strollo PJ Jr, et al. Clinical guideline for the evaluation, management and long-term care of obstructive sleep apnea in adults. J Clin Sleep Med 2009;5(3):263–76.
74. Sarrell EM, Chomsky O, Shechter D. Treatment compliance with continuous positive airway pressure device among adults with obstructive sleep apnea (OSA): how many adhere to treatment? Harefuah 2013;152(3):140–4, 184, 183.
75. Costa DJ, Mitchell R. Adenotonsillectomy for obstructive sleep apnea in obese children: a meta-analysis. Otolaryngol Head Neck Surg 2009;140(4):455–60.
76. Weatherly RA, Mai EF, Ruzicka DL, et al. Identification and evaluation of obstructive sleep apnea prior to adenotonsillectomy in children: a survey of practice patterns. Sleep Med 2003;4(4):297–307.
77. Chervin RD, Weatherly RA, Garetz SL, et al. Pediatric sleep questionnaire: prediction of sleep apnea and outcomes. Arch Otolaryngol Head Neck Surg 2007;133(3):216–22.
78. Constantin E, Tewfik TL, Brouillette RT. Can the OSA-18 quality-of-life questionnaire detect obstructive sleep apnea in children? Pediatrics 2010;125(1):e162–8.
79. Ishman SL. Evidence-based practice: pediatric obstructive sleep apnea. Otolaryngol Clin North Am 2012;45(5):1055–69.
80. Spruyt K, Gozal D. Screening of pediatric sleep-disordered breathing: a proposed unbiased discriminative set of questions using clinical severity scales. Chest 2012;142(6):1508–15.
81. McColley SA, April MM, Carroll JL, et al. Respiratory compromise after adenotonsillectomy in children with obstructive sleep apnea. Arch Otolaryngol Head Neck Surg 1992;118(9):940–3.
82. Rosen GM, Muckle RP, Mahowald MW, et al. Postoperative respiratory compromise in children with obstructive sleep apnea syndrome: can it be anticipated? Pediatrics 1994;93(5):784–8.
83. Brown KA, Morin I, Hickey C, et al. Urgent adenotonsillectomy: an analysis of risk factors associated with postoperative respiratory morbidity. Anesthesiology 2003;99(3):586–95.

84. Wilson K, Lakheeram I, Morielli A, et al. Can assessment for obstructive sleep apnea help predict postadenotonsillectomy respiratory complications? Anesthesiology 2002;96(2):313–22.
85. Nixon GM, Kermack AS, McGregor CD, et al. Sleep and breathing on the first night after adenotonsillectomy for obstructive sleep apnea. Pediatr Pulmonol 2005;39(4):332–8.
86. Statham MM, Elluru RG, Buncher R, et al. Adenotonsillectomy for obstructive sleep apnea syndrome in young children: prevalence of pulmonary complications. Arch Otolaryngol Head Neck Surg 2006;132(5): 476–80.
87. Morris LG, Lieberman SM, Reitzen SD, et al. Characteristics and outcomes of malpractice claims after tonsillectomy. Otolaryngol Head Neck Surg 2008; 138(3):315–20.
88. Bins S, Koster TD, de Heij AH, et al. No evidence for diagnostic value of Mallampati score in patients suspected of having obstructive sleep apnea syndrome. Otolaryngol Head Neck Surg 2011;145(2):199–203.
89. Teo DT, Mitchell RB. Systematic review of effects of adenotonsillectomy on cardiovascular parameters in children with obstructive sleep apnea. Otolaryngol Head Neck Surg 2013;148(1):21–8.
90. Redline S, Storfer-Isser A, Rosen CL, et al. Association between metabolic syndrome and sleep-disordered breathing in adolescents. Am J Respir Crit Care Med 2007;176(4):401–8.
91. Vgontzas AN, Bixler EO, Chrousos GP. Sleep apnea is a manifestation of the metabolic syndrome. Sleep Med Rev 2005;9(3):211–24.
92. Bhattacharjee R, Kim J, Kheirandish-Gozal L, et al. Obesity and obstructive sleep apnea syndrome in children: a tale of inflammatory cascades. Pediatr Pulmonol 2011;46(4):313–23.
93. Neligan PJ. Metabolic syndrome: anesthesia for morbid obesity. Curr Opin Anaesthesiol 2010;23(3):375–83.
94. Mador MJ, Goplani S, Gottumukkala VA, et al. Postoperative complications in obstructive sleep apnea. Sleep Breath 2013;17(2):727–34.
95. Strauss SG, Lynn AM, Bratton SL, et al. Ventilatory response to CO2 in children with obstructive sleep apnea from adenotonsillar hypertrophy. Anesth Analg 1999;89(2):328–32.
96. Brown KA, Laferriere A, Moss IR. Recurrent hypoxemia in young children with obstructive sleep apnea is associated with reduced opioid requirement for analgesia. Anesthesiology 2004;100(4):806–10 [discussion: 5A].
97. Krishna S, Hughes LF, Lin SY. Postoperative hemorrhage with nonsteroidal anti-inflammatory drug use after tonsillectomy: a meta-analysis. Arch Otolaryngol Head Neck Surg 2003;129(10):1086–9.
98. Riggin L, Ramakrishna J, Sommer DD, et al. A 2013 updated systematic review & meta-analysis of 36 randomized controlled trials; no apparent effects of non steroidal anti-inflammatory agents on the risk of bleeding after tonsillectomy. Clin Otolaryngol 2013;38(2):115–29.
99. Raghavendran S, Bagry H, Detheux G, et al. An anesthetic management protocol to decrease respiratory complications after adenotonsillectomy in children with severe sleep apnea. Anesth Analg 2010;110(4):1093–101.
100. Czarnetzki C, Elia N, Lysakowski C, et al. Dexamethasone and risk of nausea and vomiting and postoperative bleeding after tonsillectomy in children: a randomized trial. JAMA 2008;300(22):2621–30.

101. Tolska HK, Takala A, Pitkaniemi J, et al. Post-tonsillectomy haemorrhage more common than previously described–an institutional chart review. Acta Otolaryngol 2013;133(2):181–6.

102. Shargorodsky J, Hartnick CJ, Lee GS. Dexamethasone and postoperative bleeding after tonsillectomy and adenotonsillectomy in children: a meta-analysis of prospective studies. Laryngoscope 2012;122(5):1158–64.

103. Kim MS, Cote CJ, Cristoloveanu C, et al. There is no dose-escalation response to dexamethasone (0.0625-1.0 mg/kg) in pediatric tonsillectomy or adenotonsillectomy patients for preventing vomiting, reducing pain, shortening time to first liquid intake, or the incidence of voice change. Anesth Analg 2007;104(5): 1052–8 [tables of contents].

104. Arai YC, Fukunaga K, Hirota S, et al. The effects of chin lift and jaw thrust while in the lateral position on stridor score in anesthetized children with adenotonsillar hypertrophy. Anesth Analg 2004;99(6):1638–41 [tables of contents].

105. Blum RH, McGowan FX Jr. Chronic upper airway obstruction and cardiac dysfunction: anatomy, pathophysiology and anesthetic implications. Paediatr Anaesth 2004;14(1):75–83.

106. Lalwani K, Richins S, Aliason I, et al. The laryngeal mask airway for pediatric adenotonsillectomy: predictors of failure and complications. Int J Pediatr Otorhinolaryngol 2013;77(1):25–8.

107. Subramanyam R, Varughese A, Willging JP, et al. Future of pediatric tonsillectomy and perioperative outcomes. Int J Pediatr Otorhinolaryngol 2013;77(2): 194–9.

108. Gross JB, Bachenberg KL, Benumof JL, et al. Practice guidelines for the perioperative management of patients with obstructive sleep apnea: a report by the American Society of Anesthesiologists Task Force on Perioperative Management of patients with obstructive sleep apnea. Anesthesiology 2006;104(5): 1081–93 [quiz: 1117–8].

109. Koomson A, Morin I, Brouillette R, et al. Children with severe OSAS who have adenotonsillectomy in the morning are less likely to have postoperative desaturation than those operated in the afternoon. Can J Anaesth 2004;51(1): 62–7.

110. Ankichetty S, Chung F. Considerations for patients with obstructive sleep apnea undergoing ambulatory surgery. Curr Opin Anaesthesiol 2011;24(6): 605–11.

111. Blenke EJ, Anderson AR, Raja H, et al. Obstructive sleep apnoea adenotonsillectomy in children: when to refer to a centre with a paediatric intensive care unit? J Laryngol Otol 2008;122(1):42–5.

112. Kieran S, Gorman C, Kirby A, et al. Risk factors for desaturation after tonsillectomy: analysis of 4,092 consecutive pediatric cases. Laryngoscope 2013; 123(10):2554–9.

113. Don DM, Geller KA, Koempel JA, et al. Age specific differences in pediatric obstructive sleep apnea. Int J Pediatr Otorhinolaryngol 2009;73(7):1025–8.

114. Cheng J, Elden L. Outcomes in children under 12 months of age undergoing adenotonsillectomy for sleep-disordered breathing. Laryngoscope 2013;123(9): 2281–4.

115. Leonardis RL, Robison JG, Otteson TD. Evaluating the management of obstructive sleep apnea in neonates and infants. JAMA Otolaryngol Head Neck Surg 2013;139(2):139–46.

116. Robison JG, Wilson C, Otteson TD, et al. Analysis of outcomes in treatment of obstructive sleep apnea in infants. Laryngoscope 2013;123(9):2306–14.

117. Knill RL, Moote CA, Skinner MI, et al. Anesthesia with abdominal surgery leads to intense REM sleep during the first postoperative week. Anesthesiology 1990; 73(1):52–61.
118. Adesanya AO, Lee W, Greilich NB, et al. Perioperative management of obstructive sleep apnea. Chest 2010;138(6):1489–98.
119. Kheirandish-Gozal L, Kim J, Goldbart AD, et al. Novel pharmacological approaches for treatment of obstructive sleep apnea in children. Expert Opin Investig Drugs 2013;22(1):71–85.
120. Lin CM, Huang YS, Guilleminault C. Pharmacotherapy of obstructive sleep apnea. Expert Opin Pharmacother 2012;13(6):841–57.
121. Huang YS, Guilleminault C. Pediatric obstructive sleep apnea and the critical role of oral-facial growth: evidences. Front Neurol 2012;3:184.
122. Leiberman A, Tal A, Brama I, et al. Obstructive sleep apnea in young infants. Int J Pediatr Otorhinolaryngol 1988;16(1):39–44.
123. Zandieh SO, Padwa BL, Katz ES. Adenotonsillectomy for obstructive sleep apnea in children with syndromic craniosynostosis. Plast Reconstr Surg 2013; 131(4):847–52.
124. Sterni LM, Tunkel DE. Obstructive sleep apnea in children: an update. Pediatr Clin North Am 2003;50(2):427–43.
125. Strauss T, Sin S, Marcus CL, et al. Upper airway lymphoid tissue size in children with sickle cell disease. Chest 2012;142(1):94–100.
126. Guilleminault C, Huang YS, Glamann C, et al. Adenotonsillectomy and obstructive sleep apnea in children: a prospective survey. Otolaryngol Head Neck Surg 2007;136(2):169–75.
127. Gerber ME, O'Connor DM, Adler E, et al. Selected risk factors in pediatric adenotonsillectomy. Arch Otolaryngol Head Neck Surg 1996;122(8):811–4.

Ultrasound for Regional Anesthesia in Children

Santhanam Suresh, MD*, Amod Sawardekar, MD, Ravi Shah, MD

KEYWORDS

- Peripheral nerve blockade • Pediatric regional anesthesia • Peripheral nerve catheter
- Nerve stimulation • Ultrasound-guided regional anesthesia

KEY POINTS

- The use of ultrasonography has expanded the application of pediatric regional anesthesia.
- One can visualize the needle advancement and injection of local anesthetic with ultrasonography.
- Ultrasonography can aid in the placement of peripheral nerve catheters to provide prolonged analgesia.

INTRODUCTION

Advances in ultrasonography have expanded the scope of regional anesthesia practice in pediatrics. Ultrasound guidance improves the ease and safety of peripheral nerve blockade in children. It is well recognized that regional anesthesia is commonly performed in anesthetized or sedated children, contrary to adult practice.[1,2] Recent large pediatric databases (Pediatric Regional Anesthesia Network [PRAN]) elucidates the safety and efficacy of regional anesthesia in children.[3] This article is devoted to the use of ultrasound-guided pediatric regional anesthesia with its applications, techniques, and potential complications (**Table 1**).

UPPER EXTREMITY BLOCKS

Blockade of the brachial plexus can be completed at various locations and is applicable to children undergoing surgical procedures on the upper extremity. The brachial plexus can be blocked at the axillary, infraclavicular, interscalene, and supraclavicular locations. The supraclavicular brachial plexus block is the most common upper extremity block performed in children, but the increasing use of ultrasound guidance

Disclosures: None (S. Suresh, A. Sawardekar & R. Shah).
Department of Pediatric Anesthesiology, Ann & Robert H. Lurie Children's Hospital of Chicago, Feinberg School of Medicine, Northwestern University, 225 East Chicago Avenue, Box 19, Chicago, IL 60611, USA
* Corresponding author.
E-mail address: ssuresh@luriechildrens.org

Anesthesiology Clin 32 (2014) 263–279
http://dx.doi.org/10.1016/j.anclin.2013.10.008   anesthesiology.theclinics.com

Table 1
Common peripheral nerve blocks in children

Block	Indications	Dosing
Upper extremity		
Axillary	Surgery of the elbow, forearm, or hand	0.2–0.4 mL/kg 0.25% bupivacaine or 0.2% ropivacaine
Interscalene	Shoulder surgery, catheter placement for postoperative pain control	0.2–0.4 mL/kg 0.25% bupivacaine or 0.2% ropivacaine
Supraclavicular	Most upper extremity procedures	0.2–0.4 mL/kg 0.25% bupivacaine or 0.2% ropivacaine
Infraclavicular	Most upper extremity procedures, catheter placement	0.2–0.3 mL/kg 0.25% bupivacaine or 0.2% ropivacaine
Lower extremity		
Lumbar plexus	Surgery on the hip, knee, or foot	0.2–0.3 mL/kg 0.25% bupivacaine or 0.2% ropivacaine
Femoral	Surgery on the thigh or knee (eg, knee arthroscopy)	0.2–0.3 mL/kg 0.25% bupivacaine or 0.2% ropivacaine
Saphenous	Surgery on the knee, foot, or the medial aspect of the leg below the knee	0.1–0.2 mL/kg 0.25% bupivacaine or 0.2% ropivacaine
Sciatic	Surgical procedures on the foot and ankle, knee surgery (in addition to the femoral nerve block)	0.15–0.3 mL/kg 0.25% bupivacaine or 0.2% ropivacaine
Truncal		
Transversus abdominis plane block, rectus sheath	Surgery on the abdominal wall, chronic neuropathic abdominal wall pain, laparoscopic procedures, umbilical hernia repair	0.1–0.2 mL/kg 0.25% bupivacaine or 0.2% ropivacaine
Ilioinguinal/ iliohypogastric	Hernia repair, groin surgery	0.075–0.2 mL/kg 0.25% bupivacaine or 0.2% ropivacaine

when performing regional anesthesia allows the practitioner to perform brachial plexus blockade at any location safely and effectively (Santhanam Suresh MD, Personal communication). Ultrasound guidance allows the clinician to better recognize brachial plexus anatomy and improves the localization of adjacent structures during needle placement.

AXILLARY BLOCK
Anatomy and Indications

The axillary approach to the brachial plexus provides analgesia to the elbow, forearm, and hand. A single needle insertion at this location facilitates the blockade of the radial, median, and ulnar nerves. Although anatomic variations may exist, the radial nerve commonly lies posterior to the axillary artery, and the ulnar nerve is anterior

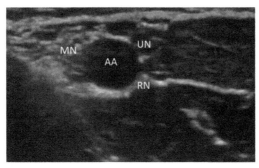

Fig. 1. Ultrasound image of the axillary neurovascular sheath. AA, axillary artery; MN, median nerve; RN, radial nerve; UN, ulnar nerve.

and inferior to the artery (**Fig. 1**). The median nerve is usually located anterior and superior to the axillary artery.[4] It is important to note that the musculocutaneous nerve is situated outside of the axillary neurovascular sheath. Specifically, it lies between the biceps brachii and coracobrachialis muscles and is often blocked separately from the radial, median, and ulnar nerves.

Technique

Ultrasound-guided axillary blocks in children are not well described in the literature, but the techniques used in adults can be applied in children.[5,6] An in-plane technique is used with the ultrasound probe placed transverse to the humerus (**Fig. 2**).[7] Multiple injections with needle repositioning allow for the circumferential spread of local anesthetic around each nerve.[8,9] Careful ultrasound-guided needle advancement should be completed because of the superficial depth of the axillary sheath.

Complications

Complications include neural injury, intravascular injection, hematoma, infection at the site of skin puncture, and skin tenderness. The use of ultrasound guidance to facilitate the needle advancement may help to reduce inadvertent intravascular puncture or injection and nerve damage.

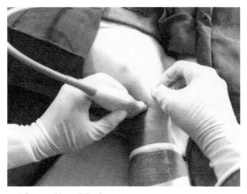

Fig. 2. Probe placement for axillary block.

INTERSCALENE APPROACH
Anatomy and Indications

Analgesia to the shoulder and proximal humerus is accomplished by blocking the brachial plexus at the interscalene groove. At this location, the trunks and roots of brachial plexus are posterior to the sternocleidomastoid muscle and lie between the anterior and middle scalene muscles (**Fig. 3**). Using this approach, the C5, C6, and C7 nerve roots are visualized between the anterior and middle scalene muscles.

Technique

The ultrasound probe is placed in the transverse oblique plane at the level of the cricoid cartilage at the lateral border of the sternocleidomastoid muscle (**Fig. 4**). Deep to the sternocleidomastoid muscle and lateral to the subclavian artery are the anterior and medial scalene muscles, which make up the interscalene groove. Contained within this groove are the hyperechoic structures that compose the neurovascular bundle of the C5, C6, and C7 nerve roots.[10] Although nerve stimulation may be used to deliver local anesthetic solution to the brachial plexus at this level, ultrasound guidance may decrease the required total volume of the local anesthetic.[11]

Complications

Successful interscalene block is accompanied by hemidiaphragmatic paralysis, recurrent laryngeal nerve block, and Horner syndrome; such associated side effects should not be mistaken for complications.[11,12] Ultrasound use may decrease the total local anesthetic needed for successful interscalene block.[13,14] The interscalene block should be used with caution in the pediatric population because of the potential risks of pneumothorax, vertebral artery injection, and intrathecal injection.[15,16]

SUPRACLAVICULAR APPROACH
Anatomy and Indications

The supraclavicular block provides analgesia to the upper arm and elbow. This block is the most common upper extremity block as recorded in the PRAN database. A simple test to check the viability of the median, radial, and ulnar nerve can be performed before the placement of this block, particularly in children who may have a compromised nerve as in elbow fractures. The trunks and divisions of the brachial plexus

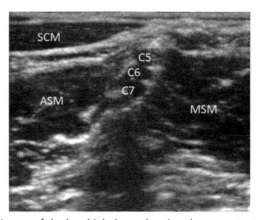

Fig. 3. Ultrasound image of the brachial plexus showing the nerve roots (C5, C6, C7). ASM, anterior scalene muscle; MSM, middle scalene muscle; SCM, sternocleidomastoid muscle.

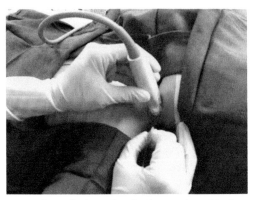

Fig. 4. Probe placement and needle insertion for interscalene block.

can be blocked at this site and are located lateral and superficial to the subclavian artery (**Fig. 5**). A simple test to check the viability of the median, radial, and ulnar nerve can be performed before the placement of this block, particularly in children who may have a compromised nerve as in elbow fractures (Thumbs Up- Radial nerve; Pincer grip of index and thumb: Median nerve; Scissoring of fingers: Ulnar nerve). The first rib is located just posterior and medial to the brachial plexus, and deep to that is the pleura.

Technique

Although few techniques have been described for pediatric patients,[10] the ultrasound probe is commonly positioned in the coronal-oblique plane, just superior to the upper border of the midclavicle. The subclavian artery is identified as a hypoechoic and pulsatile structure that lies adjacent to the brachial plexus. An in-plane approach is used to guide the needle medially toward the brachial plexus, just superior and lateral to the subclavian artery (**Fig. 6**). Directing the needle in a lateral-to-medial fashion decreases injury to vascular structures and minimizes the risk of intraneural injection.[6]

Complications

Complications include pneumothorax, hematoma, infection, hematoma, and intravascular injection. The potential for pneumothorax is present because of the lung

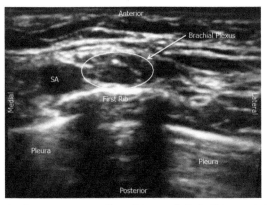

Fig. 5. Supraclavicular fossa as seen on the ultrasound. Note the proximity of the brachial plexus to the subclavian artery (SA).

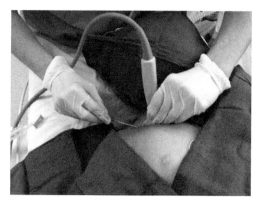

Fig. 6. Probe placement and in-plane needle insertion for the supraclavicular block.

parenchyma's location just medial to the first rib. Direct visualization of the tip and shaft of the needle with ultrasonography may help avoid this complication.

INFRACLAVICULAR APPROACH
Anatomy and Indications

The infraclavicular block, like the supraclavicular block, is used to provide analgesia for the upper arm and elbow.[3] This approach to the brachial plexus allows for blockade at the level of the cords. The cords of the plexus are located medial and inferior to the coracoid process. The axillary artery and vein are deep to the cords. The pectoralis major and minor lie superficial to the brachial plexus. The lateral cord of the plexus is seen on ultrasound as a hyperechoic structure, and the posterior cord is positioned deep to the axillary artery. The medial cord can be difficult to identify because of its anatomic location between the axillary artery and vein (**Fig. 7**).[15] This site can also be used to place catheters for prolonged analgesia in children.[16,17]

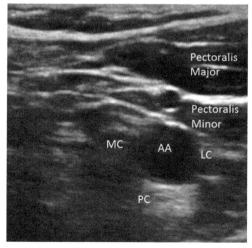

Fig. 7. Ultrasound image of the infraclavicular block; at this location, the medial (MC), posterior (PC), and lateral (LC) cords are seen around the axillary artery (AA).

Technique

A lateral approach is described to complete the ultrasound-guided infraclavicular block in pediatrics.[6] The ultrasound probe is positioned below the clavicle in a transverse orientation to identify the brachial plexus. The needle is inserted inferior to the probe and advanced using an out-of-plane technique.[18] The needle is directed laterally to the cords of the brachial plexus, avoiding vascular structures as local anesthetic is deposited into the deep portion of the neurovascular sheath. Alternatively, De José María and colleagues[15] positioned the probe parallel to the clavicle in a parasagittal plane and directed the needle in a cephalad direction toward the brachial plexus.

Complications

Infraclavicular block confers similar risks to that of the supraclavicular block, including the risk of a pneumothorax.[19] The close proximity of the cervical pleura should be noted. Additionally, the location of the axillary artery and vein make vascular puncture possible.

TRUNCAL BLOCKS

The use of ultrasonography has increased the use of truncal blocks in pediatrics. The emerging role of minimally invasive surgical techniques in children has expanded the spectrum of patients that benefit from the completion of these blocks. Ultrasound-guided techniques have increased the success rate as well as the safety of truncal blocks.

TRANSVERSUS ABDOMINIS PLANE BLOCK
Anatomy and Indications

The transversus abdominis plane (TAP) block provides analgesia to the anterior abdominal wall. It is important to note that the TAP block provides effective postoperative pain control but not surgical analgesia.[20] This block is commonly used for laparoscopic procedures to provide analgesia for port placement sites as well as for larger abdominal incisions.[21] Three muscle layers are identified lateral to the rectus abdominis: the external oblique, internal oblique, and the transversus abdominis (**Fig. 8**). The TAP lies between the internal oblique and transversus abdominis muscles. It is within this plane that the thoracolumbar nerve roots (T8–L1) traverse. These nerves deliver

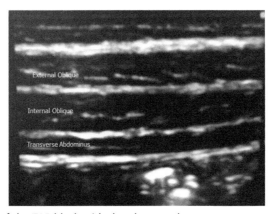

Fig. 8. Anatomy of the TAP block with the ultrasound.

sensory innervation to the skin and muscles of the anterior abdominal wall.[21] A catheter can be placed in the TAP to provide continuous analgesia in patients where the neuraxial technique is avoided.[22,23]

Technique

An in-plane approach is used with ultrasound guidance to advance the needle into the TAP where local anesthetic is delivered.[20,23] The ultrasound probe is positioned adjacent to the umbilicus and moved laterally, away from the rectus abdominis, until the 3 muscle layers of the abdominal wall are visualized (**Fig. 9**).[24,25] The needle is advanced using an in-plane technique starting from either the lateral or medial side. Injection of local anesthetic creates an elliptical pocket of local anesthetic in the TAP.

Complications

Potential complications include infection, peritoneal and/or bowel puncture, and intravascular injection.

ILIOINGUINAL/ILIOHYPOGASTRIC NERVE BLOCK
Anatomy and Indications

The ilioinguinal/iliohypogastric (IL/IH) nerves provide sensation to the inguinal area and the anterior scrotum and originate from T12 and L1 of the thoracolumbar plexus.[20] The IL/IH nerves are blocked medial to the anterior superior iliac spine as they travel across the internal oblique aponeurosis. Successful blockade of the IL/IH nerves provides equivalent relief to caudal blocks for inguinal surgery with the benefit of increased duration of analgesia.[26,27]

Technique

The ultrasound probe is placed medial to the anterior superior iliac spine, in line with the umbilicus (**Fig. 10**). Three abdominal muscle layers are identified by ultrasonography (internal oblique, external oblique, and transversus abdominis). At this level, the external oblique muscle layer can be aponeurotic and only 2 muscle layers may be recognized.[28] The IL/IH nerves appear as ovular structures between the internal oblique and transverse abdominal muscles (**Fig. 11**). The needle is inserted in-plane and advanced to the IL/IH nerves to deposit the local anesthetic. The use of ultrasound guidance has been demonstrated to reduce the volume of local anesthetic needed to produce analgesia.[29,30]

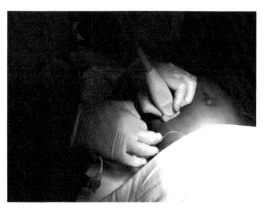

Fig. 9. Probe placement for the TAP block.

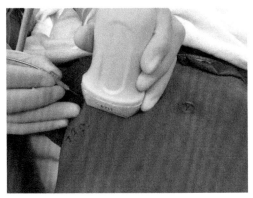

Fig. 10. Probe placement for the IL/IH block. The probe is placed between the anterior superior iliac spine and the umbilicus.

Complications

The IL/IH nerve block can rarely cause injection-site infection, intravascular injection, bowel puncture, pelvic hematoma, and femoral nerve palsy.

RECTUS SHEATH BLOCK
Anatomy and Indications

The rectus sheath block provides analgesia to the anterior abdominal wall along the midline. At this location, the rectus abdominis muscle lies on the anterior abdominal wall and is separated by the linea alba (**Fig. 12**). The thoracolumbar nerves (T7–T11) lie posterior to the rectus abdominis muscle just above the posterior sheath. The rectus sheath block is commonly used to provide postoperative pain relief for umbilical hernia and single-incision laparoscopic surgery.[31]

Technique

The ultrasound probe is placed lateral to the umbilicus so the rectus abdominis muscle is identified as the only muscle layer (**Fig. 13**). The posterior sheath lies just below the rectus abdominis and above the peritoneum (see **Fig. 12**). Using an in-plane technique, the needle is advanced in a lateral-to-medial direction to deposit local anesthetic between the rectus abdominis muscle and its posterior sheath.[32] Careful

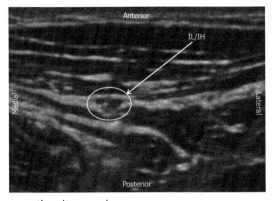

Fig. 11. IL/IH as seen on the ultrasound.

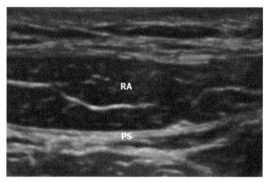

Fig. 12. Ultrasound image of the rectus sheath block. Local anesthetic should be deposited between the rectus abdominis muscle (RA) and Posterior Rectus Sheath (PS).

attention should be made to avoid injection of the local anesthetic in between the 2 layers of the posterior rectus sheath because this will result in block failure.

Complications

Complications include infection, intravascular injection, and bowel puncture.

LOWER EXTREMITY BLOCKS
Femoral Nerve Block

Anatomy and indications

The femoral nerve provides innervation to the anterior thigh and the knee. It originates from the L2, L3, and L4 nerve roots and is commonly blocked in pediatrics for surgical interventions in the knee. The femoral nerve is anatomically lateral to the femoral artery and vein. This neurovascular bundle is easily seen with ultrasonography when the probe is placed in the inguinal crease (**Fig. 14**).[33] In addition to a single-shot technique, a catheter can be safely placed to provide extended analgesia.[34,35]

Technique

With the patient in the supine position, the femoral nerve, artery, and vein are located within the inguinal crease. Once the probe is placed in the inguinal crease, the femoral artery is identified as a pulsatile structure. Lateral to this, the femoral nerve is identified

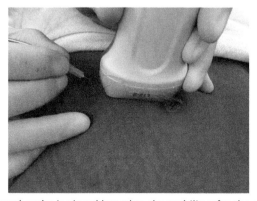

Fig. 13. The ultrasound probe is placed lateral to the umbilicus for the rectus sheath block.

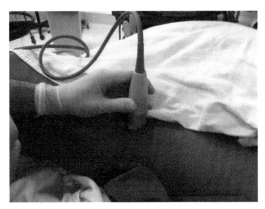

Fig. 14. Probe placement for the femoral nerve block.

and the femoral vein is visualized just medial to the artery as a collapsible vessel (**Fig. 15**). An in-plane or out-of-plane approach can be used to guide the needle to the lateral portion of the femoral nerve and circumferentially surround it with local anesthetic.[34,36] Careful visualization of the needle with advancement will avoid inadvertent vascular puncture of the femoral vessels.

Complications
Complications include infection, nerve injury, and hematoma formation caused by the femoral nerve's juxtaposition to the vein and artery.

Saphenous Nerve Block

Anatomy and indications
The saphenous nerve provides innervation to the knee and the medial portion of the leg below the knee. It is a branch of the femoral nerve and travels within the adductor canal and runs adjacent to the sartorius muscle before continuing to the medial aspect of the knee (**Fig. 16**). It can be blocked proximally to provide sensory analgesia to the anterior knee or can be blocked more distally to provide analgesia solely to the medial aspect of the lower extremity.[36]

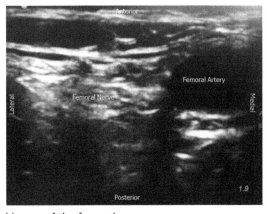

Fig. 15. Ultrasound image of the femoral nerve.

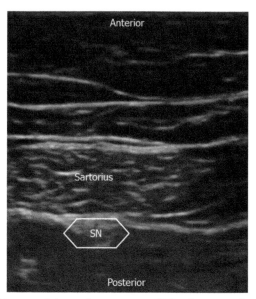

Fig. 16. Ultrasound image of the saphenous nerve (SN) adjacent to the sartorius muscle.

Technique
With patients in the supine position, the leg is abducted and laterally rotated as the probe is placed on the medial aspect of the knee. The sartorius muscle is identified, and juxtaposed to this is the saphenous nerve. The needle is directed using an in-plane technique to the saphenous nerve, where the local anesthetic is deposited (**Fig. 17**).

Complications
Complications include nerve injury, hematoma from arterial puncture, and infection.

Sciatic Nerve Block

Anatomy and indications
The sciatic nerve provides innervation to the posterior thigh and the entire leg distal to the knee (excluding the medial component). The sciatic nerve originates from the

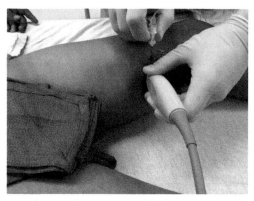

Fig. 17. Probe placement for a saphenous nerve block proximal to the knee.

nerve roots of L4 to S3. From its origin, the nerve courses through and exits the pelvis via the greater sciatic foramen and continues inferiorly to the gluteus maximus muscle. The sciatic nerve continues to course through the posterior popliteal fossa where it splits into the tibial and common peroneal nerves (**Fig. 18**). The sciatic nerve can be blocked throughout its anatomic course at the subgluteal, anterior thigh, or popliteal approaches in children.[37,38] Continuous sciatic nerve blockade, as well as a single-shot technique, can provide extended analgesia in children.[39,40]

Technique

The subgluteal approach to the sciatic nerve requires patients to lie in either the lateral decubitus position, with the hip and knee flexed, or in the prone position. In these positions, the ultrasound probe is placed between the greater trochanter and the ischial tuberosity. The gluteus maximus muscle is identified, and deep to this is the sciatic nerve. An in-plane or out-of-plane technique can be used to advance the needle with ultrasound guidance to the nerve.[41,42] Local anesthetic is injected to circumferentially surround the nerve in a single-shot technique, but a catheter can also be placed to deliver continuous nerve blockade.[43]

The use of the ultrasound has facilitated the performance of an anterior approach to the sciatic nerve blockade, during which patients may remain in the supine position.[44] This technique allows for the completion of the sciatic nerve block in nonanesthetized patients with lower extremity discomfort without moving them to the lateral or prone position. While supine, the patients' leg is abducted and laterally rotated and the probe is placed inferior to the inguinal crease. The femur is identified, and the probe is moved medially to reveal the sciatic nerve in its location deep and medial to the femur. The nerve often lies deeper in larger patients, which can make this approach technically challenging to complete in older children.

The sciatic nerve can also be blocked more distally in the popliteal fossa.[45] Patients are placed prone or can remain in the supine position, and the ultrasound probe is placed in the popliteal crease (**Fig. 19**). The popliteal artery is visualized as a pulsatile structure. Immediately adjacent to the artery is the tibial nerve. The tibial nerve can be followed proximally to the junction with the common peroneal nerve, merging together

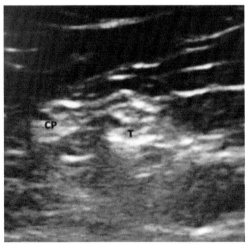

Fig. 18. Ultrasound image of the confluence of the common peroneal nerve (CP) and tibial nerve (T) from the sciatic nerve.

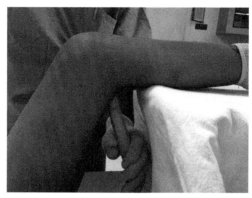

Fig. 19. Probe placement for the sciatic nerve block at the popliteal fossa while a patient is supine.

to form the sciatic nerve. The sciatic nerve can be blocked here or the tibial and common peroneal nerves can be specifically targeted at this location.

Complications
Complications include infection at the site of skin puncture, hematoma from vessel puncture, and local anesthetic toxicity.

Lumbar Plexus Block

Anatomy and indications
The lumbar plexus originates from the nerve roots from T12 to L5. Its branches include the femoral, genitofemoral, lateral femoral cutaneous, and obturator nerves. The lumbar plexus provides innervation to the lower abdomen and the upper leg and is located within the psoas muscle deep to the paravertebral muscles. The lumbar plexus can be blocked with the ipsilateral sciatic nerve to achieve complete analgesia to the lower extremity.[46]

Technique
Patients are placed in the lateral decubitus position, and the iliac crest and spinous processes are identified. The ultrasound probe is placed lateral to the midline, and the L4 or L5 transverse processes are located. Deep to the transverse process are the erector spinae and quadratus lumborum muscles. Beyond this, within the psoas major muscle, is the lumbar plexus. Because of this anatomic location, the plexus is often difficult to demarcate from the similar echogenicity to the muscle. Nerve stimulation may be used in conjunction with ultrasonography to elicit twitches of the quadriceps muscles and confirm needle positioning near the plexus.

Complications
Complications include infection, hematoma, and retroperitoneal bleeding caused by the location of the plexus.

SUMMARY

The use of ultrasonography has expanded the scope and applicability of regional anesthesia in children, which is evidenced by the progressive increase in the use of peripheral regional anesthesia in pediatric patients.[47] Ultrasonography allows for real-time visualization of needle advancement and local anesthetic spread. This visualization may decrease the total volume of local anesthetic required to achieve successful nerve blockade; however, additional data are needed to confer the benefits and risks to patients. In addition, compared with nerve stimulation, the use of ultrasound does not require the avoidance of neuromuscular blockade. Nerve stimulation continues to play a vital role in regional anesthesia,[48] and available data demonstrate the individual benefits of both the nerve stimulation and ultrasound-guided techniques.[49] Successful implementation of regional anesthesia in pediatrics is a vital component in ensuring an optimal surgical experience for children.

REFERENCES

1. Tsui B, Suresh S. Ultrasound imaging for regional anesthesia in infants, children, and adolescents: a review of current literature and its application to neuraxial blocks. Anesthesiology 2010;112:719–28.
2. Marhofer P, Sitzwohl C, Greher M, et al. Ultrasound guidance for infraclavicular brachial plexus anaesthesia in children. Anaesthesia 2004;59:642–6.
3. Polaner DM, Taenzer AH, Walker BJ, et al. Pediatric regional anesthesia network (PRAN): a multi-institutional study of the use and incidence of complications of pediatric regional anesthesia. Anesth Analg 2012;115(6):1353–64.
4. Rapp H, Grau T. Ultrasound-guided regional anesthesia in pediatric patients. Reg Anesth Pain Manag 2004;8:179–98.
5. Roberts S. Ultrasonographic guidance in pediatric regional anesthesia. Part 2: techniques. Paediatr Anaesth 2006;16:1112–24.
6. Marhofer P. Upper extremity peripheral blocks. Tech Reg Anesth Pain Manag 2007;11:215–21.
7. O'Donnell BD, Iohom G. An estimation of the minimum effective anesthetic volume of 2% lidocaine in ultrasound-guided axillary brachial plexus block. Anesthesiology 2009;111:25–9.
8. Diwan R, Lakshmi V, Shah T, et al. Continuous axillary block for upper limb surgery in a patient with epidermolysis bullosa simplex. Paediatr Anaesth 2001;11:603–6.
9. Dadure C, Motais F, Ricard C, et al. Continuous peripheral nerve blocks at home in the treatment of complex regional pain syndrome in children. Anesthesiology 2005;102:387–91.
10. Van Geffen GJ, Tielens L, Gielen M. Ultrasound-guided interscalene brachial plexus block in a child with femur fibula ulna syndrome. Paediatr Anaesth 2006;16:330–2.
11. McNaught A, Shastri U, Carmichael N, et al. Ultrasound reduces the minimum effective local anesthetic volume compared with peripheral nerve stimulation for interscalene block. Br J Anaesth 2010;06:124–30.
12. Fredrickson MJ. Ultrasound-assisted interscalene catheter placement in a child. Anaesth Intensive Care 2007;35:807–8.
13. Renes SH, Retting HC, Gielen MJ, et al. Ultrasound-guided low-dose interscalene brachial plexus block reduced the incidence of hemidiaphragmatic paresis. Reg Anesth Pain Med 2009;34:498–502.
14. Ilfeld BM, Morey TE, Wright TW, et al. Interscalene perineural ropivacaine infusion: a comparison of two dosing regimens for postoperative analgesia. Reg Anesth Pain Med 2004;29:9–16.
15. De José María B, Banus E, Navarro EM, et al. Ultrasound-guided supraclavicular vs infraclavicular brachial plexus blocks in children. Paediatr Anaesth 2008;18:838–44.

16. Mariano ER, Ilfeld BM, Cheng GS, et al. Feasibility of ultrasound-guided peripheral nerve block catheters for pain control on pediatric medical missions in developing countries. Paediatr Anaesth 2008;18:598–601.

17. Ponde VC. Continuous infraclavicular brachial plexus block: a modified technique to better secure catheter position in infants and children. Anesth Analg 2008;106:94–6.

18. Diwan R, Raux O, Troncin R, et al. Continuous infraclavicular brachial plexus block for acute pain management in children. Anesth Analg 2003;97:691–3.

19. Ilfeld BM, Morey TE, Enneking FK. Infraclavicular perineural local anesthetic infusion: a comparison of three dosing regimens for postoperative analgesia. Anesthesiology 2004;100:395–402.

20. Suresh S, Chan VW. Ultrasound guided transversus abdominis plane block in infants, children and adolescents: a simple procedural guidance for their performance. Paediatr Anaesth 2009;19(1):296–9.

21. McDonnell JG, O'Donnell B, Curley G, et al. The analgesic efficacy of transversus abdominis plane block after abdominal surgery: a prospective randomized controlled trial. Anesth Analg 2007;104(1):193–7.

22. Visoiu M, Boretsky KR, Goyal G, et al. Postoperative analgesia via transversus abdominis plane (TAP) catheter for small weight children - our initial experience. Paediatr Anaesth 2012;22:281–4.

23. Taylor L, Birmingham P, Yerkes E, et al. Children with spinal dysraphism: transversus abdominis plane (TAP) catheters to the rescue! Paediatr Anaesth 2010;20:951–4.

24. Pak T, Mickelson J, Yerkes E, et al. Transverse abdominis plane block: a new approach to the management of secondary hyperalgesia following major abdominal surgery. Paediatr Anaesth 2009;19(1):54–6.

25. Fredrickson M, Seal P, Houghton J. Early experience with the transversus abdominis plane block in children. Paediatr Anaesth 2008;18:891–2.

26. Jagannathan N, Sohn L, Sawardekar A, et al. Unilateral groin surgery in children: will the addition of an ultrasound-guided ilioinguinal nerve block enhance the duration of analgesia of a single-shot caudal block? Paediatr Anaesth 2009;19(1):892–8.

27. Hannallah RS, Broadman LM, Belman AB, et al. Comparison of caudal and ilioinguinal/iliohypogastric nerve blocks for control of post-orchiopexy pain in pediatric ambulatory surgery. Anesthesiology 1987;66:832–4.

28. Markham SJ, Tomlinson J, Hain WR. Ilioinguinal nerve block in children. A comparison with caudal block for intra and postoperative analgesia. Anaesthesia 1986;41:1098–103.

29. Willschke H, Marhofer P, Bösenberg A. Ultrasonography for ilioinguinal/iliohypogastric nerve blocks in children. Br J Anaesth 2005;95(2):226–30.

30. Smith T, Moratin P, Wulf H. Smaller children have greater bupivacaine plasma concentrations after ilioinguinal block. Br J Anaesth 1996;76:452–5.

31. Ferguson S, Thomas V, Lewis I. The rectus sheath block in paediatric anaesthesia: new indications for an old technique? Paediatr Anaesth 1996;6:463–6.

32. Willschke H, Bosenberg A, Marhofer P, et al. Ultrasonography-guided rectus sheath block in paediatric anaesthesia: a new approach to an old technique. Br J Anaesth 2006;97:244–9.

33. Oberndorfer U, Marhofer P, Bösenberg A, et al. Ultrasonographic guidance for sciatic and femoral nerve blocks in children. Br J Anaesth 2007;98(6):797–801.

34. Casati A, Baciarello M, Di Cianni S, et al. Effects of ultrasound guidance on the minimum effective anaesthetic volume required to block the femoral nerve. Br J Anaesth 2007;98:823–7.

35. Johnson CM. Continuous femoral nerve blockade for analgesia in children with femoral fractures. Anaesth Intensive Care 1994;22:281–3.
36. Simion C, Suresh S. Lower extremity peripheral nerve blocks in children. Tech Reg Anesth Pain Manag 2007;11:222–8.
37. van Geffen GJ, Scheuer M, Muller A, et al. Ultrasound-guided bilateral continuous sciatic nerve blocks with stimulating catheters for postoperative pain relief after bilateral lower limb amputations. Anaesthesia 2006;61:1204–7.
38. van Geffen GJ, Gielen M. Ultrasound-guided subgluteal sciatic nerve blocks with stimulating catheters in children: a descriptive study. Anesth Analg 2006;103: 328–33.
39. Ganesh A, Rose J, Wells L, et al. Continuous peripheral nerve blockade for inpatient and outpatient postoperative analgesia in children. Anesth Analg 2007; 105(5):1234–42.
40. Ilfeld BM, Morey TE, Wang RD, et al. Continuous popliteal sciatic nerve block for postoperative pain control at home. Anesthesiology 2002;97:959–65.
41. Chelly JE, Greger J, Casati A, et al. Continuous lateral sciatic blocks for acute postoperative pain management after major ankle and foot surgery. Foot Ankle Int 2002;23:749–52.
42. Dadure C, Bringuier S, Nicolas F, et al. Continuous epidural block versus continuous popliteal nerve block for postoperative pain relief after major podiatric surgery in children: a prospective comparative randomized study. Anesth Analg 2006;102:744–9.
43. Vas L. Continuous sciatic block for leg and foot surgery in 160 children. Paediatr Anaesth 2005;15:971–8.
44. Tsui BC, Ozelsel TJ. Ultrasound-guided anterior sciatic nerve block using a longitudinal approach: "expanding the view". Reg Anesth Pain Med 2008;33:275–6.
45. Schwemmer U, Markus CK, Greim CA, et al. Sonographic imaging of the sciatic nerve and its division in the popliteal fossa in children. Paediatr Anaesth 2004;14: 1005–8.
46. Johr M. The right thing in the right place: lumbar plexus block in children. Anesthesiology 2005;102:865–6.
47. Tsui B, Suresh S. Ultrasound imaging for regional anesthesia in infants, children, and adolescents: a review of current literature and its application in the practice of extremity and trunk blocks. Anesthesiology 2010;112:473–92.
48. Klein S, Melton S, Grill W, et al. Peripheral nerve stimulation in regional anesthesia. Reg Anesth Pain Med 2012;37:383–92.
49. Neal J, Brull R, Chan V. The ASRA evidence-based medicine assessment of ultrasound-guided regional anesthesia and pain medicine: executive summary. Reg Anesth Pain Med 2010;35:S1–9.

Perspectives on Quality and Safety in Pediatric Anesthesia

David Buck, MD, MBA*, C. Dean Kurth, MD,
Anna Varughese, MD, MPH

KEYWORDS

- Quality improvement • Pediatric anesthesiology • Safety analytics • Measurement
- Wake Up Safe

KEY POINTS

- Organizational culture underlies every improvement strategy; without a strong culture, a change, even if initially successful, is short lived.
- Changing culture and improving quality require commitment of leadership, and leaders must play an active and visible role to articulate the vision and create the proper environment.
- Quality-improvement (QI) projects require a consistent framework for improvement, because the framework provides the structure for outlining a process, identifying problems, and testing, evaluating, and implementing changes.
- Wake Up Safe is a patient safety organization composed of pediatric institutions, which strives to use QI to make anesthesia care safer.
- Root cause analysis (RCA) is a widely used methodology in safety analytics that is based on a sequence of events model of safety.

INTRODUCTION

It is the professional responsibility of pediatric anesthesiologists to deliver care to the best of their ability in the operating room.[1] In reality, however, the factors that underlie individual decisions and practices are more complex than simply "doing their best." They involve the systemic interactions of coordination of care, organizational culture, communication between nursing and surgical teams, and practice guidelines. Improving care requires an evolution in understanding how these systems interact and deliberate testing of how changes affect their performance.

It is difficult to acknowledge that pediatric care is inadequate or, worse, harmful. According to the 2012 National Healthcare Quality Report,[2] overall health care quality

Department of Anesthesiology, Cincinnati Children's Hospital, 3333 Burnet Avenue, Cincinnati, OH 45229, USA
* Corresponding author.
E-mail address: David.Buck@cchmc.org

Anesthesiology Clin 32 (2014) 281–294
http://dx.doi.org/10.1016/j.anclin.2013.11.001   anesthesiology.theclinics.com

may be improving. Even so, as of 2009, Americans received only 70% of indicated health care services needed for treating or preventing illness. Unfortunately, there is no reason to believe similar deficiencies do not exist in pediatric anesthesia.

There are meaningful, systematic ways to increase the quality of care. Intermountain Healthcare in Salt Lake City, Utah, was one of the first health care systems to pursue clinical QI.[3] Virginia Mason Medical center in Seattle, Washington, drove down waste using Lean management principles.[4] The common denominator in these organizations is the use of a structured and systematic approach to QI and a culture that supports its implementation.

At Cincinnati Children's Hospital Medical Center (CCHMC), QI has become integral to patient safety, patient and family satisfaction, efficiency, and cost. Its QI initiatives continue to grow and mature as successes and failures are learned from. Key learning areas in the QI journey have included a culture of improvement, institutional leadership, QI training, and frameworks and tools for improvement.

THE CULTURE OF IMPROVEMENT

Organizational culture underlies every improvement strategy. Without a strong culture, a change, even if initially successful, is short lived. It is not uncommon that an improvement project, successful at one institution, fails when transplanted to a new environment. The difference between success and failure may be differing organizational cultures.

Broadly, culture may be defined as "shared values and beliefs that interact with a company's people, organizational structures and control systems to produce behavioral norms."[5] A culture of safety is one that encourages open discussion of mistakes, transparency, and systems-based thinking as opposed to blaming individuals. At the personal level, this means providers feel comfortable openly reporting and talking about adverse events and near misses. At the organizational level, it means being transparent about errors and shortcomings. Some organizations have gone so far as to publish their adverse events and QI initiatives.

Organizational culture is complex and change is difficult. Poor leadership, perceived lack of ownership, constraints of external stakeholders and professional allegiances, and subcultural diversity all hinder culture change.[6] Fortunately, there are several tools and methods available to help navigate the complexity of measuring and implementing a change in culture.

It is just as important to monitor safety culture, as it is to monitor clinical metrics. Several surveys exist to measure safety culture at hospitals. For example, the Agency for Healthcare Research and Quality (AHRQ) has developed and validated a survey for hospitals on safety culture. Statements, such as the following, are assessed on a scale of 1 to 5:

- "People support one another in this unit."
- "Staff feel like their mistakes are held against them."
- "My supervisor/manager says a good word when he/she sees a job done according to established patient safety procedures."

The AHRQ also provides guidance on setting up the survey and analyzing the data. Once a baseline is determined, repeating these surveys every 6 months is recommended until the goal is achieved and then yearly thereafter.[7]

Following baseline data, a first step may be to give employees and staff the tools to discover current problems for themselves. A question often posed to employees is, "How will the next patient be harmed?" It often takes years to bring about a measurable change in culture.

LEADERSHIP IN QUALITY IMPROVEMENT

Changing culture and improving quality require commitment of leadership. Leaders must play an active and visible role to articulate the vision and create the proper environment. This means creating a culture of continuous improvement; aligning QI projects with strategic objectives; providing appropriate incentives; and ensuring adequate resources, such as time, administrative support, and information technology.

Some of the specific ways leadership promotes QI at CCHMC include

- Development of a departmental quality scorecard
- Presentation of data and goals on quality measures at quarterly staff meetings
- Highlighting QI projects at clinical steering meetings
- Participation in RCAs
- Reviewing reported adverse events and near misses
- Training new faculty and students on quality indicators and process improvement
- Linking personal and department measures with financial incentives
- Participation in organizational QI programs, both as mentors and as students[8]

Characteristics of Leadership

Certain kinds of leaders may be particularly effective at bringing about change. Management researcher Jim Collins examined more than 1400 companies looking for attributes that led companies to achieve greatness. He discovered that a particular kind of leadership, what he termed, *level 5 leadership*, is instrumental in organizational transformation. A level 5 leader is one who paradoxically has both deep personal humility and intense professional will. These leaders have exacting standards and resolve to reach long-term goals. At the same time, they are able to put the organization and greater purpose above seeking personal adulation.[9]

Taking on Leadership Roles as a Physician

The transition from practitioner to leader may be particularly difficult for physicians. Physicians traditionally function as independent practitioners. In QI, however, they may be asked to take on new roles as both team members and leaders. This transition is often difficult and may require completely new skill sets than those taught in medical school or residency.

A physician leader's role requires balancing the goals of multiple stakeholders, including the hospital, the department, and fellow colleagues. Negotiating these challenges requires an understanding of how the system functions as a whole. It also requires interpersonal skills, such as proficiency in speaking and writing, open and honest communication, negotiation, and motivation.

TRAINING IN LEADERSHIP AND QUALITY IMPROVEMENT

Leadership and QI training are shown to improve skills, knowledge, and even patient care processes.[10] Although there are not yet studies linking QI training to improved patient outcomes,[10] it is reasonable to believe that these skills and knowledge sets translate into better patient care. Many of these training programs create not only experts in QI but also leaders and teachers, further extending their influence on health care.

QI training varies among industries and organizations. Internal training includes formal hospital training programs, individual mentors, or informal on-the-job training. The Advanced Training Program in Clinical Practice Improvement, developed by Intermountain Healthcare, represents an example of an internally developed program. It sought to bridge the gap between system improvement knowledge and professional knowledge. Today, the program serves as an example for other institutions wishing to create their own QI programs.[3]

External training includes professional degree programs, such as master of business administration (MBA) and master of public health programs; online courses, such as the Institute for Healthcare Improvement (IHI) Open School; and seminars and workshops sponsored by consultants or professional societies. The IHI Open School is an example of an online educational community. The Open School features online courses, including a certificate program, forums, and a vast collection of multimedia content. It is available at no charge to students in the health professions. As an alternative to traditional MBA programs, many physicians are pursuing executive MBAs. Executive MBAs are structured to allow professionals to enroll without leaving their current job for the duration of the program. In addition, certain business schools offer MBAs with a concentration in health care management.

A typical QI training program combines practical projects with knowledge-based coursework. Studies have indicated this combination is more effective than providing either option alone.[10] Many programs emphasize testing small changes over time with objective data through plan, do, study, act (PDSA) cycles and the Model For Improvement. Other programs teach Six Sigma and Lean methodologies to improve efficiency and smooth production flow.[11] The trend in these programs is toward interdisciplinary training, integrating people from different departments and backgrounds.

At CCHMC, an internal program, the Intermediate Improvement Science Series, has been critical to the development of leaders in QI. Members from each department are nominated to attend the course, which runs 6 months, with classes 2 days per month. Over this period, attendees work with an improvement coach and their department sponsor in formulating and managing an improvement project. The improvement project is supported by workshops, seminars, and readings in the course. The classes are multidisciplinary and students learn from each other as well as previous graduates. Back in their own departments, students manage improvement projects and share their knowledge with other department members.[12,13]

CHOOSING A FRAMEWORK FOR IMPROVEMENT

QI projects require a consistent framework for improvement. The framework provides the structure for outlining a process; identifying problems; and testing, evaluating, and implementing changes. Furthermore, it provides a tool to communicate the project to others.

Examples of popular frameworks include the IHI Model for Improvement, Toyota Lean methodology, and GE Six Sigma. These frameworks share similar principles. Their origins are often in industries entirely outside of health care. As an example, the Virginia Mason Production System is a management methodology developed by Virginia Mason Medical Center that originated from Lean methodology and the Toyota Production System.[4] Additionally, frameworks may be combined; for example, Lean Six Sigma is a combination of Lean and Six Sigma.

THE MODEL FOR IMPROVEMENT

The Model for Improvement is a popular framework used at Cincinnati Children's Hospital (**Fig. 1**). It begins by asking 3 questions of change that help frame the improvement project:

- What are we trying to accomplish?
- How will we know that a change is an improvement?
- What changes can we make that will result in improvement?

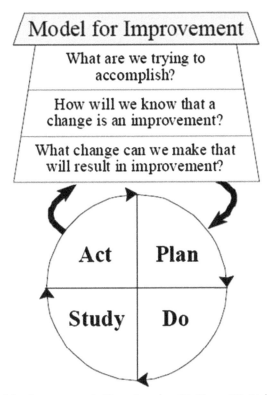

Fig. 1. The Model for Improvement. (*From* Langley GJ, Moen RD, Nolan KM, et al. The improvement guide: a practical approach to enhancing organizational performance. San Francisco (CA): Jossey-Bass; 2009; with permission.)

These questions are evaluated by designing experiments known as small tests of change, or PDSA cycles.[14] Each cycle provides learning about the process, which is used in planning the next cycle. Changes that are successful may be implemented on a wider scale or expanded to other areas. Tests of change that are not successful are modified through repeated cycles or discarded. Testing changes on a small scale through PDSA cycles mitigates the risk of implementation of a bad process. As new knowledge is gained through small tests, a theory of how the system functions is formulated. This theory aids in developing and selecting future interventions and applying them to new environments.

MEASURING QUALITY OF CARE IN PEDIATRIC ANESTHESIA
Defining Quality

In order to determine if a change is successful, appropriate quality measures must be established and tracked over time. To determine these measures, it is necessary to understand what defines quality care. The Institute of Medicine provides 6 aims of health care. These aims state that health care should be

- Safe—no patient should be harmed by health care
- Effective—evidence-based treatment should be used when available
- Patient centered—there should be a respectful approach to patient preferences, needs, and values

- Timely—delays should be reduced because these may affect satisfaction, diagnosis, and treatment
- Efficient—waste should be reduced or value increased
- Equitable—the same care should be provided regardless of personal characteristics.[15–17]

In pediatric anesthesia, it is helpful to imagine the ideal anesthetic experience for children and their families. Some examples across the intraoperative process are

- Preoperative process: timely, accurate history; thorough education; encourages questions
- Induction: no unnecessary anxiety or discomfort; appropriate parental participation
- Intraoperative experience: no serious adverse events
- Postanesthesia care unit (PACU): pain managed and treated in a timely fashion
- Postoperative course: no unexpected ICU or hospital admission.

Types of Measures

The categories of quality measures include outcome measures, process measures, structural measures, and balancing measures. Ideally, a QI project has one measure from each category, which is not always practical. For example, an outcome may be so rare that measurement is problematic. A process measure, on the other hand, may not correlate with outcomes, and should be based on evidence-based guidelines when possible. Any change, especially in a complex system like health care, may result in unintended consequences. Balancing measures look for unintended consequences and can provide a more comprehensive understanding of the effects of a change.

RUN CHARTS AND CONTROL CHARTS

After quality measures are determined, they are measured and tracked over time. Baseline data should be collected prior to testing changes and all interventions within the period of data collection should be noted.

Run charts and control charts are used to track data in QI. A run chart plots the variable over time. The mean, or median, is included on the chart as a method of centering the sample. In a control chart, upper and lower control limits are calculated to determine whether or not a process is stable, referred to as "in control."

In **Fig. 2**, a control chart plots patient and family satisfaction with pain control in a PACU. Most of the data are within the upper and lower control limits indicating this process is in control.[18]

IMPROVEMENT TOOLS

Improvement tools, such as a key driver diagram, fishbone diagram, or process flowchart, may be applied within any framework to gain additional insight into a process.

Key Drivers

Key drivers are the driving elements behind an improvement project, and they are critical to understanding the theory behind improvement. Key drivers help develop future interventions and apply successful interventions to new environments. They also help others, perhaps in different organizations, apply the improvement to their unique environment.

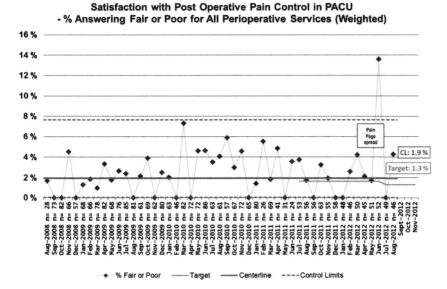

Fig. 2. A control chart for patient and family satisfaction with pain control in the PACU at Cincinnati Children's Hospital. (*Courtesy of* Department of Anesthesiology, Cincinnati Children's Hospital, Cincinnati, OH; with permission.)

Once the key drivers are identified, interventions are developed to target each key driver. The key drivers may be thought of as the "how" and the interventions thought of as the "what" of the improvement project. It may take multiple tests of change across several key drivers before an improvement is realized.

An example of key drivers for improving patient and family satisfaction with pain in the CCHMC PACU is listed in **Fig. 3**. The key drivers, such as "Parental Understanding of Pain in the PACU," are traditionally stated in the affirmative. They are specific enough that interventions can be developed. For example, "Knowledge" is too broad for a key driver. Several interventions are targeted at this key driver, including highlighting a "pain page" to parents in preoperative educational material and a preoperative pain and delirium consultation.

Flowchart

A flowchart can also be used to gain better understanding of a process. A flowchart is a graphic representation of how a process works. It should represent the current process, not a goal or ideal process. A high-level flowchart consists of 6 to 12 steps and helps give a balcony view of a process. A detailed flowchart examines the process and its complexity at a much closer level and may contain many individual steps.[19–21] The flowchart presented in **Fig. 4** is a high-level flowchart and represents the process used at CCHMC to ensure children receive muscle relaxation during intubation when appropriate. This process was the result of a QI project at CCHMC to reduce serious airway events and airway-related cardiac arrests in the operating room and PACU.

FAILURE MODES AND EFFECTS ANALYSIS

Failure modes and effects analysis (FMEA) is a proactive tool for preventing adverse events. It examines a process to determine points of failure and identify potential

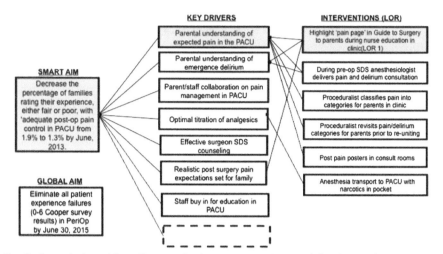

Fig. 3. Example key driver diagram for improving patient and family satisfaction in the PACU and subsequent interventions. *Abbreviations:* LOR, Level of Reliability; SDS, Same Day Surgery. (*Courtesy of* Department of Anesthesiology, Cincinnati Children's Hospital, Cincinnati, OH; with permission.)

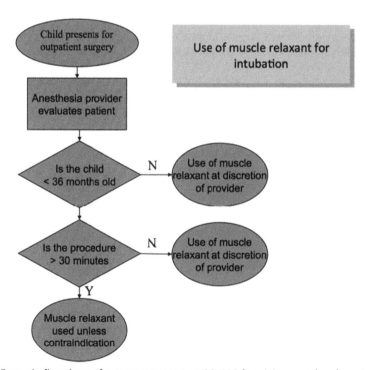

Fig. 4. Example flowchart of a current process at CCHMC for giving muscle relaxants during intubation. This process was developed to reduce serious airway events and airway cardiac arrests in the operating room and PACU. (*Courtesy of* Department of Anesthesiology, Cincinnati Children's Hospital, Cincinnati, OH; with permission.)

interventions. FMEAs work best when applied to smaller processes. Larger processes may need to be subdivided. First, each step in the process is determined. Each of these steps is then examined for potential failures. Failures may be prioritized based on likelihood of occurrence, likelihood of detection, and severity. Finally, possible interventions for the failures in each step are determined.

Fig. 5 shows an example of an FMEA examining the process of an anesthesia provider receiving narcotics from the pharmacy, administering them to a patient, and discarding waste or returning unused vials. Parts of this process that could go wrong are listed beneath each step, such as a dirty needle or syringe being used. Possible interventions are listed above each step.[22]

A key driver diagram, flowchart, and FMEA are just a sample of tools used in QI and safety analytics. The Quality and Safety Committee of the Society of Pediatric Anesthesia (SPA) and Wake Up Safe are example organizations using these tools as part of a larger framework, such as the Model for Improvement, or when conducting RCA.

QUALITY AND SAFETY COMMITTEE OF THE SOCIETY OF PEDIATRIC ANESTHESIA

The Quality and Safety Committee of the SPA is composed of more than 40 members representing the anesthesiology and pediatric anesthesiology departments of their member institutions.

The group promotes QI and patient safety in pediatric anesthesia through initiatives, such as a critical events checklist and an intraoperative handoff tool, both of which are freely available on the SPA Web site (http://www.pedsanesthesia.org/).

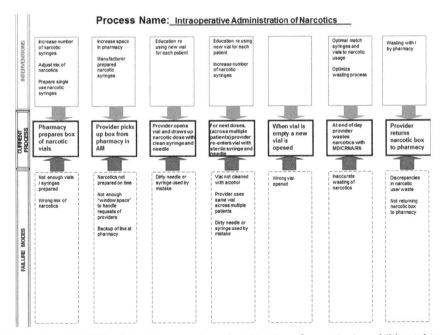

Fig. 5. Example FMEA of the intraoperative administration of narcotics in a children's hospital. (*Courtesy of* Department of Anesthesiology, Cincinnati Children's Hospital, Cincinnati, OH; with permission.)

Critical Events Checklists

Certain intraoperative events, such as air embolism or malignant hyperthermia, occur so infrequently that it is challenging for anesthesiologists to become proficient in their management. Checklists have proved an effective tool to aid providers in these rare situations. Studies in simulation have shown that checklists reduce the amount of crucial steps that are missed in intraoperative emergencies.[23]

Expanding on the work done for adult event checklists, the Quality and Safety Committee developed checklists for 17 pediatric anesthesia emergencies. Each checklist includes a brief summary of the problem and steps to take, including medications when appropriate. The checklists were developed using research by the National Aeronautics and Space Administration on checklist usability and were reviewed by human factors experts. Each checklist was then sent to a different organization for peer review and, in some cases, was tested in simulation. Recently, the Children's Hospital of Philadelphia adapted these checklists for the creation of a mobile application that includes a built-in timer, timestamps, and weight-based calculators.[19,24,25]

The checklists developed by the Quality and Safety Committee are

- Air embolism
- Anaphylaxis
- Bradycardia
- Cardiac arrest
- Difficult airway
- Fire: airway and operating room
- Hyperkalemia
- Hypertension
- Hypotension
- Hypoxia
- Local anesthetic toxicity
- Loss of evoked potentials
- Malignant hyperthermia
- Myocardial ischemia
- Tachycardia
- Transfusion and reactions
- Trauma[26]

Intraoperative Handoff Tool

It is not uncommon for multiple providers to care for children across the anesthetic course. The quality and reliability of handoffs between providers can, however, vary substantially. In an attempt to standardize the handoff process between providers, the Quality and Safety Committee developed an intraoperative handoff tool. The tool consists of a checklist incorporating key elements of a patient's intraoperative course and background. The CCHMC has had success implementing a similar checklist in operating rooms.

Categories in the intraoperative handoff tool include

- Background information
- History
- Airway
- Cardiac issues
- Medications
- Fluids
- Monitors

WAKE UP SAFE

Wake Up Safe is a patient safety organization composed of pediatric institutions that strives to use QI to make anesthesia care safer. It was established with the help of the SPA, and it currently consists of 19 pediatric institutions. The goals of the organization are to embed QI and safety analytics into pediatric anesthesia departments and institutions to decrease serious adverse events in children undergoing anesthesia.[27]

Wake Up Safe is unique in that its work encompasses all adverse events. An adverse event results in significant harm to a patient. In contrast to a serious safety event, however, which also results in harm, an adverse event does not imply that an error has occurred. This allows a broader and more accurate investigation of harm in pediatric anesthesia. In addition, Wake Up Safe investigates precursor events and near misses. Precursor events are those that have reached a patient but caused little or no harm. Near misses are events that did not reach a patient but would have caused harm if they did.

Wake Up Safe also differentiates itself from other patient safety groups by embedding organizations with capability in safety analytics and QI. QI capability is encouraged through education and the use of high-reliability processes, such as checklists, standardization, information technology, and automation.[28]

Data obtained from Wake Up Safe have offered insight into adverse safety events occurring in pediatric anesthesia. Since data collection began in July 2010, an average of 1.4 serious adverse events per 1000 anesthetics have been reported. Although it is possible that these numbers are affected by under-reporting or over-reporting, this rate corresponds closely to other rates in the literature.[28]

Respiratory events were the most common serious adverse event and often arose from complete airway obstruction treated successfully before progressing to cardiac arrest. The next most common events in decreasing order were cardiac arrest, care escalation, and cardiovascular events. In total these categories comprised 76% of all reported events. Care escalation was defined as events that did not lead to serious temporary or long-term harm but required additional treatment and resources, such as unplanned admission to a hospital or ICU. Care escalation events arose from medication errors (65%), equipment dysfunction (24%), blood reactions (9%), malignant hyperthermia (1%), and operating room fire (1%).[28]

In addition, serious adverse events have prompted Wake Up Safe to publish advisories to the pediatric anesthesia community:

- An advisory on hyperkalemic cardiac arrest was published after 4 cases of significant cardiovascular changes after large-volume intraoperative red blood cell transfusion.
- An advisory on preventing wrong-sided procedures was published after 5 such cases were reported to the organization.
- Finally, an advisory on decreasing the risk of intravenous medication errors was published after 23 adverse events, which were related to medication errors, including administering the incorrect drug, administering the incorrect dose, administering via an incorrect route, and omitting a medication, or the result of a medication reaction.

Further information and recommendations regarding these advisories can be found on the Wake Up Safe Web site (http://wakeupsafe.org/findings.iphtml).

SAFETY ANALYTICS

RCA, a widely used methodology in safety analytics, is based on a sequence of events model of safety. It looks in a linear fashion to find the most proximate error. This makes it a practical approach to adverse events and one adopted by Wake Up Safe. An RCA should be performed after an adverse event, a precursor event, or a near miss that has potential to seriously harm a patient.

After an event has occurred, a fact-finding team interviews those directly involved. This team, however, should be objective and not directly involved in the event. It may also be beneficial to interview others, such as a supervisor or colleague, to understand circumstances surrounding the event. Was there a particularly high volume that day? Was staff moved to an area they were unfamiliar with? Are they aware of existing protocols, and are they typically followed? Wake Up Safe institutions uses 3 anesthesiologists trained in safety analytics to conduct an RCA on all serious adverse events.

Similar to the fact-finding team, an RCA team is composed of members familiar with patient safety and not directly involved in the case. Members often include representatives from medical, legal, nursing, and administration. The team constructs a sequence of events from the gathered facts. For comparison, they may also establish a sequence of events of the way the process normally runs at the hospital. Flowcharts are often used to map these sequences. The team also reviews applicable policies and guidelines of the hospital.

After analysis of gathered information, the team works to establish proximate and contributing causes. The proximate cause is the cause that, when removed, would most likely have prevented the adverse event from occurring. Contributing factors are those that, if removed, would have lessened the probability of the event or lessened its severity.

Once proximate and contributing causes are established, an action plan is created to reduce the likelihood of a similar adverse event occurring. Interventions are developed for each proximate cause. The goal is to insert technologies or processes into the system to prevent the error from occurring again. The objective is not to point blame at individuals.

A specific, measurable, achievable, relevant, and timely (SMART) aim should be established for each intervention, similar to when implementing a change in a PDSA cycle. Individuals responsible for the interventions should be identified, and measures of successful implementation should be tracked.

SPREADING CHANGE AND INNOVATION

A test of change, even after it has proved effective, still requires implementation and dissemination for improvement to occur in the system of care. The spread of a change usually proves more difficult than the test. Health care is notoriously slow to adopt changes, even those that are evidence based.

Understanding the life cycle of innovation helps spread change through a department, an organization, or even a health care system. Everett M. Rogers[29] describes 5 groups of individuals in the adoption of an innovation. Communication and personal connections are critical for the flow of innovation between groups.

- Innovators are the first group to accept the innovation. They are often more adventurous and tolerant of risk.
- Early adopters are the next group to adopt the innovation. Unlike innovators, this group is socially well connected and thought of as thought leaders.
- The early majority are more risk adverse. They rely on familiarity and personal connections, including looking to early adopters.
- The late majority wait until an innovation has become the status quo.
- Laggards are the last group to accept an innovation. They are traditionalists who have skepticism for anything that is not tried and true.[29]

An often-cited phrase in QI is that not all change leads to improvement, but all improvement requires change. A systematic approach to change, such as that outlined in the Model for Improvement, increases the odds of success, minimizes risk, reduces time, and ultimately spreads innovation. The authors firmly believe these approaches have successfully increased quality of care for children at CCHMC. The spread of these tools and the open sharing of successes and failures will further the improvement of pediatric anesthesiology.

REFERENCES

1. Ahrens E. Wake up safe: root cause analysis. Red Rock Resort: Las Vegas (NV), March 18, 2013.
2. National Healthcare Quality Report 2012. Rockville (MD): U.S. Department of Health and Human Services; 2013. AHRQ Publication No. 13-0002. P H-2, H-5. Available at: http://www.ahrq.gov/research/findings/nhqrdr/nhqr12/nhqr12_prov.pdf. Accessed December 1, 2013.
3. James B, Soria N. How to run your own clinical quality improvement program. Institute for Health Care Delivery Research. Intermountain Healthcare. Salt Lake City (UT). p. 1–3. Available at: http://intermountainhealthcare.org/qualityandresearch/institute/Documents/Intermountain_miniATP_General_Program_layout_12-5-08.pdf. Accessed December 1, 2013.
4. Virginia Mason Medical Center implements lean management principles to drive out waste. Institute for Healthcare Improvement; 2011. Available at: http://www.ihi.org/knowledge/Pages/ImprovementStories/VirginiaMasonMedicalCenterImplements LeanManagementPrinciplestoDriveOutWaste.aspx. Accessed December 1, 2013.
5. Uttal B. The corporate culture vultures, fortune. 1983. p. 66–72.
6. Scott T, Mannion R, Davies H, et al. Implementing culture change in health care: theory and practice. Int J Qual Health Care 2003;15(2):111.
7. Botwinick L, Bisognano M, Haraden C. Leadership guide to patient safety. IHI Innovation Series white paper. Cambridge (MA): Institute for Healthcare Improvement, 2006. p. 10.
8. Varughese AM, Morillo-Delerme J, Kurth C. Quality management in the delivery of pediatric anesthesia care. Int Anesthesiol Clin 2006;44(1):119–39.
9. Collins J. Level 5 leadership: the triumph of humility and fierce resolve. Harv Bus Rev 2005.
10. Evidence scan: quality improvement training for healthcare professionals. The Health Foundation; 2012. p. 3–15. Available at: http://www.health.org.uk/publications/quality-improvement-training-for-healthcare-professionals/. Accessed December 1, 2013.
11. Smith B. Lean and six sigma- a one-two punch, Quality Progress. Milwaukee (WI): American Society for Quality; 2003. p. 37–41.
12. Improvement Science Education. James M. Anderson Center for Health Systems Excellence. Available at: http://www.cincinnatichildrens.org/service/j/anderson-center/education/additional-programs/. Accessed December 1, 2013.
13. Intermediate improvement science series (I2S2) course plan. Cincinnati (OH): James M. Anderson Center for Health Systems Excellence. Cincinnati Children's Hospital; 2013.
14. Langley GJ, Moen RD, Nolan KM, et al. The improvement guide: a practical approach to enhancing organizational performance. San Francisco (CA): Jossey-Bass; 2009.
15. Committee on Quality of Health Care in America, Institute of Medicine. Crossing the quality chasm: a new health system for the 21st century. Washington, DC: Institute of Medicine, National Academies Press; 2001. p. 41–53.

16. Dixon-Woods M, Bosk CL, Aveling EL, et al. Explaining Michigan: developing an ex post theory of a quality improvement program. Milbank Q 2011;89:167–205.
17. Edwards J, Davey J, Armstrong K. Returning to the roots of culture: a review and re-conceptualisation of safety culture. Saf Sci 2013;55:70–80.
18. Brassard M, Ritter D. Memory Jogger II: a pocket guide of tools for continuous improvement and effective planning. Salem (NH): GoalQPC; 2008. p. 43–4, 124–125.
19. Reinertsen JL. Physicians as leaders in the improvement of health care systems. Ann Intern Med 1998;128(10):833–8. http://dx.doi.org/10.7326/0003-4819-128-10-199805150-00007.
20. Process analysis tools: flowchart. Boston: Institute for Healthcare Improvement; 2004. p. 1–3. Available at: http://www.ihi.org/knowledge/Pages/Tools/Flowchart.aspx. Accessed December 1, 2013.
21. Science of improvement: establishing measures. Institute for Healthcare Improvement. 2011. Available at: http://www.ihi.org/knowledge/Pages/HowtoImprove/ScienceofImprovementEstablishingMeasures.aspx. Accessed December 1, 2013.
22. Failure modes and effects analysis. Boston: Institute for Healthcare Improvement; 2004. p. 1–6.
23. Arriaga AF, Bader AM, Wong JM, et al. Simulation-based trial of surgical-crisis checklists. N Engl J Med 2013;368(3):246.
24. Pediatric critical events checklist. The Children's Hospital of Philadelphia. Available at: https://itunes.apple.com/us/app/pediatric-critical-events/id709721914?ls=1&mt=8. Accessed December 1, 2013.
25. Process analysis tools: cause and effect diagram. Boston: Institute for Healthcare Improvement; 2004. p. 1–3. Available at: http://www.ihi.org/knowledge/Pages/Tools/CauseandEffectDiagram.aspx. Accessed December 1, 2013.
26. Pratap N, Pukenas E. SPA launches pediatric critical events checklists. SPA News. 26(2). Available at: http://www.pedsanesthesia.org/newsletters/2013summer/. Accessed December 1, 2013.
27. Wake up safe: about us. Wake up safe a component of The Society of Pediatric Anesthesia. Available at: http://wakeupsafe.org/aboutus.iphtml. Accessed December 1, 2013.
28. Kurth CD, Tyler D, Heitmiller E, et al. Pediatric Anesthesia Safety-Quality Improvement Program in USA.
29. Berwick D. Disseminating innovations in health care. JAMA 2003;289(15):1969–75.

Index

Note: Page numbers of article titles are in **boldface** type.

A

Acetabular surgery, reconstructive, in children with cerebral palsy, 73–75

Adenotonsillar hypertrophy, pediatric obstructive sleep apnea due to, 243–244

Adenotonsillectomy, for treatment of pediatric obstructive sleep apnea, 246–254
  anesthetic techniques, 250–252
  perioperative management, 247–250
  postoperative management, 252–254
 perioperative respiratory adverse events in children after, 51–52

Airway, anesthetic considerations in children with tumors of, 197
 difficult, managing during pediatric anesthesia and sedation outside the OR, 38–39

physiology of, pediatric, 242–243

Analgesia, for pes excavatum surgery, **175–184**

Anatomic dysfunction, pediatric obstructive sleep apnea due to, 244–245

Anesthesia. *See also* Pediatric anesthesiology.

and sedation outside the operating room, **25–43**
  anesthesia *versus* sedation, 26–27
  goals of, 26
  patient preparation, 27–28
  specific extramural sites and best practices, 28–38
    mobile sedation, 38
    procedure suite, 34–38
    radiology, 28–34
  specific issues, 38
    cardiopulmonary resuscitation, 39
    difficult airway, 38–39
    postprocedure care, 39
    quality improvement and outcome, 40–41
    risks and complications, 39–40

Anesthesiology, in children. *See* Pediatric anesthesiology.

Anesthetics, neurotoxicity of, **133–155**
  anesthesia without sensation, 133–134
  animals models of, 136–137
    immediate lessons from, 148–149
    translation to humans, 137–138
  apoptosis triggered by anesthetics, 136
  apoptotic neuronal cell death, 135–136
  effects on learning and behavior in young children, 138–146
  historical perspective, 134–135
    deleterious effects of anesthetics on developing brain, 135
    nociceptive response of immature brain to surgery, 134–135

Anesthesiology Clin 32 (2014) 295–308
http://dx.doi.org/10.1016/S1932-2275(13)00114-6
anesthesiology.theclinics.com

Moving?

Make sure your subscription moves with you!

To notify us of your new address, find your **Clinics Account Number** (located on your mailing label above your name), and contact customer service at:

Email: journalscustomerservice-usa@elsevier.com

800-654-2452 (subscribers in the U.S. & Canada)
314-447-8871 (subscribers outside of the U.S. & Canada)

Fax number: 314-447-8029

**Elsevier Health Sciences Division
Subscription Customer Service
3251 Riverport Lane
Maryland Heights, MO 63043**

*To ensure uninterrupted delivery of your subscription, please notify us at least 4 weeks in advance of move.

Printed and bound by CPI Group (UK) Ltd, Croydon, CR0 4YY

07/10/2024

01040499-0014